Holland • Frei

CANCER 6
MEDICINE
REVIEW

EDITORS

DONALD W. KUFE, MD
Professor of Medicine
Dana-Farber Cancer Institute
Harvard Medical School
Boston, Massachusetts

RAPHAEL E. POLLOCK, MD, PHD
Head, Division of Surgery
Professor and Chair, Department of Surgical Oncology
Senator A.M. Aiken Jr. Distinguished Chair
University of Texas
MD Anderson Cancer Center
Houston, Texas

RALPH R. WEICHSELBAUM, MD
Chair, Department of Radiation and Cellular Oncology
University of Chicago Hospitals
Director, Chicago Tumor Institute
Chicago, Illinois

ROBERT C. BAST JR, MD
Internist and Professor of Medicine
Vice President for Translational Research
Harry Carothers Wiess Chair for Cancer Research
University of Texas
MD Anderson Cancer Center
Houston, Texas

JAMES F. HOLLAND, MD, SCD (HC)
Distinguished Professor of Neoplastic Diseases
Director Emeritus, Derald H. Ruttenberg Cancer Center
Mount Sinai School of Medicine
New York, New York

EMIL FREI III, MD
Physician-in-Chief, Emeritus
Dana-Farber Cancer Institute
Richard and Susan Smith Distinguished Professor of Medicine
Harvard Medical School
Boston, Massachusetts

Holland • Frei

CANCER6
MEDICINE
REVIEW

A companion to
Holland-Frei
Cancer Medicine-6

2003
BC Decker Inc
Hamilton • London

BC Decker Inc
P.O. Box 620, LCD 1
Hamilton, Ontario L8N 3K7
Tel: 905-522-7017; 800-568-7281
Fax: 905-522-7839; 888-311-4987
E-mail: info@bcdecker.com
www.bcdecker.com

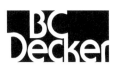

03 04 05 06 / WCL / 9 8 7 6 5 4 3 2 1

ISBN 1-55009-221-9
Printed in Canada

Sales and Distribution

United States
BC Decker Inc
P.O. Box 785
Lewiston, NY 14092-0785
Tel: 905-522-7017; 800-568-7281
Fax: 905-522-7839; 888-311-4987
E-mail: info@bcdecker.com
www.bcdecker.com

Canada
BC Decker Inc
20 Hughson Street South
P.O. Box 620, LCD 1
Hamilton, Ontario L8N 3K7
Tel: 905-522-7017; 800-568-7281
Fax: 905-522-7839; 888-311-4987
E-mail: info@bcdecker.com
www.bcdecker.com

Foreign Rights
John Scott & Company
International Publishers' Agency
P.O. Box 878
Kimberton, PA 19442
Tel: 610-827-1640
Fax: 610-827-1671
E-mail: jsco@voicenet.com

Japan
Igaku-Shoin Ltd.
Foreign Publications Department
3-24-17 Hongo
Bunkyo-ku, Tokyo, Japan 113-8719
Tel: 3 3817 5680
Fax: 3 3815 6776
E-mail: fd@igaku-shoin.co.jp

UK, Europe, Scandinavia, Middle East
Elsevier Science
Customer Service Department
Foots Cray High Street
Sidcup, Kent
DA14 5HP, UK
Tel: 44 (0) 208 308 5760
Fax: 44 (0) 181 308 5702
E-mail: cservice@harcourt.com

*Singapore, Malaysia,Thailand, Philippines,
Indonesia, Vietnam, Pacific Rim, Korea*
Elsevier Science Asia
583 Orchard Road
#09/01, Forum
Singapore 238884
Tel: 65-737-3593
Fax: 65-753-2145

Australia, New Zealand
Elsevier Science Australia
Customer Service Department
STM Division
Locked Bag 16
St. Peters, New South Wales, 2044
Australia
Tel: 61 02 9517-8999
Fax: 61 02 9517-2249
E-mail: stmp@harcourt.com.au
www.harcourt.com.au

Mexico and Central America
ETM SA de CV
Calle de Tula 59
Colonia Condesa
06140 Mexico DF, Mexico
Tel: 52-5-5553-6657
Fax: 52-5-5211-8468
E-mail: editoresdetextosmex@prodigy.net.mx

Argentina
CLM (Cuspide Libros Medicos)
Av. Córdoba 2067 - (1120)
Buenos Aires, Argentina
Tel: (5411) 4961-0042/(5411) 4964-0848
Fax: (5411) 4963-7988
E-mail: clm@cuspide.com

Brazil
Tecmedd
Av. Maurílio Biagi, 2850
City Ribeirão Preto – SP – CEP: 14021-000
Tel: 0800 992236
Fax: (16) 3993-9000
E-mail: tecmedd@tecmedd.com.br

PREFACE

We have attempted to provide a useful companion work for the new sixth edition of *Cancer Medicine*. This textbook is the most up-to-date and complete reference book that is available on the biology, diagnosis, epidemiology, and treatment of cancer. Because of its vast scope, readers may wish to test their proficiency in one or more of the areas covered in this work. We hope that *Holland-Frei Cancer Medicine-6 Review* will provide such an opportunity.

The organization of the *Review*, with questions that are grouped by chapter, will allow the reader to devote energies to those specific areas he or she needs to review. Moreover, the style of several possible responses—with only one being the correct response—is analogous to the type of questions on the American Board of Internal Medicine Examination in Oncology as well as the In-service Examination in Surgical Oncology. Therefore, the *Review* should aid the student in board examination preparation.

We would like to express our gratitude to those individuals who were called upon to deliver questions for the editors' review. One of the very strengths of *Holland-Frei Cancer Medicine-6 Review* is that many of the questions were written by the chapter authors themselves (individuals with world-renowned expertise in the field), who are well aware of the key issues in their own field. The question-writing contributors should be praised for their interest in enhancing the educational value of *Cancer Medicine-6*.

The authors also gratefully acknowledge the dedication of the production staff at BC Decker Inc. Without their support, the successful completion of *Holland-Frei Cancer Medicine-6 Review* would have been impossible.

We appreciate any comments and suggestions from our readers as we look forward to future editions of the *Review*.

The Editors

CONTRIBUTORS

Stuart Aaronson, MD

James L. Abbruzzese, MD, FACP

Aviva Abosch, MD, PhD

Scott I. Abrams, PhD

David H. Abramson, MD

Sunil J. Advani, MD

Jaffer A. Ajani, MD

Karen Albritton, MD

Edward P. Ambinder, MD

Kenneth C. Anderson, MD

Michael Andreeff, MD, PhD

Anne L. Angiolillo, MD

Narin Apisarnthanarax, MD

Richard Aplenc, MD, MSCE

James O. Armitage, MD

Anna Bafico, PhD

Joseph Bailes, MD

Anna D. Barker, PhD

Lawrence W. Bassett, MD, FACR

Robert C. Bast Jr, MD

Norman Beauchamp Jr, MD

Robert S. Benjamin, MD

Jonathan S. Berek, MD, MMSc

Ross S. Berkowitz, MD

Mark Bernstein, MD

Steven H. Bernstein, MD

Donald Berry, PhD

Joseph R. Bertino, MD

William L. Bigbee, PhD

Charles D. Blanke, MD

Archie Bleyer, MD

Gerald P. Bodey, MD

Ernest C. Borden, MD

Marcia S. Brose, MD, PhD

Thomas A. Buchholz, MD

Aman U. Buzdar, MD

Mitchell S. Cairo, MD

Alan C. Carver, MD

Barrie R. Cassileth, PhD

A. Philippe Chahinian, MD

William H. Chambers, PhD

Richard Champlin, MD

Yung-Chi Cheng, MD

Haesun Choi, MD

Theodore D. Chung, PhD

John A. Cidlowski, PhD

Margie L. Clapper, PhD

Gary L. Clayman, DDS, MD, FACS

Lewis Clayman, DMD, MD

James E. Cleaver, PhD

Steven K. Clinton, MD, PhD

Carmel J. Cohen, MD

Harvey J. Cohen, MD

Jeffrey I. Cohen, MD

Peter D. Cole, MD

R. Edward Coleman, MD

Michael Colvin, MD

Ana Maria Comaru-Schally, MD, MS

Karen E. Conner, BA, MS IV

James L. Connolly, MD

Christopher L. Corless, MD, PhD

Joseph W. Costa Jr, DMD

R. Lee Cothran, MD

Kenneth H. Cowan, MD, PhD

Christopher H. Crane, MD

Carlo M. Croce, MD

Chistopher P. Crum, MD

Anthony V. D'Amico, MD

Chau T. Dang, MD

Lisa M. DeAngelis, MD

Alberto S. DeLeo, MD

Laurie D. DeLeve, MD, PhD

Samuel R. Denmeade, MD

Maria T. DeSancho, MD

Mark W. Dewhirst, DVM, PhD

Robert B. Diasio, MD

Eduardo M. Diaz Jr, MD, FACS

Kip W. Dolphin, MD

Brian J. Druker, MD

Ira J. Dunkel, MD

Madeleine M. Duvic, MD

Ann M. Dvorak, MD

Harold F. Dvorak, MD

Joseph Paul Eder, MD

Patricia J. Eifel, MD

Lawrence H. Einhorn, MD

Suhendan Ekmekcioglu, PhD

Ezekiel J. Emanuel, MD, PhD

Paul F. Engstrom, MD

Warren E. Enker, MD

Agamemnon Epenetos, PhD, FRCP

Jeremy J. Erasmus, MC

Carmen P. Escalante, MD

Richard Essner, MD, FACS

Alison A. Evans, ScD

Douglas B. Evans, MD

Michael S. Ewer, MD, MPH

Harmon J. Eyre, MD

Mark K. Ferguson, MD

Karen K. Fields, MD

Olivera J. Finn, PhD

Marshall S. Flam, MD

Kathleen M. Foley, MD

Judah Folkman, MD

Yuman Fong, MD

Richard S. Foster, MD

Arthur E. Frankel, MD

Janet L. Franklin, MD

Arnold S. Freedman, MD

Emil Frei III, MD

Valentin Fuster, MD

Robert F. Gagel, MD

Robert Gallo, MD

Chirag D. Gandhi, MD

Guillermo Garcia-Manero, MD

Paul S. Gaynon, MD

Mark C. Gebhardt, MD

Teresa Ann Gilewski, MD

Ann Marie Gillenwater, MD

Timothy D. Gilligan, MD

Edward L. Giovannucci, MD, DPH

Donald P. Goldstein, MD

Harvey M. Golomb, MD

David W. Goodrich, PhD

Jane Gooen-Piels, PhD

Richard G. Gorlick, MD

Richard Gralla, MD

F. Anthony Greco, MD

John Greene, MD

Elizabeth Ann Grimm, PhD

Elizabeth G. Grubbs, MD

Paul E. Grundy, MD

David E. Gutstein, MD

Karin M.E.H. Gwyn, MD

John D. Hainsworth, MD

William N. Hait, MD

Stanley R. Hamilton, MD

Axel-R Hanauske, MD, PhD

Nasser Hanna, MD

Curtis C. Harris, MD

Harold A. Harvey, MD

Tayyaba Hasan, PhD

Michael C. Heinrich, MD

Clyde A. Helms, MD

Brian E. Henderson, MD

Connie Henke Yarbro, MS, RN, FAAN

Ronald B. Herberman, MD

Arthur L. Herbst, MD

Teru Hideshima, MD, PhD

James F. Holland, MD, ScD (hc)

Jimmie C. Holland, MD

Richard T. Hoppe, MD

Gabriel N. Hortobagyi, MD

Arti Hurria, MD

Christopher J. Hurt

Mark Hurwitz, MD

John T. Isaacs, PhD

Ahmedin Jemal, MD

Anuja Jhingran, MD

Steven Joffe, MD, MPH

Ellen Jones, MD, PhD

Hamilton Jordan

V. Craig Jordan, OBE, PhD, DSc

John A. Kalapurakal, MD

Raghu Kalluri, MD

Barton A. Kamen, MD, PhD

Hagop M. Kantarjian, MD

Philip W. Kantoff, MD

Richard M. Kaufman, MD

Harmeet Kaur, MD

Michael J. Keating, MD

Nancy E. Kemeny, MD

Samuel Kenan, MD

Merrill S. Kies, MD

Youn H. Kim, MD

John M. Kirkwood, MD

Catherine E. Klein, MD

Elise C. Kohn, MD

Ritsuko Komaki, MD

Christina A. Kousparou, PhD

Robert J. Kreitman, MD

Donald W. Kufe, MD

Joanne Kurtzberg, MD

Razelle Kurzrock, MD

Beverly Lange, MD

George E. Laramore, MD, PhD

Richard A. Larson, MD

Denise A. Levitan, MD, PhD

Chuan Y. Li, PhD

Edward H. Lin, MD

Lance A. Liotta, MD

Scott M. Lippman, MD

Janina A. Longtine, MD

Evelyne M. Loyer, MD

Donald F. Lynch Jr, MD

Henry T. Lynch, MD

Tobey J. MacDonald, MD

Paul F. Mansfield, MD

Richard G. Margolese, MD

Neyssa Marina, MD

John M. Maris, MD

Maurie Markman, MD

Peter M. Mauch, MD

H. Page McAdams, MD

Kenneth S. McCarty Jr, MD, PhD

Kenneth S. McCarty Sr, PhD

Beryl McCormick, MD

Lorraine I. McKay, PhD

Catherine M. McLachlin, MD

Anna T. Meadows, MD

Jeffrey I. Mechanick, MD

Curtis J. Mettlin, PhD

William H. Meyer, MD

Matthew Meyerson, MD

Elizabeth C. Miller, MS, RD

Franco Minardi, MD

David L. Mitchell, MS, PhD

Anne C.E. Moor, PhD

Charles S. Morrow, MD, PhD

Donald L. Morton, MD, FACS

Natalia Moryl, MD

Jeffrey Moscow, MD

Arno S. Mundt, MD

Hyman B. Muss, MD

Piero Mustacchi, MD, ScD (Hon)

James Nachman, MD

Lee M. Nadler, MD

Rita Nanda, MD

Victor A. Neel, MD, PhD

Alfred I. Neugut, MD, PhD

Craig R. Nichols, MD

Mark Nichols, PhD

Larry Norton, MD

William D. Odell, MD, PhD, MACP

William K. Oh, MD

Takao Ohnuma, MD, PhD

Olufunmilayo I. Olopade, MD, FACP

Bernhard Ortel, MD

Brian O'Sullivan, MD, FRCPI

Edward Pan, MD

Alberto S. Pappo, MD

Arthur B. Pardee, PhD

David M. Parham, MD

Ben Ho Park, MD, PhD

Harvey I. Pass, MD

Edward F. Patz Jr, MD

Sherrie L. Perkins, MD, PhD

Elizabeth J. Perlman, MD

Marco A. Pierotti, MD

James F. Pingpank, MD

Peter W.T. Pisters, MD, FACS

David Piwnica-Worms, MD, PhD

Giuseppe Pizzorno, PhD, PharmD

William K. Plunkett Jr, PhD

Brian Pogue, PhD

Raphael E. Pollock, MD, PhD

Kornelia Polyak, MD, PhD

Jerome B. Posner, MD

Kalmon D. Post, MD

Michael D. Prados, MD

Leonard Prosnitz, MD

Martin N. Raber, MD

Hannah Rabinowich, PhD

Elizabeth Raetz, MD

Kristjan T. Ragnarsson, MD

Jamal Rahaman, MD

Kanti R. Rai, MD

Noopur Raje, MD, MB, BS

Jacob H. Rand, MD

R. Lor Randall, MD, FACS

Mark J. Ratain, MD

Gregory H. Reaman, MD

John C. Reed, MD, PhD

Marvin S. Reitz Jr, PhD

Susan R. Rheingold, MD

Jerome P. Richie, MD

Frederick Rickles, MD

Paula Trahan Rieger, RN, MSN

Michael L. Ritchey, MD

Leslie L. Robison, PhD

Miguel A. Rodriguez-Bigas, MD

Carlos Rodriguez-Galindo, MD

John C. Roeske, PhD

Kenneth V.I. Rolston, MD, FACP

Brian R. Rood, MD

Gerald Rosen, MD

Julie Ross, PhD
Bruce J. Roth, MD
Jack A. Roth, MD
Jacob H. Rotmensch, MD
Eric K. Rowinsky, MD
Janet D. Rowley, MD, DSc
Eric H. Rubin, MD
John C. Ruckdeschel, MD
Raymond W. Ruddon, MD, PhD
Anita L. Sabichi, MD
Thaddeus Samulski, PhD
Edward A. Sausville, MD
Kadri Sayed, MD
David T. Scadden, MD
Andrew V. Schally, PhD, DSc, MDhc
Amy C. Schefler, BA
Charles A. Schiffer, MD
Jeffrey Schlom, PhD
Stuart J. Schnitt, MD
Robert A. Schnoll, PhD
David E. Schteingart, MD
Kitt Shaffer, MD, PhD
Brenda Shank, MD, PhD
Steven I. Sherman, MD
Suzanne Shusterman, MD
Elin R. Sigurdson, MD
Richard T. Silver, MD
Paul M. Silverman, MD
Robert Smith, PhD
Thomas C. Smyrk, MD
Arthur J. Sober, MD
Morando Soffritti, MD
K. Eric Sommers, MD
Stephen T. Sonis, DMD
Gabriella Sozzi, PhD
Michael B. Sporn, MD
Dempsey Springfield, MD
Graeme S. Steele, MD
David P. Steensma, MD
Craig W. Stevens, MD, PhD
Richard M. Stone, MD
Walter J. Storkus, PhD
Erich M. Sturgis, MD
Max W. Sung, MD

Antonella Surbone, MD
Stephen G. Swisher, MD
Joseph M. Taraska, JD
Ayalew Tefferi, MD
Lisa A. Teot, MD
Richard L. Theriault, DO, MBA, DSc, FACP
David C. Thomas, MD
Michael J. Thun, MD, MS
Swan N. Thung, MD
Robert Timmerman, MD
Jeffrey A. Toretsky, MD
Guillermo L. Tortolero-Luna, MD, PhD
Douglas S. Tyler, MD
Ara A. Vaporciyan, MD
James W. Vardiman, MD
Andrew J. Vickers, MD
Bert Vogelstein, MD
Daniel D. Von Hoff, MD, FACP
Zeljko Vujaskovic, MD, Phd
Helen Hai-Ling Wang, MD, PhD
Barbara Weber, MD
Jane C. Weeks, MD, MSc
Ralph R. Weichselbaum, MD
Lawrence Weiss, MD
Ainsley Weston, PhD
J. Taylor Wharton, MD
Theresa Whiteside, MD, PhD
Charles B. Wilson, MD, DSc, MSHA
Stephanie R. Wilson, MD
Suzanne L. Wolden, MD
Robert A. Wolff, MD
Robert C. Wollman, MD
S. Diane Yamada, MD
James C. Yao, MD
Kathy Yao, MD
Edward T.H. Yeh, MD
Tina W.F. Yen, MD
Sai-Ching Jim Yeung, MD, PhD
David Yousem, MD
Michael R. Zalutsky, PhD
Hassane M. Zarour, MD
Marvin Zelen, PhD
Anthony L. Zietman, MD

CONTENTS

Preface v

Contributors vii

Cardinal Manifestations and Informatics 1
    Questions 2
    Answers 3

Scientific Foundations 5
    Questions 6
    Answers 22

Cancer Diagnosis 32
    Questions 33
    Answers 39

Therapeutic Modalities 43
    Questions 44
    Answers 60

Multidisciplinary Management 72
    Questions 73
    Answers 80

Cancer Management 85
    Questions 86
    Answers 122

Pediatric Oncology 146
    Questions 147
    Answers 155

Complications 160
    Questions 161
    Answers 172

CARDINAL MANIFESTATIONS
AND INFORMATICS

DIRECTIONS: Numbering for questions and answers reflects the corresponding chapter in *Cancer Medicine-6*. Each question contains suggested responses. Select the best response to each question. Answers for Cardinal Manifestations and Informatics begin on page 3.

1.1   **Malignant tumors can be differentiated from benign tumors by**
a.   A faster growth rate
b.   Heterogeneity of cell types
c.   Density of growth factor receptors
d.   Tissue invasion

1.2   **Which one of the following mechanisms is thought to have a key role in carcinogenesis?**
a.   Amplication of tumor suppressor genes
b.   Decreased cyclin activity
c.   Repression of proto-oncogenes
d.   Methylation of tumor suppressor genes

1.3.   **Which one of the following statements is true?**
a.   Carcinoma in situ of the bronchus metastasizes more frequently than does ductal carcinoma in situ of the breast.
b.   Sarcoma metastases are exclusively hematogenous.
c.   Lymph node metastases from breast cancer can regress after resection of the primary tumor.
d.   Bone tumors metastasize to lungs and lung tumors metastasize to bones, but bone tumors and lung tumors do not metastasize to bone and lung, respectively.

1.4   **Carcinomas in situ of mucosal surfaces are usually asymptomatic. When invasive cancers develop, which location of carcinoma is likely to be asymptomatic and to be discovered last?**
a.   Common bile duct
b.   Right upper lobe bronchus
c.   Cecum
d.   Jejunum
e.   Sigmoid colon

1.5   **Weight gain as a presenting complaint of cancer is common in which of the following tumors?**
a.   Gastric carcinoma
b.   Astrocytoma of the temporal lobe
c.   Small cell carcinoma of the lung
d.   Ovarian cancer
e.   Retroperitoneal lymphoma

1.6   **Which of the following environmental exposures is considered *not* to induce cancer?**
a.   Bacterial infection
b.   Hypoxia
c.   Viral infection
d.   Thermal radiation
e.   Ultraviolet radiation

ONCOLOGY AND INFORMATICS

162.1   **1. The Internet does *not* provide access to which of the following?**
a.   Bulletin boards
b.   E-mail
c.   Discussion groups
d.   Server-only networking schemes
e.   Client-server networking schemes

162.2   **Which of the following statements best describes desirable attributes of the electronic medical record?**
a.   It supports a single simplified view of the data.
b.   It offers continuous access for authorized users.
c.   It supports direct data entry by unit clerks and nurses only.
d.   It guarantees confidentiality and privacy but not audit trails.
e.   It does not require the measurement of health status and functional levels.

162.3   Which of the following statements about oncology informatics is false?
   a.   Moore's law states that the performance of computer technology doubles every 18 months.
   b.   Metcalfe's law states that the power of a network rises by the square of the number of computers attached to it.
   c.   The majority of oncologists use electronic medical records in their offices.
   d.   The Internet has become the "library of choice" for oncologists.
   e.   The Surveillance, Epidemiology, and End Results (SEER) database is useful for finding outcome data for cancer patients.

ANSWERS

1.1   Answer: (d)   Growth rate of benign tumors is usually slower than that of their malignant counterparts, but this characteristic does not distinguish between them exclusively. Both benign and malignant tumors may contain multiple cell types: benign and malignant teratomas, osteochondromas, and carcinosarcomas. Growth factor receptors are present in some instances of both benign and malignant tumors. Mutant truncated receptors that signal despite the absence of growth factor are more common in malignant tumors. Benign tumors compress adjacent tissues but do not invade outside their capsule. Malignant tumors may compress adjacent tissues forming a pseudocapsule, but they also invade as a primary characteristic. Invasion may occur through the interstices between adjacent cells, and also represents proteolytic activity destroying basement membranes, collagen, and adjacent cell membranes. The placenta is a special benign tissue that does invade the uterine wall.

1.2   Answer: (d)   Amplified tumor suppressor genes should inhibit tumor growth. Mutant *P53*, which is inactive as a tumor suppressor gene, gives the illusion of an amplified tumor suppressor gene. Cyclin activity may be normal or increased in cancer cells. Activation, not repression of proto-oncogenes, leads to oncogenic activity. Methylation of cytosine residues often accounts for silencing of normal expression. Excessive methylation of cancer cell deoxyribonucleic acid has been observed, including methylation of tumor suppressor genes.

1.3   Answer: (c)   Carcinoma in situ of the bronchus, the breast, and, indeed, any mucosal surface, by definition has failed to penetrate the basement membrane. Such tumors do not have access to lymphatic or capillary vessels. Metastasis that is attributed to carcinoma in situ probably represents a geographic miss in finding a coexistent invasive component. Although uncommon, sarcomatous metastasis in regional lymph nodes occurs with much greater frequency than does metastasis in remote nodes, supporting the proposition that they are lymphogenous in pathogenesis. Bone tumors can metastasize to bones, although it is often difficult to distinguish such lesions from multifocal primary tumors. Lung neoplasms metastasize to lungs with high frequency. In a randomized trial of the National Surgical Adjuvant Breast Project, eventual palpable axillary node recurrence in patients who did not undergo axillary node resection at the time of simple mastectomy was only half the expected frequency based on axillary node involvement found in the randomized dissected group, supporting the concept that regression of axillary metastasis had occurred.

1.4   Answer: (c)   The narrower the conduit, the earlier the obstructive signs can appear, particularly in an unpaired organ. Invasive cancers distort luminal size by fibrosis and accumulation of tumor cells. Painless jaundice is an early finding in common bile obstruction by tumor, whether from external compression of pancreatic cancer or intrinsically from luminal narrowing from common bile duct cancer. Carcinoma of the right or left hepatic duct, as in carcinoma of a single ureter, can only be discovered late because of compensation by the unimpaired fellow duct. Invasive bronchial carcinoma leads to early cough, disorder of bronchial ciliary function, and pneumonia. Carcinomas that narrow the jejunum or sigmoid lead to small or large intestinal compromise and obstruction with disordered intestinal function. Carcinoma of the cecum, because of the liquid content and because of its large diameter, is characteristically discovered late, often because of bleeding or symptomatic hepatic metastases rather than gastrointestinal symptoms.

1.5   Answer: (d)   Although ascites occurs in gastric carcinoma, presenting complaints are much more commonly anorexia, weight loss, and digestive complaint or pain. Astrocytoma of the temporal lobe would not be expected to distort endocrine function or to cause weight gain. It would more likely present with sensory or motor seizure activity or headache. Small cell carcinoma of the lung can produce the syndrome of inappropriate antidiuretic hormone secretion, but weight gain is not common, despite mild edema. Retroperitoneal lymphoma may present with fever, bilateral ureteral obstruction, and intestinal dysfunction or pain, but rarely ascites. Ovarian cancer commonly presents as constipation, increasing abdominal girth, and weight gain owing to ascites.

1.6   Answer: (b)   *Helicobacter pylori* has been linked epidemiologically to gastric cancer. Several cancers are associated with viral infection including carcinoma of the cervix, Burkitt's lymphoma, acute T-cell leukemia, Kaposi's sarcoma, and carcinoma of the liver. Heat, as applied with body warming canisters in certain cultures, has led to carcinomas of the chronically burned skin. Other types of acute burns can also lead to squamous carcinomas of the skin. Ultraviolet radiation is the principal carcinogen, leading to basal cell carcinomas, squamous carcinomas, and melanoma, which taken together are the most common cancers in the United States. Although the centers of tumors are hypoxic, there are no data suggesting that those who live at high altitudes, where oxygen levels are low, have an increase in cancer frequency.

ONCOLOGY AND INFORMATICS

162.1   **Answer: (d)**   Networking schemes include server-server, client-server, and client-client varieties.

162.2   **Answer: (b)**   Electronic medical records should support a simultaneous multiple-user view of the data; offer continuous access for authorized users; support direct data entry by physicians, unit clerks, and nurses; and guarantee confidentiality, privacy, and audit trails; they do require the measurement of health status and functional levels.

162.3   **Answer: (c)**   A minority of oncologists use electronic medical records in their practices today. It is estimated that < 10% are active users. However, it is predicted that within 5 years a majority of oncologists will be using electronic medical records as a routine part of their practice.

SCIENTIFIC FOUNDATIONS

DIRECTIONS: Numbering for questions and answers reflects the
corresponding chapter in *Cancer Medicine-6.*
Each question contains suggested responses.
Select the best response to each question.
Answers for Scientific Foundations begin on page 22.

CANCER BIOLOGY

2.1 The most sensitive and specific method to detect a germline mutation in a cancer-predisposing gene using genomic deoxyribonucleic acid (DNA) from blood is
    a. Southern blot restriction fragment length polymorphism (RFLP)
    b. Northern blot
    c. Sequencing of reverse transcriptase polymerase chain reaction (RT-PCR) amplified fragments
    d. Sequencing of PCR amplified fragments
    e. Single nucleotide polymorphism (SNP) oligoarray

2.2 Techniques that enable the comprehensive and unbiased analysis of gene expression profiles include all of the following *except*
    a. Copy DNA (cDNA) microarray hybridization
    b. Expressed sequence tag (EST) sequencing
    c. RT-PCR
    d. Serial analysis of gene expression (SAGE)
    e. Oligonucleotide array hybridization

2.3 The method of choice for the identification of novel protein markers for cancer diagnosis from serum or other body fluid is
    a. Enzyme-linked immunosorbent assay (ELISA)
    b. Immunoblotting
    c. Immunoprecipitation
    d. Mass spectrometry

3.1 Which of the following characteristics of cell proliferation distinguish normal from neoplastic cells?
    a. Only normal cells fail to grow exponentially over time.
    b. Neoplastic cells display shorter cell cycle time compared with their normal counterparts.
    c. Neoplastic cells display an increased growth fraction or a higher percentage of cells in the cell cycle at a given time.
    d. Neoplastic cells spend less time in the S phase (deoxyribonucleic acid [DNA] synthesis phase) compared with their normal counterparts.
    e. Mitosis requires less time in neoplastic cells compared with normal cells.

3.2 Which of the following changes in the retinoblastoma gene product is oncogenic?
    a. Overproduction of retinoblastoma protein
    b. Activating mutation that prevents normal regulation of the retinoblastoma protein's effect on stimulating proliferation
    c. Mutation that prevents phosphorylation of retinoblastoma protein
    d. Mutation that allows overphosphorylation of retinoblastoma protein
    e. Overabundance of messenger ribonucleic acid coding for the retinoblastoma gene product

3.3 Overexpression of the *BCL2* gene is thought to lead to cancer because
    a. Normal cell death is prevented
    b. Cells are more likely to enter the cell cycle
    c. Cell cycle time is shortened
    d. Cells become more sensitive to external growth factors
    e. Growth-promoting signals are enhanced

3.4 The "start," or restriction point, in the cell cycle precedes mitosis and commits the cell irreversibly to cell division. Which one of the following is correct?
    a. The "start" point refers to a point in G_0 (resting phase of the cycle), which, when passed, commits the cell to division.
    b. It refers to initiating synthesis of genes during the S phase of the cell cycle.
    c. It refers to a point late in G_1 in a cell cycle that commits the cell to DNA synthesis (to the S phase).
    d. It refers to a point late in G_1, which, if passed, commits the cell to division.
    e. In normal cells, alkylating agents rarely cause cycle arrest in G_2.

3.5 Which of the following statements regarding molecular control of the cell cycle is *not* correct?
    a. Cyclin-dependent kinases (CDKs), along with cyclins, which are the regulatory subunits of CDKs, are primarily responsible for the transit of cells through the various stages of the cell cycle.
    b. The CDK/cyclin-driven cell cycle progression is under the control of inhibitors, that is, under negative control.
    c. The retinoblastoma *(RB)* gene product transcriptionally activates genes that inhibit CDK function.
    d. The *RB* gene is the gatekeeper for the restriction point. When *RB* becomes phosphorylated, the gate opens, and the cell proceeds through its cycle.
    e. Certain oncogenic viral protein products, for example, human papillomavirus type E7, may complex with and inactivate Rb protein and, thus, have an effect comparable to deletion of a tumor suppressor gene.

4.1   **Defects in apoptosis mechanisms can play roles in which of the following aspects of tumor biology?**
     a.   Cell accumulation
     b.   Metastasis
     c.   Chemoresistance
     d.   Growth factor independence
     e.   All of the above

4.2   **Apoptosis is caused by**
     a.   Depletion of cellular adenosine triphosphate
     b.   Plasma membrane leakage
     c.   Endonuclease activation
     d.   Caspase activation
     e.   Defective cell division

4.3   **Which of the following statements about mitochondria and apoptosis regulation is *not* true?**
     a.   BCL2 family proteins control the release of apoptogenic proteins from mitochondria.
     b.   Multiple stimuli can trigger mitochondrial release of apoptogenic proteins, including growth factor deprivation, irradiation, and deoxyribonucleic acid–damaging anticancer drugs.
     c.   Mitochondria are required for apoptosis.
     d.   Multiple proteins are released from mitochondria during apoptosis, including cytochrome c, AIF, SMAC, and Endo G.

4.4   **Which of the following is *not* an example of a caspase-activation pathway?**
     a.   Tumor necrosis factor/*fas* family death receptors
     b.   The mitochondrial release of cytochrome
     c.   Granzyme B injection into target cells by cytolytic T cells
     d.   Complement-mediated cytotoxicity
     e.   *P53*-mediated induction of proapoptotic *BCL2* family genes

4.5   **Signal transduction pathways that impinge on the core apoptosis machinery include**
     a.   Retinoids and retinoid receptors
     b.   Nuclear factor κB
     c.   AKT
     d.   Estrogens, androgens, and other steroids
     e.   All of the above

5.1   **Small molecule inhibitors of what class of signal transduction proteins have shown efficacy in the treatment of chronic myelogenous leukemia (CML)?**
     a.   Growth factors
     b.   Tyrosine kinases
     c.   Ras
     d.   Transcription factors
     e.   None of the above

5.2   **Which of the following describes the method of use of a monoclonal antibody to the ErbB2/HER2/neu receptor approved as a first-line therapy for metastatic breast cancer?**
     a.   Alone
     b.   In combination with paclitaxel
     c.   In combination with doxorubicin
     d.   All of the above
     e.   None of the above

5.3   **A dominant hereditary cancer syndrome owing to mutational activation of the c-*met* receptor tyrosine kinase is**
     a.   Li-Fraumeni syndrome
     b.   Multiple endocrine neoplasia (MEN) IIA
     c.   Hereditary renal papillary carcinoma
     d.   Adenoma polyposis coli
     e.   MEN IIB

6.1   **What is a retroviral oncogene?**
     a.   A variant of a viral gene
     b.   A cellular gene with transforming potential
     c.   A gene without transforming activity

    d.   A transposon gene incorporated randomly in the viral genome

    e.   A gene able to induce oncogenic transformation following its random insertion in human deoxyribonucleic acid

6.2   **What is the mechanism of action of oncogenically activated growth factor receptors?**

    a.   They transmit information from the cell to the outside environment.

    b.   They interact with a growth factor in the cytoplasm.

    c.   Their activity is strictly dependent on binding with a growth factor present outside of the cell.

    d.   They signal cell growth by an autocrine loop.

    e.   The oncogenic growth factor receptors constitutively promote a growth factor signal cascade.

6.3   **What is *apoptosis*?**

    a.   A process of cell death regulated by specific genes

    b.   A mechanism of cell death that can occur randomly

    c.   A mechanism that leads to cell survival in specific conditions

    d.   A process that determines a cell volume enlargement

    e.   A kind of tissue necrosis

6.4   **What are the features of the oncogenic chimeric protein derived from *bcr-abl* gene fusion?**

    a.   The *bcr-abl* fusion creates a new protein with similar tyrosine kinase activity but abnormal cellular localization.

    b.   The *bcr-abl* enzymatic activity is always switched on.

    c.   Abnormal activation of *abl* renders it independent by the interaction with proteins carrying SH2 and SH3 domains.

    d.   The fused gene *bcr-abl* is inappropriately expressed in chronic myelogenous leukemia (CML).

    e.   The *bcr-abl* fused protein is no longer capable of binding retinoic acid.

6.5   **Which of the following statements is appropriate regarding the current model of tumor development and progression?**

    a.   The *P53* gene is involved in early phases of colorectal cancer development.

    b.   The *FHIT* gene plays a pivotal role in lymphoma development.

    c.   The *bcr-abl* gene fusion leads to CML initiation.

    d.   Only oncogenes lead to neoplasia initiation.

    e.   The genes *ras* and *P53* are not involved in the progression of hematologic malignancies.

7.1   **Familial forms of cancer such as Li-Fraumeni syndrome, familial adenomatous polyposis (FAP), and Lynch syndrome involve mutations of tumor suppressor genes and display which kind of inheritance pattern?**

    a.   Autosomal dominant

    b.   Autosomal recessive

    c.   X-linked

    d.   None of the above

7.2   **You perform a genetic test for an *APC* gene mutation on an 8-year-old boy in a family who has had several cases of FAP. The test comes back negative (no mutation found). What do you tell the child and his parents?**

    a.   The child does not have an *APC* gene mutation and he has no risk of developing colorectal cancer.

    b.   The child does not have an *APC* gene mutation and he has the same risk of developing colorectal cancer as a member of the general population (5% lifetime).

    c.   The child probably has no *APC* gene mutation and is likely not to develop FAP.

    d.   The test is inconclusive, and the child should be managed as if he has a 50% risk of developing FAP.

7.3   **A family with a history of multiple cancers consistent with the Li-Fraumeni syndrome comes to you for prenatal genetic counseling. The mother has been tested and found to carry a germline mutation of *P53* at codon 273, converting an arginine to a histidine. The fetus is tested, and the result is negative (no mutation at codon 273). What do you tell the parents?**

    a.   The fetus does not have a heritable *P53* gene mutation and has no risk of developing leukemias and other cancers present in this family.

    b.   The child does not have a *P53* gene mutation and has the same risk of developing cancers as a member of the general population.

    c.   The child probably has no *P53* gene mutation and is likely not to develop the Li-Fraumeni phenotype.

    d.   The test is inconclusive, and the child should be managed as if he or she has a 50% risk of developing the syndrome.

8.1   **The Philadelphia chromosome contains which of the following fusion genes?**

    a.   *PML-RARA*

    b.   *MLL-ELL*

    c.   *BCR-ABL*

    d.   *AML1-ETO*

8.2   **The novel therapy for chronic myelogenous leukemia, imatinib mesylate (Gleevec), belongs to which of the following drug classes?**
a.   Monoclonal antibody
b.   Tyrosine kinase inhibitor
c.   Farnesyl transferase inhibitior
d.   Vascular epithelial growth factor (VEGF) inhibitor

8.3   **The following cytogenetic abnormalities all portend a poor prognosis in patients with acute myelogenous leukemia (AML)** *except*
a.   del(5q)
b.   del(7q)
c.   t(11;19)(q23;p13.1)
d.   t(15;17)(q22;q12–21)

8.4   **The t(8;14)(q24;q32) is characteristic of which of the following lymphomas?**
a.   Burkitt's lymphoma
b.   Anaplastic large cell lymphoma
c.   Follicular lymphoma
d.   Mantle cell lymphoma

8.5   **Which of the following is an oncogene involved in the progressive accumulation of genetic mutations resulting in colorectal tumorigenesis?**
a.   *ras*
b.   *APC*
c.   *TP53*
d.   *DCC*

8.6   **Which of the following sets of tumors have been shown to carry identical translocations yet result in two completely different phenotypes?**
a.   Neuroepitheliomas and Ewing's sarcoma
b.   Ewing's sarcoma and desmoplastic small round cell tumor
c.   Myxoid liposarcoma and lipoma
d.   All of the above

8.7   **Recurring chromosomal aberrations in solid tumors have not been as well characterized as those that occur in hematologic malignancies because**
a.   It is difficult to obtain chromosome preparations from solid malignancies because of extensive fibrosis and necrosis
b.   Until recently, many investigators did not fully realize the relevance of chromosome changes in malignant cells
c.   Karyotypes of solid tumors frequently reveal high modal numbers, making it difficult to distinguish between primary and secondary genetic changes
d.   Of all of the above reasons

9.1   **All of the following are typical properties of cancer cells growing in cell culture** *except*
a.   Loss of anchorage dependence
b.   Resistance to apoptosis
c.   Increased requirement for serum or growth factors in the culture medium
d.   Loss of normal cell-matrix interactions
e.   Increased agglutinability to plant lectins

9.2   **Alterations of E-cadherin expression and function have been observed in a number of human cancers. Down-regulation of E-cadherin correlates with**
a.   Increased tumor invasiveness
b.   Decreased metastases
c.   Enhanced patient survival
d.   Improved cell-matrix interaction
e.   Normal cell-cell adhesiveness

9.3   **Methylation of deoxyribonucleic acid (DNA)**
a.   Usually occurs on adenine-rich sequences
b.   Usually results in increased gene expression
c.   Is often aberrant in cancer tissue
d.   Has not been observed in oncogene-induced malignant transformation
e.   Is never seen in regulatory regions of human genes

10.1   **Angiogenesis and metastasis have in common which of the following?**
     a.   Growth factor receptor activation
     b.   Matrix metalloproteinase production and activation
     c.   Integrin engagement
     d.   Locomotion
     e.   All of the above

10.2   **Tumors have divergent metastatic potential for which of the following reasons?**
     a.   Patient gender and tumor genotype
     b.   Patient gender and human leukocyte antigen (HLA) type
     c.   Tumor genotype and local microenvironment
     d.   Patient gender, tumor genotype, and HLA type
     e.   Local microenvironment only

10.3   **Which of the following statements is *not* true?**
     a.   Tumor cells disseminate equally in all organs.
     b.   Invasion and metastasis are late events in tumor progression.
     c.   Homing events are involved in organ preference of metastasis.
     d.   A frequent site of metastasis is the first capillary bed encountered by the circulating cancer cell.
     e.   Metastasis is a highly inefficient process.

10.4   **Which of the following have *not* been examined clinically as potential molecular targets for cancer invasion?**
     a.   Integrins
     b.   Matrix metalloproteinases
     c.   Serine and tyrosine kinases
     d.   Locomotion
     e.   None of the above

11.1   **Which one of the following statements about the antiangiogenic action of thalidomide is *not* correct?**
     a.   Thalidomide decreases circulating levels of vascular endothelial growth factor (VEGF) and basic fibroblast growth factor (bFGF).
     b.   Thalidomide decreases circulating endothelial cells up to tenfold.
     c.   Thalidomide suppresses angiogenesis in experimental models such as the rabbit cornea.
     d.   Thalidomide inhibits angiogenesis through inhibition of tumor necrosis factor (TNF)-α.

11.2   **Poorly vascularized tumors are**
     a.   Less responsive to angiogenesis inhibitors than are rapidly growing tumors
     b.   Generally more responsive to angiogenesis inhibitors than are rapidly growing tumors
     c.   About equally responsive to angiogenesis inhibitors as are rapidly growing tumors

11.3   **Interferon-α is an angiogenesis inhibitor because**
     a.   It is immunosuppressive
     b.   It inhibits overexpression of bFGF by human tumor cells
     c.   At high doses it is cytotoxic
     d.   Of none of the above reasons

11.4   **Which one of the following statements about antiangiogenic chemotherapy is *not* true?**
     a.   It targets endothelial cells directly or indirectly.
     b.   It is also called low-dose chemotherapy.
     c.   It has also been called metronomic therapy.
     d.   It is more toxic than chemotherapy.

11.5   **Which of the following is *not* true of the way *P53* normally suppresses tumor angiogenesis?**
     a.   It up-regulates thrombospondin 1.
     b.   It induces degradation of histoplasma inhibitory factor (HIF)-1 α.
     c.   It suppresses transcription of VEGF.
     d.   It becomes mutated or deleted.
     e.   It down-regulates bFGF binding protein expression.

11.6   **Which one of the following statements is correct?**
     a.   Microvessel density is useful as a prognostic indicator of risk of mortality or metastasis in certain tumors.
     b.   Microvessel density is useful for predicting efficacy of antiangiogenic therapy.

    c.   Microvessel density correlates with tumor flow.

    d.   Microvessel density correlates with success of chemotherapy.

CANCER IMMUNOLOGY

12.1   **One reason why tumor cells and autologous antigen-presenting cells (APCs) that have taken up tumor antigens display non-identical sets of epitopes recognized by tumor-reactive CD8+ T cells is the differential expression by tumor cells and APCs of which of the following?**

    a.   Human leukocyte antigen (HLA) class I genotypes

    b.   Immunoproteasome

    c.   Integrin molecules

    d.   Fibronectin

    e.   CD4 molecules

12.2   **Melanoma antigens have been most extensively evaluated over the past decade because**

    a.   Melanoma represents the highest incidence form of cancer

    b.   Of the ease of isolation of specific T cells or antibodies that recognize melanoma antigens

    c.   Of the higher rate of mutations in melanoma versus other types of cancer

    d.   Leukopenia commonly observed in patients with melanoma allows a greater source of T cells

    e.   All melanomas express the identical set of tumor antigens

12.3   **The category of tumor antigen theoretically *least* likely to promote pathologic autoimmunity if employed in a vaccine formulation is**

    a.   Cancer-testis antigens

    b.   Melanoma antigens

    c.   Epithelial tumor antigens

    d.   Cell-cycle regulatory antigens

    e.   Idiotypic tumor antigens

12.4   **Single epitope vaccines in the cancer setting are likely to yield modest clinical benefit because**

    a.   Tumors are antigenically heterogeneous

    b.   Tumor lesions frequently contain antigen-loss variants

    c.   Single epitope vaccines fail to be recognized by both cytotoxic T lymphocytes and T helper cells required for optimal clinical benefit

    d.   They require the selection of patients based on HLA typing

    e.   Of all of the above reasons

13.1   **Tumor markers are molecules that signal the malignant process. These molecules can be (More than one may be correct.)**

    a.   Deoxyribonucleic acid (DNA)

    b.   Ribonucleic acid (RNA)

    c.   Proteins

    d.   Phospholipids

    e.   All of the above

13.2   **For use as an ideal cancer screening marker in a clinically asymptomatic population, the most important performance characteristic of the marker is**

    a.   Use of biologic specimens that can be obtained noninvasively

    b.   Very high disease specificity

    c.   Very high test sensitivity

13.3   **Carcinoembryonic antigen (CEA) is a useful marker in colon cancer for (More than one may be correct.)**

    a.   Early detection and screening

    b.   Diagnosis

    c.   Prognosis

    d.   Metastasis

13.4   **At present, serum immunoassay for the level of cancer antigen 125 (CA 125) is the best-established screening and diagnostic marker for ovarian cancer. Its greatest utility is for (More than one may be correct.)**

    a.   Identifying women at elevated risk for ovarian cancer as a result of inheritance of germline mutations in *BRCA1* or -2 genes

    b.   Detection of early stage, and highly curable, disease

    c.   Monitoring the response to chemotherapy

    d.   Prognosis

13.5 **New genomic and proteomic technologies have contributed new tools and approaches for (More than one may be correct.)**
    a. Discovery of new early detection and screening markers
    b. Molecular diagnostics
    c. Molecular classification of disease and prognostics
    d. Novel therapeutics
    e. All of the above

14.1 **Tumor-specific transplantation antigens (TSTAs) expressed on murine tumors are responsible for**
    a. Deletion of T lymphocytes
    b. Increased natural killer (NK) cell activity in the spleen
    c. Immunization of mice and protection against the challenge with tumor cells
    d. Tumor growth
    e. Loss of class I major histocompatibility complex (MHC) antigens from the surface of tumor cells

14.2 **Antitumor effector cells can mediate tumor rejection in vivo by which one of the following mechanisms?**
    a. Cytotoxicity
    b. Complement activation
    c. Elimination of regulatory T cells
    d. Proliferation
    e. Antigen cross-presentation

14.3 **Human NK cells present in the circulation or body fluids of patients with cancer have which of the following characteristics?**
    a. Expression of T-cell receptor
    b. Impairment in cytotoxic activity and a proneness to undergo apoptosis
    c. CD3+, CD56+, and CD16– by flow cytometry
    d. Expression of very high levels of immunoglobulin
    e. Lack of responsiveness to interleukin-2

14.4 **Immunotherapy of cancer is based on which of the following rationales?**
    a. Tumor cells are not recognized by the host immune system.
    b. Activated T cells are necessary for tumor growth.
    c. Activation of immune effector mechanisms could result in tumor elimination.
    d. Activation of macrophages in tissues is responsible for the development of tumor sensitivity to immune effector cells.
    e. Enhanced antibody production leads to tumor demise.

14.5 **Tumor escape from the immune response of the host could involve which one of the following?**
    a. Gain of MHC class II molecules
    b. Gain of MHC class I molecules
    c. Overexpression of interferon-γ
    d. Ability of the tumor to suppress antitumor effector cell function
    e. Production by the tumor of FasL

15.1 **Failure of cytolytic T cells (CTLs) to recognize tumor cells is often the result of tumor cells losing expression of**
    a. Major histocompatibility complex (MHC) class I
    b. Transforming growth factor (TGF)-β
    c. ICAD
    d. FADD

15.2 **Tumor cells secrete immunosuppressive factors that inhibit the normal expression of immune effector function. The factors commonly include**
    a. Interleukin-2 (IL-2) and interferon-γ
    b. TGF-β and IL-10
    c. Tumor necrosis factor (TNF) and TGF-α
    d. IL-10 and interferon-γ

15.3 **Activation-induced cell death (AICD) associated with T-cell interactions with tumor cells represents a mechanism of elimination of T cells by**
    a. Induction of apoptosis of activated T cells on subsequent encounter with antigen
    b. Ligation of CD4 or CD28 co-stimulatory molecules
    c. Binding of Fas (CD95) on T cells and FasL (CD95L) on tumor cells
    d. Induction of apoptosis of activated T cells on subsequent encounter with antigen, and ligation of CD4 or CD28 co-stimulatory molecules

e. Induction of apoptosis of activated T cells on subsequent encounter with antigen and binding of Fas (CD95) on T cells and FasL (CD95L) on tumor cells

f. Ligation of CD4 or CD28 co-stimulatory molecules and binding of Fas (CD95) on T cells and FasL (CD95L) on tumor cells

15.4 **Evidence for suppression of immune effector cells has been documented by demonstrating a reduction in expression of components of intracytoplasmic signal transduction pathways including**

a. IL-8

b. BCL2

c. T cell antigen receptor (TCR) ζ chain

d. Granzyme B

e. Cytolysin

15.5 **Tumor cells suppress expression of effector function of NK cells and CTLs as a consequence of abnormally high levels of membrane complement regulatory proteins including**

a. CD36, CD55, CD59

b. CD46, CD55, CD59

c. Decorin

d. Cytolysin

CANCER ETIOLOGY

16.1 **Which extracolonic cancer is *not* considered an integral tumor in hereditary nonpolyposis colorectal cancer (HNPCC), also know as Lynch syndrome?**

a. Endometrial cancer

b. Ovarian cancer

c. Lung cancer

d. Pancreatic cancer

e. Upper uroepithelial tract cancer

16.2 **The natural history of HNPCC is characterized by which of the following? (More than one may be correct.)**

a. Early-onset colorectal cancer (CRC) with an excess of metachronous CRC

b. An increased risk of carcinoma of the ovary, which is the second most common cancer in HNPCC

c. A threefold increased incidence rate of colonic polyps throughout the lifetime of the patient when compared with that of the general population

d. Poorly differentiated and mucinous features, with an exaggerated lymphoid response of the tumor

e. A survival advantage in patients with CRC when compared by stage with non-HNPCC controls with CRC

f. All of the above

16.3 **Cowden disease is an autosomal dominant inherited rare disorder that is characterized by which of the following features? (More than one may be correct.)**

a. Multiple hamartomas including gastrointestinal hamartomatous polyps and benign and malignant neoplasms of the breast, thyroid, uterus, and skin

b. Facial trichilemmoma, acrokeratosis, or papillomatous papules in virtually all patients

c. An inordinately high risk of colorectal cancer

d. All of the above

16.4 **Mutated *BRCA1* and *BRCA2* genes predispose their carriers to the hereditary breast/ovarian cancer syndrome (HBOC). Which of the following does *not* characterize HBOC?**

a. An excess of breast and ovarian cancer

b. An excess of male breast cancer in *BRCA2* mutation carriers

c. An excess of pancreatic carcinoma in *BRCA2* carriers

d. An excess of hepatocellular carcinoma in both *BRCA1/2* carriers

e. An excess of bilateral breast cancer in *BRCA1/2* carriers

16.5 **Genetic counseling is considered to be mandatory for patients with hereditary forms of cancer when they are considering germline mutation testing. Which one of the following is *not* true of the genetic counseling process?**

a. Genetic counseling can most effectively be performed through a letter or pamphlet sent to the patient describing all features of the particular disorder where a mutation has been identified.

b. Genetic counselors, whenever possible, should be involved in the genetic counseling process.

  c. Physicians who are knowledgeable about the pertinent issues that should be covered in genetic counseling may provide this service.

  d. Genetic counseling should include details about the natural history of the particular disorder, availability of screening and management strategies, and the potential for emotional distress.

17.1 **What class of chemicals is referred to as the "food mutagens?"**
 a. Polycyclic aromatic hydrocarbons
 b. Heterocyclic amines
 c. Aromatic amines
 d. Aflatoxins
 e. Tobacco-specific nitrosamines

17.2 **There are several mechanisms of deoxyribonucleic acid (DNA) repair. Most mechanisms of DNA repair involve multienzyme complexes. Which mechanism of DNA repair involves only a DNA alkyltransferase?**
 a. Nucleotide excision repair
 b. Mismatch repair
 c. Double-strand break repair
 d. Direct DNA repair
 e. Base excision repair

17.3 **Which of the following is the term for the amount of a chemical carcinogen that reaches a target tissue in a form that becomes activated to a chemical species capable of causing a lesion in DNA?**
 a. The cancer dose
 b. The carcinogen dose
 c. The biologically effective dose
 d. The initiation dose
 e. The cancer promoter

17.4 **Which of the following is true? Caretaker genes**
 a. Are tumor suppressor genes
 b. Are directly involved in neoplastic initiation
 c. Control cellular proliferation and death
 d. Are oncogenes
 e. Maintain genomic stability

17.5 **Results from molecular epidemiology studies can be assessed for causation by**
 a. The consistency of the association between carcinogen exposure and cancer
 b. The "weight of the evidence" principle using criteria proposed by Bradford-Hill
 c. The biologic plausibility of the association
 d. The specificity of the association
 e. The temporality of the association
 f. All of the above

18.1 **Among the various exogenous hormones studied with regard to breast cancer, the highest risk per year of use is associated with**
 a. Oral contraceptives
 b. Estrogen replacement therapy
 c. Stilbestrol therapy
 d. Combined estrogen and progesterone replacement therapy
 e. Tamoxifen

18.2 **Which of the following is *not* an established risk factor for breast cancer?**
 a. Dietary fat
 b. Age at menopause
 c. Postmenopaual obesity
 d. Age at menarche
 e. Family history of breast cancer

18.3 **Germline mutations have been consistently associated with familial breast cancer in all of the following genes *except***
 a. *BRCA1*
 b. *ATM*
 c. *TP53*
 d. *BRCA2*

18.4 **Which of the following are *not* associated with a decreased risk of endometrial cancer?**
a. Obesity
b. Oral contraceptive use
c. Parity
d. Age at menopause
e. Progesterone

18.5 **Major determinants of prostate cancer risk include**
a. Race
b. Age
c. Family history of prostate cancer
d. Intake of vitamin E and selenium

19.1 **Radiation kills cells by**
a. Apoptosis
b. Reproductive failure
c. Heat
d. Apoptosis and reproductive failure
e. All of the above

19.2 **Relative to the power of polycyclic hydrocarbons to induce transformation,**
a. Radiation is a more potent inducer
b. Radiation is a less potent inducer
c. Radiation is an equally potent inducer
d. Radiation's potency as an inducer is unknown

19.3 **Radiation mediates cellular changes by**
a. Inducing genomic instability
b. A bystander effect
c. Causing mutations
d. Inactivation of tumor suppressor genes
e. All of the above methods

19.4 **The organ with the greatest risk of radiation-induced cancer in males is**
a. Bone marrow
b. The esophagus
c. The colon
d. The cervix
e. None of the above

19.5 **The risk of death as a result of radiation exposure from chest radiography is**
a. > the risk of death from smoking 1 pack of cigarettes per day
b. > the risk of death from rock climbing
c. > age-adjusted mortality at age 55 years
d. Approximately 1 in 1,000,000
e. None of the above

20.1 **The most important solar wavelengths for skin cancer induction are**
a. Ultraviolet (UV) A
b. UVB
c. UVC

20.2 **The photoproducts produced by sunlight in DNA result in the production of which characteristic mutations that can be recognized in *P53*?**
a. Transversions that change purines to pyrimidines
b. Deletions of two or more bases
c. Conversion of cytosine to thymidine at dipyrimidine sites
d. Transitions at individual cytosines

20.3 Xeroderma pigmentosum is a sun-sensitive disease with elevated rates of cancer owing to mutations that mainly affect which pathway for processing UV damage?
  a. Photolyase
  b. DNA polymerase-δ
  c. Nucleotide excision repair
  d. Patched-smoothened-hedgehog gene

20.4 The *P53* gene develops mutations in sun-exposed areas of the skin that are thought to be precursors of which form of cancer?
  a. Basal cell carcinoma (BCC)
  b. Squamous cell carcinoma (SCC)
  c. Spitz nevi
  d. Melanoma

21.1 The tumor most specifically related to asbestos exposure is
  a. Laryngeal cancer
  b. Lung cancer
  c. Mesothelioma
  d. Gastrointestinal cancer
  e. Renal cancer

21.2 The most powerful agent demonstrated to be carcinogenic for the pleura by experimental studies is
  a. Asbestos
  b. Glass fiber
  c. Rock wool
  d. Ceramic fiber
  e. Erionite

21.3 Which of the following statements is *false*?
  a. Tobacco smoke increases the incidence of lung cancer.
  b. Asbestos exposure increases the incidence of lung cancer.
  c. The association of tobacco smoke and asbestos exposure increases the incidence of lung cancer.
  d. Tobacco smoke increases the incidence of mesothelioma.
  e. Asbestos exposure increases the incidence of mesothelioma.

22.1 Retrovirus infections cause which of the following kind of mutations?
  a. Point mutations
  b. Insertional mutations
  c. Chromatid exchange
  d. Deletions
  e. Homologous recombination

22.2 The retroviral large terminal repeat sequence contains all of the following *except*
  a. A ribonucleic acid (RNA) polymerase promoter
  b. A polyadenylation signal
  c. A transcriptional termination signal
  d. Transcriptional enhancers
  e. The RNA packaging signal

22.3 In which one of the following diseases have retroviruses *not* been implicated?
  a. Leukemias
  b. Immunodeficiency diseases
  c. Central nervous system diseases
  d. Liver cancer
  e. Mammary tumors

23.1 Epstein-Barr virus has been associated with each of the following malignancies *except*
  a. Kaposi's sarcoma
  b. Hodgkin's disease
  c. Nasopharyngeal carcinoma
  d. Burkitt's lymphoma
  e. T-cell lymphoma

23.2 **Kaposi's sarcoma–associated herpesvirus is strongly associated with each of the following malignancies** *except*
   a. Body cavity lymphomas
   b. Kaposi's sarcoma in non–acquired immunodeficiency syndrome (AIDS) patients
   c. T-cell lymphomas
   d. Kaposi's sarcoma in AIDS patients
   e. Castleman's disease

23.3 **Which of the following is** *incorrect* **about Kaposi's sarcoma–associated herpesvirus?**
   a. Kaposi's sarcoma–associated herpesvirus has been transmitted by kidney transplantation.
   b. Kaposi's sarcoma–associated herpesvirus can be transmitted vertically from mother to child.
   c. Nearly all persons seropositive for Kaposi's sarcoma–associated herpesvirus develop Kaposi's sarcoma.
   d. Kaposi's sarcoma–associated herpesvirus is more common in African men than in American men.
   e. Kaposi's sarcoma–associated herpesvirus has been detected in the peripheral blood of patients with Kaposi's sarcoma.

23.4 **Which of the following diseases associated with Epstein-Barr virus is very responsive to antiviral (acyclovir) therapy?**
   a. Epstein-Barr virus–associated hemophagocytic syndrome
   b. Oral hairy leukoplakia
   c. Epstein-Barr virus–associated lymphoproliferative disease
   d. Infectious mononucleosis
   e. Epstein-Barr virus–associated Hodgkin's disease

24.1 **Which of the following is (are) associated with a risk of cervical neoplasia?**
   a. The presence of a squamocolumnar junction
   b. Infection by cancer-associated human papillomavirus (HPV) types
   c. Sexual activity
   d. Persistent HPV infection
   e. All of the above
   f. None of the above

24.2 **Potential uses of HPV testing include which of the following?**
   a. Monitoring of male sexual partners
   b. Management of high-grade cervical intraepithelial neoplasia
   c. Triage of low-grade cervical intraepithelial neoplasia
   d. Triage of nondiagnostic epithelial atypias in the Papanicolaou smear
   e. All of the above

24.3 **Recent studies with HPV 16–derived vaccines have successfully achieved which of the following?**
   a. Regression of cervical cancer
   b. Prevention of persistent HPV infection
   c. Prevention of HPV 16 –related preinvasive disease
   d. Prevention of persistent HPV infection and of HPV 16–related preinvasive disease
   e. All of the above are correct

25.1 **Which of the following hepatitis viruses have been determined to be the direct causative agent for hepatocellular carcinoma (HCC)? (More than one may be correct.)**
   a. Hepatitis A virus
   b. Hepatitis B virus (HBV)
   c. Hepatitis C virus (HCV)
   d. Hepatitis D virus
   e. Hepatitis E virus

25.2 **Which of the following treatments have been shown to lead to reduction in the risk of developing HCC? (More than one may be correct.)**
   a. Interferon-α for the treatment of chronic hepatitis B
   b. Lamivudine or adefovir dipivoxil for the treatment of chronic hepatitis B
   c. Hepatitis B vaccine for the prevention of hepatitis B
   d. Interferon-α for chronic hepatitis C
   e. Ribavirin and interferon-α for hepatitis C

25.3 Which of the following screening programs for HCC in high-risk populations results in survival prolongation? (More than one may be correct.)
   a. Ultrasonography of the liver every 6 months
   b. Serum α-fetoprotein (AFP) every 6 months
   c. Neither of the above has been proven effective

26.1 Which of the following describe(s) schistosomal cystitis? (More than one may be correct.)
   a. Granulomatous reaction to viable schistosomal ova plugged in the vesical venules
   b. Granulomatous reaction to nonviable or broken-down schistosomal ova trapped in bladder capillaries
   c. Precancerous condition because it gives rise to bladder papillomas and polyps
   d. Precancerous condition if squamous metaplasia is present
   e. Associated with increased urinary excretion of "*N*-nitroso" compounds

CANCER EPIDEMIOLOGY, PREVENTION, AND SCREENING

27.1 The cancer incidence rate in a country is
   a. The number of new cases occurring in that country each year
   b. The fraction of new patients who die each year
   c. The rate at which new cancers are diagnosed per 100,000 people per year
   d. The rate at which new patients die each year

27.2 Cancer incidence and death rates in the United States are currently age adjusted (age standardized) to the age distribution of the US population in
   a. 1970
   b. 1980
   c. 1990
   d. 2000
   e. None of the above

27.3 The proportion of people in the United States who die from cancer is approximately
   a. 15%
   b. 25%
   c. 35%
   d. 45%

27.4 The introduction and wide dissemination of a new screening test such as prostate-specific antigen (PSA) has the largest immediate impact on
   a. The incidence rate
   b. The death rate
   c. The relative survival
   d. The relative risk

27.5 For which major cancer is the incidence rate higher in Whites but the death rate higher in African Americans?
   a. Lung and bronchus cancers
   b. Colon and rectal cancers
   c. Breast cancer in women
   d. Prostate cancer

28.1 Hypermethylation of the promoter of a number of "lung cancer genes" has been identified recently as a common cause of
   a. Aberrant transcriptional induction
   b. Transcriptional silencing
   c. Protein truncation
   d. Gene mutation

28.2 All of the following genes contribute to the biologic activity of nicotine (dependence, metabolism, enzymatic induction) *except*
   a. Cytochrome P-450 2D6
   b. Cytochrome P-450 1A1
   c. Glutathione S-transferase M1
   d. Dopamine D2 receptor

28.3 **Which of the following is *not* a component of the "5As" model for a physician-based smoking cessation intervention?**
a. Arranging a follow-up visit to determine the patient's progress with cessation efforts
b. Assisting the patient with cessation by providing nicotine-replacement therapy as needed
c. Assembling a workstation to train nurses in treating nicotine addiction
d. Asking all patients who are seen about their tobacco use
e. Assessing the patient's readiness to quit smoking

28.4 **Efficacious methods for cessation treatment include**
a. Use of the transdermal nicotine patch
b. Skills building to avoid relapse
c. Use of bupropion
d. Physician counseling
e. All of the above

29.1 **When conducting human trials of novel oncology therapies, randomized intervention trials are frequently the study type of choice. However, when evaluating nutrition and cancer hypotheses, randomized trials often have all of the following shortcomings *except***
a. The study usually cannot be blinded
b. Poor compliance is common
c. Subject recall is biased
d. The studies are expensive

29.2 **A postmenopausal woman wishes to make lifestyle and diet changes that are likely to reduce her risk of breast cancer. Based on the evidence to date, which of the following is the best advice for this woman?**
a. Consume a diet with at least 30 g/d of soy isoflavones, exercise regularly, and eat a diet rich in fruits and vegetables.
b. Avoid weight gain, drink a minimal amount of alcohol, if any, and consume a diet rich in fruits and vegetables.
c. Reduce dietary fat and sugar intake, and ensure adequate dietary selenium.
d. Consume a diet high in fiber and vitamin E and exercise regularly.

29.3 **A patient asks your advice on ways to reduce cancer risk through nutrition. This patient is 35 years old and has a family history of several types of cancer. What would you recommend?**
a. Buy reduced-fat items at the grocery store.
b. Take a daily multivitamin and consume more fruits and vegetables.
c. Refer the patient to a registered dietitian (RD) for individual counseling.
d. Eliminate charbroiled and smoke-cured meats.

30.1 **Chemoprevention trials in breast cancer have shown that**
a. Contralateral breast cancer occurs at a rate of 0.8% yearly, and a slightly increased rate of ovarian cancer exists with fenretinide treatment
b. Tamoxifen chemoprevention trials currently show the same risk of contralateral secondary tumors in patients who are treated with a placebo
c. Women entering the tamoxifen chemoprevention trial must demonstrate a fourfold increase in risk before starting the study
d. Fenretinide and tamoxifen have been shown in laboratory studies to be more effective alone than in combination to suppress mammary carcinogenesis
e. Fenretinide can cause ocular toxicity

30.2 **Regarding the use of tamoxifen as a chemopreventive agent, which of the following most accurately describes its mechanism of action?**
a. Tamoxifen has a strong estrogen-inducing effect on human mammary tissue.
b. Tamoxifen has neither antiestrogen nor estrogen agonist effects on breast tissue.
c. Tamoxifen has no role in the treatment of estrogen receptor–negative carcinomas.
d. Tamoxifen suppresses insulin-like growth factor 1 in breast cancer.
e. Tamoxifen does not induce synthesis of transforming growth factor β (TGF-β).

30.3 **The action of retinoids as chemoprevention agents is most likely based on**
a. Action through the steroid receptor family
b. Control of normal differentiation and proliferation of a number of cells, except those of mesenchymal origin
c. Control of carcinogenesis
d. Control of cell growth
e. Interference with the antiestrogenic effects of tamoxifen

31.1 When evaluating cancer screening, one of several measures of a screening test's accuracy is sensitivity. Which of the following statements is correct with respect to what sensitivity measures?
    a. Sensitivity is the overall average score of the test's accuracy.
    b. Sensitivity is the proportion of individuals with a positive test among all who test positive for the disease.
    c. Sensitivity is the proportion of individuals with a positive test among all who are tested and have the disease.
    d. Sensitivity is the proportion of individuals that test positive.

31.2 The positive predictive value (PPV) is the proportion of all positive screening tests that result in a diagnosis of cancer. Which of the following most influences the magnitude of the positive PPV?
    a. Sensitivity
    b. Specificity
    c. The false-positive rate and the false-negative rate
    d. The false-positive rate and the prevalence of disease

31.3 A prospective randomized clinical trial (RCT) with a mortality end point is favored over an observational study to evaluate the efficacy of a screening test because it eliminates
    a. Lead-time bias
    b. Length bias
    c. Self-selection bias
    d. All of the above

31.4 Which of the following has been shown to be an effective screening test for breast cancer?
    a. Mammography
    b. Clinical breast examination
    c. Ultrasonography
    d. Magnetic resonance imaging (MRI)

31.5 Which of the following screening tests has been shown to reduce both colorectal cancer incidence and mortality?
    a. Fecal occult blood test (FOBT)
    b. Endoscopy
    c. FOBT and endoscopy
    d. Neither FOBT or endoscopy

CLINICAL TRIALS AND OUTCOMES ASSESSMENT

33.1 The most important quantities for designing and monitoring clinical trials are
    a. Prior probabilities
    b. Posterior probabilities
    c. Predictive probabilities
    d. *p* Values
    e. Confidence intervals

33.2 Hierarchic models are useful in statistical analysis because they
    a. Make a minimal number of assumptions
    b. Implicitly assume that hazards are constant over time
    c. Mean that confidence levels are the same as posterior probabilities of the corresponding intervals
    d. Consider different levels of experimental units and allow for borrowing information across the various units within each level of the hierarchy
    e. Allow for continuation of a trial beyond its originally scheduled termination point

33.3 The virtue of decision analysis for designing clinical trials is that it considers
    a. The effective treatment of patients in the trial
    b. The scientific issue of learning about the various treatments; it therefore promotes the effective treatment of patients who present after the trial
    c. The consequences of carrying out a trial with a particular design
    d. The uncertainty present before the trial concerning the effectiveness and toxicity of the various treatments
    e. All of the above

33.4   **Which of the following is a type of adaptation within a clinical trial that is facilitated by a bayesian approach?**
a.   Early stopping of the trial on the basis of negative results
b.   Early stopping of the trial on the basis of positive results
c.   Continuation of the trial beyond its planned end point because the results are equivocal
d.   Adding and dropping of treatment arms
e.   All of the above

33.5   **Biomarkers can enhance the worth of using an adaptive design in phases II and III by**
a.   Giving early information about the ultimate end point using models for the relationship between biomarkers and the ultimate end point
b.   Eliminating the need for phase I trials
c.   Eliminating the need to observe the ultimate end point
d.   Making irrelevant any relationship between treatment and biomarkers
e.   Doing all of the above

34.1   **What is the difference, if any, between a cost-benefit analysis and a cost-effectiveness analysis?**
a.   A cost-benefit analysis looks at an intervention in isolation, whereas a cost-effectiveness analysis compares two interventions.
b.   A cost-benefit analysis evaluates commercial investments, whereas a cost-effectiveness analysis evaluates investments in medical interventions.
c.   A cost-benefit analysis measures benefits in financial terms, whereas a cost-effectiveness analysis measures benefits in units of medical effect.
d.   A cost-benefit analysis examines short-term costs and benefits, whereas a cost-effectiveness analysis examines short- and long-term effects.
e.   The two terms are synonymous.

34.2   **What is the difference between "efficacy" and "effectiveness?"**
a.   Efficacy measures outcomes under carefully controlled conditions, whereas effectiveness measures outcomes in the routine care setting.
b.   Efficacy considers only effects on survival, whereas effectiveness considers all outcomes.
c.   Efficacy considers short- and long-term effects, whereas effectiveness considers only short-term effects.
d.   Efficacy is a statistical measure, whereas effectiveness is a clinical measure.
e.   The two terms are synonyms.

34.3   **Although randomized trials are the best strategy for assessing the impact of alternative interventions on survival, cost consequences of alternative treatment strategies can be adequately estimated from retrospective reviews of billing data. True or false?**

34.4   **What is the threshold, in dollars per year of life saved, above which a medical intervention would _not_ be considered cost-effective?**
a. $100
b. $1,000
c. $10,000
d. $100,000
e. $1,000,000

34.5   **What is the difference between clinical practice guidelines and critical pathways?**
a.   Guidelines are developed by national organizations, whereas critical pathways are developed by practices or individual institutions.
b.   Guidelines dictate what the treatment should be, whereas critical pathways specify how a particular treatment should be given.
c.   Guidelines describe the care to be provided by physicians, whereas critical pathways describe the care to be provided by ancillary personnel.
d.   Guidelines are designed to achieve optimal benefits for patients, whereas critical pathways are designed to save resources.
e.   The two terms are synonymous.

ANSWERS

CANCER BIOLOGY

2.1   **Answer: (d)**   Northern blot and RT-PCR use ribonucleic acid (RNA) as starting material; this approach would require that the gene of interest be expressed in the blood (which may or may not be true depending on the gene). Southern blot RFLP is highly specific for the detection of mutations if there is a restriction enzyme that is able to differentiate between the wild-type and mutant forms. In addition, Southern blot requires relatively large amounts of DNA. SNP oligoarrays are highly sensitive and specific for the detection of known mutations but are not able to identify previously unknown mutants. PCR performed on genomic DNA is currently the simplest and most sensitive technique to detect mutations in DNA.

2.2   **Answer: (c)**   Although RT-PCR is extremely sensitive for detecting the expression of a specific gene, it requires the design of primers specific for the gene of interest, and it is difficult to perform in a comprehensive way. cDNA and oligoarray hybridizations and SAGE can measure the expression of thousands of genes simultaneously. The disadvantage of arrays to SAGE is the requirement of knowing the sequence of genes to be analyzed (because the cDNAs or oligonucleotides have to be placed on the arrays), but their major advantage is that they are relatively easy to perform in high throughput and are less expensive.

2.3   **Answer: (d)**   ELISA, immunoblotting, and immunoprecipitation all require the availability of a specific antibody for the protein of interest; therefore, they cannot be used for the discovery of new diagnostic markers. Mass spectrometry allows the unbiased comparison of samples from normal healthy and cancer patients and, based on this analysis, the identification of cancer-specific markers.

3.1   **Answer: (c)**   All tumor cells are believed to multiply exponentially in the initial period following the transformation event. A flattening out of the growth rate over time occurs due to an increase in cell loss, nutritional depletion of tumor cells, or lengthening of cell cycle time. However, the percentage of cells not in the cell cycle (ie, in the G_0 phase) is higher in normal cells than in cancer cells. In other words, tumor cells are more likely to enter G_1 phase and less likely to exit the cell cycle, which leads to an increased growth fraction in cancer cells. Conversely, cancer cells do not grow faster (have shorter cell cycle times) or require less time to complete DNA synthesis or undergo mitosis. Another assessment of the growth fraction is the labeling index, which is a measure of the number of cells synthesizing DNA at any given time; this index typically employs thymidine incorporation to label such S-phase cells by autoradiography.

3.2   **Answer: (d)**   Tumor cells are less likely, compared with their normal counterparts, to remain at the G_1–S cell cycle boundary (ie, be on hold before DNA synthesis). In nontumorigenic cells, the retinoblastoma protein is produced throughout the cell cycle; however, phosphorylation by enzymes such as G_1 cyclin kinase complexes inactivates this protein, thereby releasing cells from G_1 arrest. p53 protein phosphorylation also aids in allowing release from the pre-DNA synthesis phase. As such, both retinoblastoma and p53 protein are tumor suppressor proteins whose normal function provides an important control against overproliferation. Inactivation of the normal suppressor function of these proteins, as might occur by an inability to become dephosphorylated, or by deletion or truncation, could result in loss of normal regulation mitigating against proceeding through the cell cycle, which would thereby lead to neoplastic transformation.

3.3   **Answer: (a)**   In addition to inactivation of tumor suppressor genes and activating mutations in growth-promoting proto-oncogenes, potentially oncogenic genes also include those that code for proteins that prevent or interfere with the normal process of programmed cell death. The *BCL2* gene product may interact with mitochondrial or other intercellular membranes, thereby preventing an oxygen-dependent apoptotic signal. For example, the translocation between chromosomes 14 and 18, characteristic of many follicular lymphomas, allows overexpression and thereby places the *BCL2* gene under the control of the immunoglobulin heavy chain gene promoter.

3.4   **Answer: (d)**   The restriction point or start site in the cell cycle was originally discovered when normal cells, at low serum concentrations, accumulated at a point during late G_1 phase. The addition of serum to the culture allowed the cells to proceed through the cycle. Once past the restriction point, the cells were committed to DNA synthesis and usually cell division. The restriction point is not a component of the "go" or S phase of the cell cycle.

3.5   **Answer: (c)**   The molecular control of the cell cycle is becoming increasingly understood. The control of transit through the cell cycle is mediated by CDK along with their regulatory subunit cyclins. The CDK/cyclin system is under the regulatory control of inhibitors such as Rb and other tumor suppressor gene products. Phosphorylation by kinases activates many of these products. For example, the Rb gene product must become phosphorylated in order to open the restriction point gate and allow for transit of the cell into the S phase. Products of oncogenic viruses can bind and functionally deplete the cells of the Rb gene product. *P53*, another tumor suppressor gene, transcriptionally activates genes such as *WAF1/CIP/p21*, which regulate CDK activity.

4.1   **Answer: (e)**

4.2   **Answer: (d)**

4.3   **Answer: (c)**

4.4   **Answer: (d)**

4.5   **Answer: (e)**

5.1   **Answer: (b)**   Imatinib (Gleevec), a low molecular weight tyrosine kinase inhibitor, blocks adenosine triphosphate (ATP) from binding to the Abl tyrosine kinase, which is activated in the Bcr-Abl translocation in CML. Remarkable responses have been observed in patients with this disease as well as in those with gastrointestinal stromal tumors, which contain activating mutations of the c-kit receptor tyrosine kinase.

5.2   **Answer: (b)**   In preclinical animal models, a humanized monoclonal antibody directed against this tyrosine kinase receptor inhibited growth of tumors overexpressing the amplified normal gene. This antibody also enhanced the responsiveness of such tumor cells to taxanes, anthracyclines, and platinum compounds and has been approved as a first-line therapy in combination with paclitaxel.

5.3   **Answer: (c)**   This hereditary syndrome is characterized by multiple bilateral renal papillary tumors. Several different mutations in the c-*met* tyrosine kinase domain, which lead to constitutive activation of kinase activity, have been identified as being genetically transmitted in affected family members. Activating mutations of c-*met* commonly occur in spontaneously occurring renal papillary carcinomas as well. Each of the other syndromes listed is due to genetic transmission of a different cancer gene.

6.1   **Answer: (b)**

6.2   **Answer: (e)**

6.3   **Answer: (a)**

6.4   **Answer: (b)**

6.5   **Answer: (c)**

7.1   **Answer: (a)**   Although there are rare forms of inherited cancer that display an autosomal recessive phenotype (Fanconi's and Bloom syndromes), most familial forms of cancer are inherited in an autosomal dominant fashion. This may seem counterintuitive because biallelic inactivation of tumor suppressor genes is needed for the initiation and progression of carcinogenesis. However, in familial cancer syndromes, one inactivated allele is inherited; therefore, only one additional "hit" is necessary to fulfill Knudson's hypothesis. In essence, the germline transmission of the inactivated tumor suppressor allele has accelerated the process of tumorigenesis by requiring only one additional somatic mutation rather than two, as occurs in patients with sporadic (noninherited) forms of cancer.

7.2   **Answer: (d)**   A negative result on a genetic test such as that described above is generally uninterpretable. The negative result could be owing to the fact that the child did not inherit the mutation or because the test used could not detect the mutation that was present. Current conventional genetic tests vary widely in their sensitivities, depending on the gene in question and the type of mutation. In FAP only about 75% of mutations are detectable with commercially available tests.

7.3   **Answer: (b)**   If one knows the precise mutation in the family, and this mutation can be detected in the mother, then the same technology can be used to rigorously test for the presence of the mutation in any other family member. The sensitivity and specificity of the test are theoretically 100% under these circumstances, and quite different from the case in question 7.2, in which it is not known if the particular family's mutation is detectable by available technology.

8.1   **Answer: (c)**   The Philadelphia chromosome is a translocation involving chromosome 9 and 22 [t(9;22)(q34;q11)]. The genetic consequence of the t(9;22) is to move the *ABL* gene, a nonreceptor tyrosine kinase on chromosome 9, next to the *BCR* (*b*reakpoint *c*luster *r*egion) gene on chromosome 22. The leukemogenic nature of the BCR-ABL protein results from the fact that its *ABL*-derived tyrosine kinase function is constitutively activated.

8.2   **Answer: (b)**   Imatinib mesylate is a tyrosine kinase inhibitor that prevents *BCR-ABL*–mediated transfer of phosphate to its substrate.

8.3   **Answer: (d)**   The t(15;17)(q22;q12–21) results in the *PML-RARA* fusion gene. Patients have classic acute promyelocytic leukemia (APL) with characteristic AML-M3 morphology, which includes a dramatic accumulation of promyelocytes in the bone marrow and presence of Auer rods within the cytoplasm of the promyelocytic blasts.

      The *RARA* gene encodes the retinoic acid receptor alpha protein. The *PML-RARA* fusion gene is thought to interfere with wild-type *RARA* function in a dominant manner. These patients have a dramatic response to all-*trans* retinoic acid (ATRA) therapy, which acts as a differentiating agent. The prognosis in APL, treated optimally with ATRA and an anthracycline-containing chemotherapy regimen, is more favorable than in other subtypes of AML.

8.4   **Answer: (a)**   In all cases of Burkitt's lymphoma the *myc* gene, located on chromosome 8q24, is involved in translocations with immunoglobulin genes. In 70 to 80% of cases, the translocations involve the heavy chain on 14q32, whereas the remaining translocations involve the κ chain on 2p12 or the λ chain locus on 22q11. Anaplastic large cell lymphoma is associated with a t(2;5)(p23,q35). A t(14;18)(q32;q21) is seen in 80 to 90% of cases of follicular lymphoma, and a t(11;14)(q13;q32) is found in over 70% of cases of mantle cell lymphoma.

8.5　　**Answer: (a)**　All four genes have been implicated in colorectal tumorigenesis. However, *ras* is an oncogene, whereas *APC, TP53,* and *DCC* are all tumor suppressor genes.

8.6　　**Answer: (a)**　Neuroepitheliomas and Ewing's sarcomas both carry a t(11;22)(q24;q12), resulting in the fusion of the human *FLI1* gene on chromosome 11 with the coding sequence of the *EWS* gene on chromosome 22. The discovery of the identical translocation in neuro-epithelioma and Ewing's sarcoma has changed the treatment modality in neuroepithelioma. Use of therapy similar to that used for Ewing's sarcoma has resulted in a marked improvement in the response of these tumors to therapy. Desmoplastic round small cell tumors are characterized by a t(11;22)(p13;q12), resulting in the fusion of the *EWS* and *WT1* genes, whereas Ewing's sarcomas are characterized by the fusion of the *FLI1* and *EWS* genes. The t(12;16), resulting in the fusion of the *CHOP* gene on chromosome 12 to *FUS* on chromosome 16, is characteristic of myxoid liposarcomas and is used diagnostically to distinguish these tumors from lipomas, which involve the translocation of HMGIC at 12q15 to multiple different translocation partners.

8.7　　**Answer: (d)**

9.1　　**Answer: (c)**　See Table 9-1.

9.2　　**Answer: (a)**　Down-regulation of E-cadherin correlates with increased invasiveness, metastasis, and poor prognosis in cancer patients. (Because E-cadherin is involved in cell adhesion, its down-regulation would result in decreased cell-matrix interaction and cell-cell adhesiveness.)

9.3　　**Answer: (c)**　Methylation of CpG islands is another mechanism for regulatory gene expression. In general, though not always, hyper-methylated DNA sequences are less expressed, and hypomethylated sequences are more expressed. Alterations in DNA methylation patterns have been observed in tumor cell lines, animal tumor models, and primary human cancers. Hypermethylation of DNA has been postulated to be involved in the loss of tumor suppressor gene function. Aberrantly methylated CpG sequences have been detected in serum and tissue of patients with colorectal, nonsmall cell lung, liver, and prostate cancers. Data suggest that oncogene-induced malignant transformation is mediated through alterations in DNA methylation.

10.1　　**Answer: (e)**　Angiogenesis and metastasis are both composed of invasive behavior, using the same "hardware" and "software." Activation of growth factor receptor signaling is common to both, with many of the same growth factors involved. Proteinase secretion and activation are necessary for vascular development and remodeling, as well as malignant invasive behavior. Integrin engagement is used by both endothelial cells and tumor cells in adhesive activity and in cross-talk with growth factor receptors and is a critical component of one mechanism of cell survival. Locomotion, motile behavior, is part of the process of vascular remodeling as it is involved in inflammation and metastatic behavior as well.

10.2　　**Answer: (c)**　Tumor genotype, molecular phenotype, and local microenvironment interactions are critical in regulation of individual tumor metastatic potential. Although there may be differential metastatic dissemination of certain cancer cell types in women and men, a clear etiologic role of gender has not been demonstrated as a general phenomenon. Immune surveillance is an important part of tumor dissemination and one that is still an active direction for study. No HLA haplotypes have had a consistent or broad impact on cancer dissemination.

10.3　　**Answer: (b)**　Invasive behavior has been demonstrated to begin prior to frank malignant transformation and demonstration of an invasive front. Tumor-associated vascular blushes have been seen near areas of atypical ductal hyperplasia not immediately proximate to the carcinoma in situ. Patients with presumed in situ cancer can later succumb to metastatic disease that is histologically and molecularly identical to the in situ cancer, indicating that an occult dissemination process had not been observed in the assessment and diagnosis of the initial case.

10.4　　**Answer: (e)**　All have been tested clinically. Humanized monoclonal antibodies against the integrin αvβ3 have been studied in phase I and II clinical trials and have shown some potential for disease stabilization. Several inhibitors of the matrix metalloproteinase family have been tested in phase I to III clinical trials; none have reached US New Drug Administration status or obtained US Food and Drug Administration approval because of toxicity and/or lack of activity. Multiple small molecule and monoclonal antibody inhibitors of kinase action are at various steps of clinical evaluation and approval (trastuzumab [Herceptin], gefitinib [Iressa], imatinib [Gleevec]). Reagents to block protein kinase C and cyclin-dependent kinases are in investigational status (UCN-01 and flavopiridol). Many of these have antimotility activity, as does the calcium influx inhibitor CAI.

11.1　　**Answer: (d)**

11.2　　**Answer: (b)**

11.3　　**Answer: (b)**

11.4　　**Answer: (d)**

11.5　　**Answer: (d)**

11.6　　**Answer: (a)**

CANCER IMMUNOLOGY

12.1   **Answer: (b)**   The immunoproteasome catalyzes a differential set of peptide epitopes than the "conventional" proteasome and is differentially expressed by tumor cells and APCs. As a result, APCs may process and present not only most tumor-expressed epitopes but additional novel epitopes that a tumor does not normally express. The HLA genotypes of a tumor and autologous APCs are identical. Integrin and fibronectin molecules are involved with intercellular adhesion and are unrelated to the range of epitopes presented by tumor cells or APCs. CD4 molecules are expressed by the T helper cells and are not involved with CD8+ T-cell recognition of tumor cells or APCs.

12.2   **Answer: (b)**   Patients with melanoma display significant spontaneous and therapeutically induced regressions of their disease, and have circulating in their blood elevated levels of T cells and antibodies that recognize melanoma-associated antigens. This has facilitated molecular and biochemical procedures to identify melanoma antigens and has made the study of melanoma more prevalent over the past 10 years. Melanoma is not the most common form of cancer and does not display a higher rate of mutations when compared with other types of cancer. Leukopenia is not commonly observed in these patients. Lastly, melanomas express many common antigens and also a range of unique (idiotypic) antigens that may result from mutation events. Hence, they do not express identical sets of tumor antigens.

12.3   **Answer: (e)**   Since vaccines are designed to elicit specific high-affinity T cells and antibodies that could attack normal tissues that coexpress tumor antigens, pathologic autoimmunity would be theoretically least likely in a case in which the antigen is unique (idiotypic) to the cancer and is not shared with normal tissues. Each of the other categories of tumor antigens cited are expressed by tumors and other normal somatic cells in the body, which could invite attack from the immune system if stimulated by effective vaccine formulations.

12.4   **Answer: (e)**   Single epitope vaccines may prove limited in their clinical efficacy in treating all patients with a given histotype of cancer because of each of these reasons. As the cancer evolves and is subjected to immune regulation, this selective pressure results in the gradual outgrowth of tumor cell variants that fail to express the class of antigens recognized by T cells and antibodies. Single epitope vaccines will also fail to stimulate coordinate CD4+ and CD8+ T-cell responses that are believed optimal for the clearance of disease. Furthermore, peptide epitopes are tailored to specific HLA-presenting molecules to which they can bind; hence, only those patients that express the matched HLA type would likely benefit from a single epitope vaccine.

13.1   **Answer: (e)**   All four of these classes of biologic molecules have been identified as tumor markers.

13.2   **Answer: (b)**   As cancer in the general population is of low prevalence, it is most important that primary screening markers have a very low false-positive rate (ie, that individuals with a positive test actually have disease) because more expensive and invasive clinical tests must be performed in individuals with a positive test to determine if a malignancy is actually present. The other listed criteria are also important for a useful test, but very high test specificity is the key performance characteristic.

13.3   **Answer: (c) and (d)**   CEA lacks requisite specificity and has relatively poor sensitivity as a primary screening and diagnostic marker. It is most useful in monitoring of colorectal cancer patients for early indication of recurrence following surgical resection of the primary tumor to detect potentially curable recurrent disease. Serum CEA levels also appear to be useful as a prognostic marker; higher preoperative CEA levels are associated with poorer 5-year survival, and very high levels are highly indicative of liver metastases. CEA appears to provide useful prognostic information specifically in colon cancer patients who develop liver metastasis following initial curative resection.

13.4   **Answer: (c) and (d)**   Screening for *BRCA* germline mutations presently requires genomics-based methods. As with many single markers in most malignancies, CA 125 lacks both sensitivity and specificity for early-stage ovarian cancer. It does have proven clinical utility in monitoring therapeutic response and recurrence.

13.5   **Answer: (a), (b), and (c)**   These technologies have demonstrated utility in improved detection of early-stage disease using profiling approaches, as well as in clinically useful discrimination of molecular subclasses of disease. Although not presently well developed, these approaches also offer substantial promise for the identification of new cancer markers and ultimately better characterization of signaling pathways and identification of new therapeutic targets.

14.1   **Answer: (c)**   In a series of classic transplantation experiments performed in syngeneic mice, it has been demonstrated that immunization of the animals with the heat-killed (unable to grow) tumor cells protected the mice from a challenge with viable tumor cells, which killed the nonimmunized mice. Based on these experiments, it has been concluded that tumor cells expressing TSTAs are capable of inducing protective immune responses.

14.2   **Answer: (a)**   Although the mechanisms responsible for in vivo elimination of tumor cells are complex, it has been shown in several tumor model systems that killing of tumor cells (cytotoxicity) by activated T cells capable of secreting perforin and granzyme B is at least in part responsible for tumor regression. Effector T cells can mediate tumor antigen–specific and –nonspecific cytotoxicity against tumor targets. NK cells are also involved in mediating antitumor cytotoxicity.

14.3 **Answer: (b)**   Recent evidence indicates that NK cells in the circulation of patients with cancer bind annexin V and have lower levels of FcγRIII-associated ζ- chain than do NK cells of normal donors. These features suggest that NK cells in patients with cancer are prone to apoptosis and thus may be defective in their antitumor functions.

14.4 **Answer: (c)**   Immunotherapy of cancer exists in various forms, and it includes cytokine-mediated, antibody-mediated, and cell-mediated responses to administered biologic agents. Any one of these mechanisms or, more likely, several mechanisms together can bring about tumor regression in those individuals who are responsive to immunotherapy. Unfortunately, complete responses to either specific or nonspecific immunotherapy are rare, and so far no firm correlations have been made between clinical and immune responses to immunotherapies in patients with cancer.

14.5 **Answer: (d)**   Human tumors have the well-known potential to produce a wide variety of immunosuppressive molecules that are present in the circulation of patients with cancer and contribute to tumor-related immune suppression. Tumors escape from the immune system because they have evolved mechanisms to actively interfere with functions of the immune cells, specifically, tumor-specific T cells.

15.1 **Answer: (a)**   T cells recognize peptide antigens present in a groove of MHC class I or II molecules. CTLs target antigens present in the context of MHC class I molecules. It is common for tumor cells to loose expression of MHC class I molecules; this can manifest via a variety of mechanisms. The loss of expression represents a means for selection of tumor cells that can evade T-cell responses. TGF-β is an immunosuppressive cytokine, and ICAD and FADD are involved in the process of apoptosis.

15.2 **Answer: (b)**   Tumors secrete a variety of immunomodulatory factors and cytokines, and the local intratumoral microenvironment represents a hazardous environment for infiltrating immune cells. The suppressive factors produced by tumors also have systemic immunosuppressive effects. It is commonly observed that TGF-β and IL-10 are associated with the suppressive effects of tumors.

15.3 **Answer: (e)**   By definition, in a normally functioning immune system, AICD refers to the induction of apoptosis of previously activated T cells on subsequent encounter with antigen and represents a mechanism for regulating expression of immune responses. AICD is mediated mainly via CD95:CD95L interactions but can also involve TNF and TRAIL. In contrast, co-stimulatory signals induced via binding of CD4 or CD28 protect T cells from AICD.

15.4 **Answer: (c)**   There is evidence for reduced expression of the ζ chain in T cells and natural killer (NK) cells from cancer patients in comparison to these cells from individuals without cancer. The ζ chain is part of a complex of molecules linked to cell surface receptors, such as TCR, that cooperate in transducing signals for activation of the immune cell functions following binding of their relevant ligands. IL-8 is a cytokine with many effects on the immune system, but it is particularly important for recruiting inflammatory cells. BCL2 is an anti-apoptotic regulator for cells. Granzyme B and cytolysin are components of lytic granules released by NK cells and CTLs as part of their mechanism of lysis of tumor cells.

15.5 **Answer: (b)**   Although CD36, CD46, CD55, and CD59 all are complement regulatory proteins, there is little evidence for CD36 modulation of responses to tumor cells. Decorin binds and inactivates TGF-β. Cytolysin is the effector molecule that is inhibited by complement regulatory proteins.

CANCER ETIOLOGY

16.1 **Answer: (c)**   Lung cancer has been investigated in the United States and Europe in patients with the diagnosis of HNPCC. Despite the high population risk of lung cancer, there was a significant deficit for this disease, even when correcting for cigarette-smoking behavior.

16.2 **Answer: (a), (d), and (e)**   For reasons that remain obscure, HNPCC patients may manifest colonic polyps but they do not exceed the number, location, or variety found in the general population. Endometrial, not ovarian, carcinoma is the second most common cancer in HNPCC.

16.3 **Answer: (a) and (b)**   In spite of the presence of hamartomatous polyps in the gastrointestinal tract, colorectal cancer has not shown an excess occurrence in this disease.

16.4 **Answer: (d)**   The tumor spectrum has increased significantly, particularly with respect to *BRCA2*. However, to date, there is no evidence that hepatocellular carcinoma is an integral component of HBOC.

16.5 **Answer: (a)**   Patients must be aware of the pros and cons of genetic counseling, and they should be able to ask questions about any of the clinical, surveillance, and management measures and gene testing for the particular hereditary syndrome involved in their family. A letter or pamphlet is insufficient given the fact that the patient may not fully comprehend the significance of a positive or negative finding in a mutation. For example, a negative finding is not a true negative unless a bona fide germline cancer-causing mutation has been certified as present in the family.

17.1   **Answer: (b)**   Whereas exposure to polycyclic aromatic hydrocarbons and aflatoxins may occur as the result of their presence in foods, the heterocyclic amines are formed in the cooking of food through the pyrolysis of amino acids, creatinine, and glucose.

17.2   **Answer: (d)**   Most mechanisms of DNA repair require highly coordinated multiprotein complexes to accomplish a step-by-step DNA-repair process. However, DNA alkyltransferases (eg, O6-methyltransferase) are suicide enzymes that catalyze the translocation of an alkyl moiety from an alkylated base to a cysteine residue at their active site. Thus, one molecule of the enzyme is capable of repairing a single alkyl lesion in the absence of strand scission.

17.3   **Answer: (c)**   The biologically effective dose of a carcinogen provides an integrated measure of the amount of chemical reaching a target tissue, as well as the propensity of the individual to biologically activate the chemical into a reactive species that causes DNA damage.

17.4   **Answer: (e)**   Caretaker genes are involved in maintaining genomic stability and influence an individual's cancer susceptibility. Examples include DNA repair genes.

17.5   **Answer: (f)**

18.1   **Answer: (d)**   Several epidemiologic studies and a recently reported Women's Health Institutes (WHI) trial document the highest risks with combined estrogen and progesterone therapy.

18.2   **Answer: (a)**   Although initial case-control studies suggested that dietary fat was an important risk factor for breast cancer, recent prospective studies such as the Nurses Health Study have not replicated this finding. Dietary fat intervention is part of the randomized WHI trial.

18.3   **Answer: (b)**   Mutations in the *ATM* gene have not yet been definitively associated with breast cancer.

18.4   **Answer: (d)**   Age at menopause has not been associated with a decreased risk of endometrial cancer, whereas all of the other four are known to be protective.

18.5   **Answer: (d)**   Vitamin E and selenium are currently under study as potential chemoprevention agents, but they have not yet been validated consistently in epidemiologic studies.

19.1   **Answer: (d)**

19.2   **Answer: (b)**

19.3   **Answer: (e)**

19.4   **Answer: (a)**

19.5   **Answer: (d)**

20.1   **Answer: (b)**   At 280 to 320 nm, UVB corresponds to the absorption peak of deoxyribonucleic acid (DNA). UVC is shielded by the ozone layer, and UVA is important in skin aging but less in cancer.

20.2   **Answer: (c)**   Mutations occur at the 3' cytosine of a TC or CC sequence.

20.3   **Answer: (c)**   Photolyase does not exist in human cells, DNA polymerase-δ is a normal replication enzyme, and the patched-smoothened-hedgehog gene is responsible for basal cell nevus syndrome.

20.4   **Answer: (b)**   Patches of *P53* mutant cells in the skin are considered precursors of SCC. BCC arises from mutations in the patched-smoothened-hedgehog gene, and melanoma and Spitz nevi may be related to solar exposure but in ways, as yet, poorly explained.

21.1   **Answer: (c)**   Even though lung cancer is the tumor to which asbestos-exposed people are at greatest risk, many other agents can increase its incidence. On the contrary, mesothelioma is the tumor most specifically related to asbestos exposure. Data on other types of tumor are not clear cut.

21.2   **Answer: (e)**   Experiments performed on rats have demonstrated that, at equivalent doses, erionite is the most powerful carcinogenic agent for the pleura. The incidence of mesothelioma is lower, although still high, with different kinds of asbestos studied (such as crocidolite and chrysotile) and with man-made mineral fibers.

21.3   **Answer: (d)**   Both tobacco smoke and asbestos exposure increase the incidence of lung cancer, with a multiplicative effect in the case of associated exposure; on the contrary, only asbestos exposure, and not tobacco smoke, increases the incidence of mesothelioma.

22.1   **Answer: (b)**

22.2   **Answer: (e)**   The RNA packaging signal is located between the long terminal repeat and the *GAG* gene.

22.3   **Answer: (d)**   Human T-cell lymphotropic virus causes leukemia and tropical spastic paraparesis, feline leukemia virus can cause immuno-deficiency, and murine mammary tumor virus causes mammary tumors.

23.1   **Answer: (a)**   Epstein-Barr virus deoxyribonucleic acid (DNA) and proteins have been detected in about 50% of cases of Hodgkin's disease, in virtually all anaplastic nasopharyngeal carcinoma, in most African Burkitt's lymphomas, and in some T-cell lymphomas. Epstein-Barr virus is not associated with Kaposi's sarcoma. Human herpesvirus 8, known as Kaposi's sarcoma–associated herpesvirus, is strongly linked with Kaposi's sarcoma.

23.2   **Answer: (c)**   Kaposi's sarcoma–associated herpesvirus DNA has been detected in tumors from patients with classic or HIV-associated Kaposi's sarcoma. The virus has also been detected in body cavity lymphomas, also referred to as *primary effusion lymphomas*. Kaposi's sarcoma–associated herpesvirus has been detected in biopsies from patients with multicentric Castleman's disease, especially the plasma cell variant. The virus has not been consistently detected in T-cell lymphomas.

23.3   **Answer: (c)**   Kaposi's sarcoma–associated herpesvirus is not thought to be pathogenic in most healthy individuals; however, the virus is strongly associated with Kaposi's sarcoma in immunocompromised persons. Kaposi's sarcoma–associated herpesvirus has been transmitted by renal allografts and from mother to child. Antibodies to the virus are detected more commonly in African and Mediterranean populations than in the United States. Viral DNA has been detected in mononuclear cells in 50% of patients with Kaposi's sarcoma.

23.4   **Answer: (b)**   Acyclovir inhibits the replication of Epstein-Barr virus DNA. Biopsies from patients with oral hairy leukoplakia show evidence of active virus replication, and treatment with acyclovir is often effective; however, the disease frequently recurs when treatment is stopped. In contrast, lesions from Epstein-Barr virus–associated Hodgkin's disease and lymphoproliferative disease often show little active virus replication, and acyclovir has generally not been effective. Controlled studies have shown no significant clinical benefit in the treatment of patients with infectious mononucleosis with acyclovir, and the antiviral has not been effective for treatment of virus-associated hemophagocytic syndrome.

24.1   **Answer: (e)**   The squamocolumnar junction of the cervix is uniquely susceptible to HPV infection and its sequelae, including preinvasive and invasive neoplasia. Over 95% of cervical epithelial neoplasms are associated with sexually transmitted HPVs, and the risk of developing a neoplasm is as high as 20% in persistently infected individuals.

24.2   **Answer: (d)**   HPV testing is not useful for managing male partners, most of whom do not harbor visible lesions. Over 80% of clear-cut low- and high-grade cervical intraepithelial neoplasms are HPV positive (including cancer-associated HPVs), and this information is of little use clinically. However, because the negative predictive value of HPV testing is so high, nondiagnostic atypias that are HPV negative may be managed conservatively, without necessitating colposcopy.

24.3   **Answer: (d)**   The viruslike particle–derived vaccines appear highly effective in preventing infection and thus in preventing cervical neoplasia. However, they are not effective at reversing cervical neoplasia once it has developed.

25.1   **Answer: (b)**   Although hepatitis B and C viruses have in epidemiologic studies been associated with HCC, only the HBV has been shown to integrate into the genome of hepatic parenchymal cells, inducing loss of growth regulation by a variety of mechanisms. These include expression of the viral hepatitis B X-protein, which activates proto-oncogenes, or mutations in codon 249 of the *P53* tumor suppressor gene.

     No studies have definitively shown a direct effect of the HCV in HCC; the association is most likely owing to increased hepatic parenchymal cell regeneration and cirrhosis.

     Co-infection and superinfection of patients with chronic hepatitis B infection with the hepatitis D virus have been shown to produce exacerbation of chronic hepatitis and accelerated progression to cirrhosis. No direct transforming effects of the hepatitis D virus have been reported.

     Hepatitis A and E are enterically transmitted viruses that produce a self-limiting disease course and have not been associated with HCC.

25.2   **Answer: (a), (c), and (d)**   The effectiveness of interferon-α in the secondary prevention of HCC in patients with chronic HBV infection has been reported in at least two studies. In the first study, 101 male patients with chronic HBV infection were randomized to placebo or interferon-α treatment. Follow-up was between 1.1 and 11.5 years after the end of therapy. HCC was detected in 1 of 67 treated patients compared with 4 of 34 placebo controls ($p = .013$). In another study the cumulative occurrence rate of HCC in 313 patients (94 treated with interferon-α, 219 not treated) was assessed at the end of 3, 5, and 10 years. Rates for treated versus untreated patients were 4.5% versus 13.3% at 3 years, 7.0% versus 19.6% at 5 years, and 17.0% versus 30.8% at 10 years ($p = .0124$).

     Universal hepatitis B vaccination has reduced the prevalence rate of infection with HBV. In Alaska the prevalence of positive serum hepatitis B surface antigen has decreased by 99% and in Taiwan from 0.8 to 0.7% in children. In Taiwan the annual incidence of HCC in children has since decreased from 0.70 (1981–1986) to 0.36 per 100,000 children (1990–1994).

Treatment of chronic hepatitis C with interferon-α has been shown to be associated with a reduced incidence of HCC. In an international survey, the overall relative HCC risk was three times higher in untreated patients compared with interferon-treated anti-HCV-positive patients and more than six times higher in untreated versus treated anti-HCV-positive/anti-HBc-negative patients. In a report by the International Interferon-α Hepatocellular Carcinoma Study Group, which involves 21 centers, data on HCC occurrence were collected from 637 patients, 356 of whom did not receive treatment and 281 of whom received interferon-α. For anti-HCV-positive patients without HBV markers, 29 of 129 (22%) untreated and 6 of 116 (5%) treated patients developed HCC.

The combination of interferon-α and ribavirin has been shown to produce sustained responses in 30 to 40% of patients, which was an improvement over the 6 to 15% of sustained responses in patients treated with interferon-α alone in an earlier study. However, studies evaluating the efficacy of the combination treatment in the secondary prevention of HCC have yet to be reported.

Lamivudine and adefovir dipivoxil, nucleoside analogs that have been shown to be effective for the treatment of chronic hepatitis B infection, improve hepatic inflammation and reduce hepatic fibrosis. At this time, neither lamivudine nor adenovir dipivoxil have been proven to reduce the incidence of subsequent HCC.

25.3 **Answer: (c)** Screening programs in high-risk populations (adults with chronic HBV infection over the age of 35 years) have resulted in the increased detection of HCC. In 1.3 million people in China screened with a combination of ultrasonography and serum AFP every 6 months, 500 cases of HCC were detected. Survival benefit will depend on the efficacy of available treatment modalities for early-stage HCC and the means to carry out interventions expeditiously. A randomized study demonstrating the survival benefit for the screened population as compared with controls has yet to be performed.

26.1 **Answer: (a), (d), and (e)**

CANCER EPIDEMIOLOGY, PREVENTION, AND SCREENING

27.1 **Answer: (c)** The cancer incidence rate is the rate at which new cancers are diagnosed in the population each year, expressed per 100,000 people per year. When age-adjusted, cancer incidence rates can be compared across different populations, whereas the number of cases depends on the size and age of the population.

27.2 **Answer: (d)** Beginning with 1999, data on incidence and mortality are standardized to the age distribution of the US population in 2000. However, these rates are not directly comparable with rates based on other standard populations. For example, rates from other countries are age standardized to the age distribution of the world population.

27.3 **Answer: (b)** Presently 23% (approximately 25%) of people in the United States die from cancer. This percentage has increased over time owing to the decline in cardiovascular death rates and to the aging of the population.

27.4 **Answer: (a)** The introduction of the PSA test in the late 1980s caused a huge and immediate increase in the incidence rate of prostate cancer in the United States. Any effects on the death rate and relative survival, if these exist, take longer to determine.

27.5 **Answer: (c)** Breast cancer in women is the only major cancer for which incidence is higher in white women (presumably because of greater screening and/or risk factors) but mortality is higher in African American women (because of factors that adversely affect survival).

28.1 **Answer: (b)** Hypermethylation of the promoter region of a gene results in transcriptional silencing and loss of gene function. Aberrant methylation of the promoter region of *P16, DAPK*, and *APC* has been identified in lung tumors. Recent findings suggest that hypermethylation of the *P16* promoter may serve as an early biomarker of lung cancer risk.

28.2 **Answer: (c)** The gene that has not been associated with the biologic activity of nicotine is glutathione S-transferase M1. Nicotine metabolism is altered in *CYP2D6* ultrarapid metabolizers. Nicotine is a potent inducer of the *CYP1A1* gene. Lastly, polymorphisms in the dopamine D2 receptor have been linked to nicotine dependence.

28.3 **Answer: (c)** The 5As model involves (1) asking patients about their smoking status, (2) assessing their willingness to quit, (3) advising patients who smoke to quit, (4) assisting them to quit via proven treatments, and (5) arranging follow-up appointments to track progress of cessation. The model does not, however, recommend workstations for nurse training.

28.4 **Answer: (e)** The Agency for Healthcare Research and Quality sanctions the transdermal nicotine patch, behavioral counseling that involves skills building to avoid relapse, bupropion, and physician counseling as methods for treating nicotine addiction.

29.1 **Answer: (c)** Recall bias is more common in case-control studies in which subjects who have cancer and subjects who do not have cancer are asked questions about past diet habits, and the results are compared. The other answers are true. Dietary changes usually cannot be blinded because the subject is aware that he/she is eating more or less of a certain food. It is difficult to implement dietary changes; therefore, compliance in diet studies is often poor. Because diet changes must be maintained for long periods of time and a large number of subjects are needed to determine an effect, intervention studies are often very expensive.

29.2 **Answer: (b)** Although several of these recommendations are potentially beneficial, the majority of the scientific literature suggests that the advice in option (b) is best. There is not enough evidence on soy isoflavones to recommend a specific amount to intake per day. Sugar intake, independent of total calories, has not been thoroughly investigated and remains controversial. Finally, the relationship between vitamin E and breast cancer has only recently been evaluated and was not discussed in this chapter.

29.3 **Answer: (c)** Although all of these recommendations may be helpful, a nutrition assessment by an RD is the most appropriate recommendation. An RD is an expert in converting peer-reviewed scientifically based food and nutrition research into realistic applications for patients. RDs can identify problematic dietary patterns and recommend practical solutions based on an individual's health status and diet habits.

30.1 **Answer: (e)** Fenretinide, a retinoid derivative, is administered with a monthly 3-day drug holiday to prevent ocular toxicity. Contralateral breast cancers occur at a rate of 0.8% per year in patients who receive fenretinide. This drug may suppress the rate of ovarian cancer. Tamoxifen has been shown to have superior results over a placebo in preventing breast cancer. Women entering the tamoxifen chemoprevention trial must demonstrate a twofold increase in developing breast cancer.

30.2 **Answer: (d)** Tamoxifen has been shown to have both estrogen agonist and antagonist properties. In human breast cancer, tamoxifen has predominantly an antiestrogen effect and is generally used in patients whose tumors are known to be estrogen receptor positive. Tamoxifen induces the synthesis of TGF-α and induces insulin-like growth factor 1, which is a mutagen for breast cancer. These properties of tamoxifen may explain its efficacy, albeit limited, in estrogen receptor–negative tumors.

30.3 **Answer: (a)** The intracellular receptors for retinoids and thyroid hormone both belong to the steroid receptor family. These receptors are involved in the selective regulation of transcription of specific genes that control cell growth and differentiation. Retinoids are also responsible for maintaining normal differentiation and proliferation of mesenchymal cells, as well as arresting the process of carcinogenesis. Retinoids are necessary for stem cells to mature and differentiate. Retinoids and tamoxifen have a synergistic effect in chemoprevention.

31.1 **Answer: (c)** Among all tested individuals with the disease, a screening test identifies them as either likely having cancer (positive) or likely not having cancer (negative). Sensitivity is the proportion of all individuals with the disease (true-positives and false-negatives) who were correctly identified by the screening test (true-positives only) within a specified period of time, usually the screening interval. Sensitivity is calculated as follows:

True-positives ÷ (True-positives + False-negatives)

31.2 **Answer: (d)** In cancer screening, the PPV (True-positives ÷ [True-positives + False-positives]) is commonly used as an indicator of test effectiveness, that is, the proportion of individuals with cancer among all individuals with a positive test. The greatest influence on PPV apart from the definition of a false-positive derives from the specificity of the screening test

True-negatives ÷ (True-negatives + False-positives)

and the magnitude of the underlying prevalence of disease in the population undergoing screening. Even if sensitivity and specificity are equal in two groups undergoing screening, the group with the greater prevalence of disease will have a more favorable PPV.

31.3 **Answer: (d)** In an RCT, the distorting effects of self-selection are bypassed through random assignment to either an experimental group invited to receive screening or an uninvited group. The mortality end point is not subject to the effects of lead-time or length bias or overdiagnosis.

31.4 **Answer: (a)** At this time only mammography is recommended for primary screening for breast cancer. Randomized trials have shown reduced breast cancer mortality owing to screening with and without clinical breast examination. Although some have proposed that ultrasonography can be used as a stand-alone screening test, at this point evidence indicates its value as an adjunct to mammography. MRI may prove useful for women at high risk or who have very dense breasts, but it must still be regarded as experimental.

31.5 **Answer: (c)** The goal of screening for colorectal cancer is both the detection of early-stage adenocarcinomas and the detection and removal of adenomatous polyps, which are accepted as being potential precursors for colorectal cancer. Reduction in colorectal cancer morbidity and mortality through screening is achieved through a combination of (1) more favorable stage at diagnosis of occult disease and (2) disease prevention resulting from the removal of precursor lesions. The potential for FOBT to contribute to reduced incidence is the result of positive test results (indicating either bleeding polyps or false-positives) that result in endoscopy that leads to removal of adenomatous polyps.

CLINICAL TRIALS AND OUTCOMES ASSESSMENT

33.1 **Answer: (c)** Predictive probabilities refer to future results for a given trial design. In the context of monitoring trials, they can be calculated for any particular decision regarding continuation of the trial. Predictive probabilities incorporate posterior probabilities and, therefore, also prior probabilities; however, they also include the sampling variability present in future observations. Depending on one's statistical persuasion, one may object to all three of (a), (b), and (c) because they are bayesian entities, and therefore give one of the frequentist answers,

(d) and (e). However, these two answers are flawed in that they do not combine future uncertainty with that present in parameter values before a trial (design) or with the information that has accrued at a point during a trial (monitoring).

33.2   **Answer: (d)**   Levels of experimental units can be samples over time for a patient, of patients within a center, of centers within a trial, of trials within a country, and so on. Borrowing strength across units within the same level of the hierarchy depends on the observed data, with comparable data implying a greater strength.

33.3   **Answer: (e)**   The focus of a decision analysis is the worth of any particular action. *Worth* is measured in terms of maximizing effective treatment of patients (whether within or outside of the trial) or monetary gain (in the case of a pharmaceutical company) or both. Answers (a), (b), and (c) refer to such worth. Answer (d) refers to a separate issue but one that is also critical in decision making. One conducts a clinical trial to learn, that is, to remove uncertainty; but learning has costs, in terms of both ineffective treatment and monetary price. A decision analysis weighs the advantages with the costs in the context of the current state of information.

33.4   **Answer: (e)**   The bayesian approach is flexible in all the ways indicated. However, operating characteristics (such as false-positive rates) of the final design can and should be evaluated. If the adaptation employed is sufficiently complicated, finding operating characteristics requires simulation methods.

33.5   **Answer: (a)**   The possibility of a relationship between biomarkers and the ultimate end point (such as survival) can be considered explicitly via modeling. However, such modeling should not imply a relationship; rather, it merely allows for the possibility of one. This possibility is supported or not by the data from the trial. An implication is that information about biomarkers alone is not sufficient to conclude efficacy for the ultimate end point. The latter (usually) requires the observation of some ultimate events. Moreover, modeling should allow for the possibility of different relationships between biomarkers and the ultimate end point, depending on treatment. Adaptive designs may have limited usefulness in trials in which only a small number of events are expected by the time accrual has ended.

34.1   **Answer: (c)**   All economic analyses examine the difference in cost among alternative strategies; they differ in how they measure the benefits resulting from those strategies. Cost-benefit analyses measure benefits in financial terms by assigning a dollar value to the health outcome. The cost-benefit ratio is calculated by dividing the incremental cost of the more expensive strategy by the incremental benefit, measured in units of currency. Cost-effectiveness analyses, in contrast, measure the benefits of health care interventions in units of medical effect, usually years of life saved or quality-adjusted life years. For example, the cost-effectiveness of combination chemotherapy compared with single-agent therapy for a given disease would be calculated by dividing the additional cost (in dollars) per patient treated, divided by the increase in life expectancy or quality-adjusted life expectancy.

34.2   **Answer: (a)**   Efficacy, defined as the results of an intervention in carefully selected patients treated under controlled conditions, is best measured by a phase III trial. Effectiveness, in contrast, is a measure of the impact of routine medical interventions in all patients. It is assessed by observing the outcomes of care, typically in a cohort study design.

34.3   **Answer: False**   Randomization enhances the validity of conclusions regarding the effects of treatment on quality of life and economic outcomes just as it does for survival and other biologic outcomes. If costs, for example, are related to pretreatment characteristics and those characteristics also influence treatment choice, then it may be difficult or impossible to determine the independent impact of treatment choice on cost in a nonrandomized study design.

34.4   **Answer: (d)**   A range for this threshold has been established by examining cost-effectiveness ratios for interventions that are generally regarded by society as reasonable and those that are generally regarded as inordinately expensive for the degree of benefit produced. The conclusion is that interventions costing under approximately $50,000 per year of life saved are cost-effective, and those costing over $100,000 are cost-ineffective. Cost-effectiveness ratios falling between these levels are in a gray zone. In general, cancer therapies that result in clinically meaningful improvements in patient outcomes have been shown to be cost-effective regardless of the cost of the treatment.

34.5   **Answer: (b)**   Guidelines dictate what the treatment should be, for example, whether adjuvant therapy should be given and what the regimen(s) should be. Critical pathways, in contrast, specify how that therapy should be delivered, including the frequency of follow-up visits and testing, the tasks to be assumed by physicians and nurses, and so forth. Both are designed to eliminate variation in patterns of care that represent deviations from what is believed to be the most effective and cost-effective approach.

CANCER DIAGNOSIS

DIRECTIONS: Numbering for questions and answers reflects the corresponding chapter in *Cancer Medicine-6*. Each question contains suggested responses. Select the best response to each question. Answers for Cancer Diagnosis begin on page 39.

CANCER PATHOLOGY

35.1 In breast cancer, all of the following are components of grading *except*
a. Nuclear pleomorphism
b. Tumor necrosis
c. Tubule formation
d. Mitotic rate

35.2 Vascular permeability factor/vascular endothelial growth factor (VPF/VEGF), specifically VEGF-A, is a cytokine with which of the following properties?
a. It renders the microvasculature permeable to plasma and plasma proteins.
b. It is expressed by most malignant tumor cells.
c. It stimulates endothelial cell migration and division.
d. It rearranges endothelial cell gene expression.
e. Its expression is modulated by cytokines, oxygen concentration, oncogenes, and tumor suppressor genes.
f. All of the above properties pertain to VEGF-A.

35.3 Which of the following is a useful application of immunohistochemistry in the evaluation of human tumors?
a. Categorization of undifferentiated malignant tumors
b. Determination of the site of origin of metastatic tumors
c. Discrimination between adenocarcinoma and mesothelioma
d. Categorization of non-Hodgkin's lymphomas
e. All of the above

35.4 A 27-year-old woman is found to have atypical squamous cells; high-grade squamous intraepithelial lesion (ASC-H) is not excluded by the results of her annual routine Papanicolaou (Pap) smear. At this point, her physician should
a. Continue to recommend that she undergo an annual routine Pap smear
b. Recommend more frequent Pap smears, such as every 4 to 6 months
c. Recommend colposcopy
d. Recommend cone biopsy
e. Recommend simple hysterectomy

35.5 Several diagnostic assays are available to detect the Philadelphia chromosome (t[9;22][q34;q11]) in blood or bone marrow cells from patients with chronic myelogenous leukemia. The most sensitive technique for follow-up of these patients for minimal residual disease after therapy is
a. Complete karyotype
b. Southern blot hybridization
c. Fluorescence in situ hybridization on interphase nuclei
d. Western blot test
e. Reverse-transcriptase polymerase chain reaction (RT-PCR)

IMAGING

36.1 Which of the following noninvasive modalities uses ionizing radiation to image patients? (More than one may be correct.)
a. Computed tomography (CT)
b. Magnetic resonance imaging (MRI)
c. Ultrasonography
d. Positron emission tomography (PET)
e. Chest radiography

36.2 PET imaging with fluorodeoxyglucose (FDG) theoretically takes advantage of which biologic property to image tumors? (More than one may be correct.)
a. Apoptosis
b. Angiogenesis
c. Glucose metabolism
d. Purine metabolism

36.3 **FDG-PET has been used in which of the following clinical scenarios (at least for some tumors)? (More than one may be correct.)**
  a. Differentiating benign from malignant abnormalities
  b. Staging tumors
  c. Screening for cancer
  d. Predicting recurrence versus fibrosis

36a.1 **Overall median survival for patients with cancer of unknown primary site (CUP) is**
  a. 1 month
  b. 4 months
  c. 12 months
  d. 2 years
  e. 5 years

36a.2 **The histology of most CUP cases is**
  a. Adenocarcinoma
  b. Squamous cell carcinoma
  c. Sarcoma
  d. Undifferentiated
  e. Large cell carcinoma

36a.3 **New imaging methods that hold promise for determination of primary site in CUP include**
  a. Interventional neuroradiology
  b. Focused ultrasonography
  c. Magnetic resonance imaging (MRI) and positron emission tomography (PET) scanning
  d. High-resolution computed tomography (CT) scanning
  e. Digital subtraction angiography

36a.4 **Comparison between studies of CUP is difficult because**
  a. They are generally poorly designed
  b. It is a rare condition, so patient numbers are low
  c. Not many studies have been done on this frustrating topic
  d. Studies often use very different selection criteria and imaging strategies
  e. Most studies of CUP are outdated

36a.5 **Common sites of involvement in CUP include all of the following *except***
  a. Skin
  b. Bone
  c. Central nervous system
  d. Cervical nodes
  e. Liver

36b.1 **If an intra-axial brain lesion does not enhance, which of the following is most likely to be present?**
  a. Glioblastoma multiforme
  b. Metastasis
  c. Hemangioblastoma
  d. Low-grade astrocytoma
  e. None of the above

36b.2 **Which of the following suggests that a brain tumor may be of a high grade?**
  a. Cyst formation
  b. Infratentorial location
  c. Cytotoxic edema
  d. Gray matter involvement
  e. None of the above

36b.3 **The most common extra-axial neoplasm is**
  a. The seminoma
  b. The hamartoma
  c. The meningioma
  d. The chordoma
  e. None of the above

36b.4 Multiple hemangioblastomas are seen in association with
   a.   von Hippel-Lindau disease
   b.   Bourneville's disease
   c.   Turcot's syndrome
   d.   Sturge-Weber syndrome
   e.   None of the above

36b.5 A midline cystic lesion with involvement of the strap muscles is characteristic of
   a.   A branchial cleft cyst
   b.   A plunging ranula
   c.   A thyroglossal duct cyst
   d.   A cystic hygroma
   e.   None of the above

36c.1 The optimal imaging modality to evaluate the local extent of a superior sulcus tumor is
   a.   Magnetic resonance imaging (MRI)
   b.   Computed tomography (CT)
   c.   Positron emission tomography (PET)
   d.   Radionuclide bone scan
   e.   Plain radiography

36c.2 Which one of the following statements is *not* true regarding the staging evaluation of a patient with nonsmall cell lung cancer?
   a.   An adrenal mass with CT density attenuation < 10 Hounsfield units (HU) is typically benign.
   b.   Whole body fluorodeoxyglucose (FDG)-PET imaging allows staging of intra- and extrathoracic disease using a single study.
   c.   FDG-PET imaging has higher sensitivity and specificity than does CT in detecting adrenal metastases.
   d.   FDG-PET imaging often alters management in patients staged with conventional anatomic imaging.
   e.   Radionuclide bone scan should be performed routinely in all patients with potentially resectable nonsmall cell lung cancer.

36c.3 Which one of the following statements is *not* correct in the staging of a patient with small cell lung cancer (SCLC)?
   a.   A traditional TNM (tumor, node, mestastasis) system is typically used to describe disease extent.
   b.   CT or MRI of the brain is often performed in asymptomatic patients to detect occult metastases.
   c.   Routine CT or MRI of the abdomen is typically performed to detect liver and abdominal node metastases.
   d.   FDG-PET imaging may simplify staging but has not been extensively used or evaluated.
   e.   Radionuclide bone scanning and MRI are usually performed to detect bone metastases only if the patient has extensive disease.

36c.4 In the imaging evaluation of a mediastinal mass, which is true?
   a.   Contrast resolution with CT is superior to MRI.
   b.   MRI can be useful in demonstrating vascular structures without contrast enhancement.
   c.   CT and MRI can usually differentiate thymomas from lymphomas.
   d.   CT imaging can often distinguish a fibrotic mass from a persistent or recurrent tumor after treatment of mediastinal lymphoma.
   e.   CT imaging is the preferred modality for evaluating neurogenic tumors within the mediastinum.

36d.1 What is the best imaging technique in staging endometrial and cervical carcinomas?
   a.   Computed tomography (CT)
   b.   Magnetic resonance imaging (MRI)
   c.   Ultrasonography
   d.   Intravenous pyelography

36d.2 What is the most sensitive and specific technique to evaluate a possible adrenal adenoma?
   a.   Positron emission tomography
   b.   Enhanced CT with dynamic technique
   c.   Chemical-shift MRI
   d.   Ultrasonography

36d.3 What is the primary imaging modality to evaluate hypervascular liver tumors?
   a.   CT without contrast
   b.   CT with multiphasic technique
   c.   MRI with dynamic technique
   d.   T2-weighted sequence of MRI

36d.4 **The presence of which of the following in a patient is the absolute contraindication for performing an MRI?**
   a. Orthopedic screws
   b. Biliary stent
   c. Pacemaker
   d. Sutures

36e.1 **What should be the initial imaging modality used for evaluation of a suspected osseous lesion?**
   a. Magnetic resonance imaging (MRI)
   b. Radiography
   c. Computed tomography (CT)
   d. Ultrasonography
   e. Positron emission tomography (PET)

36e.2 **What imaging modalities may be used for biopsy guidance?**
   a. Fluoroscopy
   b. CT
   c. MRI
   d. Ultrasonography
   e. All of the above

36e.3 **Which of the following imaging modalities is (are) most useful for characterization of tumor mineralization?**
   a. MRI
   b. CT
   c. Radiography
   d. Ultrasonography
   e. CT and radiography
   f. MRI and ultrasonography

36e.4 **What is the best approach to percutaneous sampling of a musculoskeletal mass?**
   a. Always take the approach that looks easiest on the images.
   b. Try to cross as many anatomic compartments as possible to decrease the risk of bleeding.
   c. Always use a large-gauge needle as a definitive diagnosis can never be made from a fine-needle aspiration (FNA) biopsy.
   d. Consult with the surgeon and oncologist regarding the biopsy approach as the path traversed by the needle may significantly alter further treatment.

36e.5 **Which of the following musculoskeletal masses may be definitively diagnosed by MRI without the need for biopsy?**
   a. Soft tissue lymphoma
   b. Intramuscular metastasis
   c. Lipoma
   d. Rhabdomyosarcoma

36f.1 **Concerning *diagnostic* mammography, which one of the following statements is *not* true?**
   a. A family history of breast cancer is one of the indications for the study.
   b. It is used to evaluate clinical findings.
   c. It is indicated after an abnormal screening mammography.
   d. A radiologist should be present during the performance of the examination.
   e. A radiopaque marker *(BB)* should be placed over palpable masses prior to the examination.

36f.2 **Concerning the American College of Radiology Breast Imaging Reporting and Data System (BI-RADS), which one of the following statements is *not* correct?**
   a. The breast tissue composition indicates the relative sensitivity of the examination.
   b. "Benign findings" means short-term (6-mo) follow-up is recommended.
   c. "Highly suggestive of malignancy" means ≥ 95% probability of malignancy.
   d. "Incomplete assessment" means that further work-up is needed prior to a final assessment.
   e. "Suspicious abnormality" means that biopsy should be considered.

36f.3 **Concerning abnormal findings on mammography, which one of the following statements is *not* correct?**
   a. Fine linear branching calcifications are suspicious.
   b. The differential for an architectural distortion is radial scar, previous biopsy, and carcinoma.
   c. Compared with shape and margins, density is a better predictor of malignancy for masses.
   d. A segmental distribution (within a duct and its branches) is suspicious.
   e. Masses with obscured margins should be further evaluated with spot compression views.

36f.4 **Concerning breast ultrasonography, which one of the following statements is *not* correct?**
a. Fibroglandular tissue is more echogenic than fat.
b. Simple cysts characteristically have a round to oval shape and an anechoic interior.
c. Fibroadenomas typically are oval, wider than tall, and have circumscribed margins.
d. Cancers are typically hyperechoic (more echogenic than surrounding tissue).
e. It plays an important role in imaging-guided biopsies.

36f.5 **Concerning image-guided breast biopsies, which one of the following statements is *not* correct?**
a. The desirable positive predictive value for biopsy is ≥ 10% (≥ 10 cancers/100 biopsies).
b. Compared with open biopsy, an advantage of needle biopsy is lower cost.
c. An advantage of needle biopsy (fine-needle aspiration or core needle biopsy) is no change in future mammograms.
d. Stereotactic equipment is used to guide needle biopsy of calcifications.
e. A core needle biopsy diagnosis of atypical ductal hyperplasia mandates excisional biopsy.

36g.1 **Regarding microbubble contrast agents, which of the following statements is *false*?**
a. They oscillate when exposed to a low mechanical index (MI) ultrasound field.
b. They disrupt the signal when exposed to a high MI ultrasound field.
c. They enhance the Doppler signal from blood.
d. They are composed of tiny bubbles of gas in a supporting shell.
e. They are optimally imaged with power and color Doppler imaging.

36g.2 **Detection of a liver tumor on ultrasonography is mainly dependent on**
a. The size of the tumor
b. The location of the tumor
c. The vascularity of the tumor
d. The inherent contrast difference between the tumor and the background liver
e. The technique used

36g.3 **The most important goal of intraoperative liver ultrasonography in a patient with metastases is**
a. Localization of tumors prior to resection
b. Detection of additional tumors not seen on preoperative imaging
c. Localization of the major liver vasculature prior to resection
d. Demonstration of the relationship of tumors to major liver fissures
e. Demonstration of the relationship of tumors to major blood vessels

36h.1 **In which one of the following patients would a bone scan be most useful?**
a. Woman with stage II breast cancer
b. Man with prostate cancer and prostate-specific antigen (PSA) of 8
c. Woman with lung cancer and hilar metastases
d. Asymptomatic woman with cervical cancer and pelvic node metastases
e. Man with squamous cell carcinoma of the oropharynx

36h.2 **Treatment for which one of the following malignancies is *not* covered by Medicare?**
a. Lung cancer
b. Malignant melanoma
c. Head and neck cancers
d. Multiple myeloma
e. Esophageal cancer

36h.3 **Which one of the following statements concerning the use of positron emission tomography (PET) in lung cancer is *not* true?**
a. Diagnosis, staging, and restaging are indications covered by Medicare.
b. The specificity of PET in detecting lung cancer in a nodule indeterminate by computed tomography (CT) is greater than the sensitivity.
c. The accuracy of PET in staging the mediastinum is greater for PET than for CT.
d. PET detects previously unsuspected metastatic disease in 10 to 15% of patients.
e. False-positive PET results in the evaluation of pulmonary nodules are most commonly caused by the presence of granulomatous inflammatory processes.

36i.1 **Which of the following is an example of molecular imaging in clinical practice today?**
   a.   Noncontrast computed tomography (CT)
   b.   Myocardial perfusion imaging with thallium 201 (^{201}Tl)
   c.   18-fluorodeoxyglucose positron emission tomography (^{18}FDG-PET)
   d.   Gadolinium diethylenetriamine pentaacetic acid (Gd-DTPA)-enhanced magnetic resonance imaging (MRI)
   e.   None of the above

36i.2 **Which of the following are in vivo reporter genes that can be imaged?**
   a.   Herpes simplex virus 1 thymidine kinase
   b.   Firefly luciferase
   c.   Somatostatin receptor type 2
   d.   All of the above

ANSWERS

CANCER PATHOLOGY

35.1   **Answer: (b)**

35.2   **Answer: (f)**   VEGF-A is a multifunctional cytokine that is expressed by nearly all malignant tumors. Its expression is regulated by cytokines, oxygen concentration, oncogenes, and tumor suppressor genes. It renders tumor vessels and normal venules permeable to plasma and plasma proteins, stimulates endothelial cell migration and division, and alters the pattern of endothelial cell gene expression.

35.3   **Answer: (e)**   Immunohistochemistry provides a wide range of information about tumors.

35.4   **Answer: (c)**   Although several management options exist for patients whose smears are interpreted as atypical squamous cells of undetermined significance (ASCUS)—including human papillomavirus deoxyribonucleic acid (HPV DNA) testing (the preferred approach for those women whose original Pap smear is liquid-based), repeat cytology, and colposcopy—the recommended management of women with ASC-H is referral for colposcopic evaluation. When no lesion is identified after colposcopy in women with ASC-H, it is recommended that, when possible, a review of the cytology, colposcopy, and histology results be performed. If a diagnosis of ASC-H is upheld, cytologic follow-up at 6 and 12 months and HPV DNA testing at 12 months is acceptable. Women who are found to have ASC or greater on their repeat cervical cytology tests or who subsequently test positive for high-risk HPV DNA should be referred for colposcopy again.

35.5   **Answer: (e)**   Although all of the methods listed allow one to detect either the characteristic chromosomal translocation, its associated chimeric messenger ribonucleic acid, or its fusion protein product, PCR-based assays are the most sensitive method for detecting the presence of the translocation. The PCR technique allows an exponential amplification of the target DNA or complementary DNA. PCR assays for chromosomal translocations can detect as few as 1 in 100,000 to 1 in 1,000,000 cells.

IMAGING

36.1   **Answer: (a), (d), and (e)**   CT, PET, and chest radiography all use ionizing radiation to image patients, with radiation doses dependent on the modality and parameters for that study (eg, kV, mA, number of images, injected dose for PET). MRI uses magnetic fields, and ultrasonography uses sound waves to produce the images; thus, there is no radiation dose to the patient with these modalities.

36.2   **Answer: (c)**   FDG is a D-glucose analogue and uses a fundamental property of tumors, increased glucose metabolism, for imaging purposes. Because malignant cells are typically more metabolically active than are normal cells, they demonstrate increased uptake and trapping of FDG. Thus, areas of high metabolic activity can be visualized by PET and are suggestive of a malignant process.

36.3   **Answer: (a), (b), and (d)**   PET imaging has been used to help differentiate benign from malignant abnormalities seen on conventional imaging, to stage tumors, and to predict recurrent disease. There are no studies to date that have used PET as a screening tool.

36a.1   **Answer: (b)**   Overall median survival for patients with CUP is dismal, only about 4 months. However, certain subsets of patients may live significantly longer, particularly those for which a specific treatment can be found. Occasional CUP patients survive longer than expected even with nonspecific treatment.

36a.2   **Answer: (a)**   Most CUP cases show adenocarcinomatous histology, which is difficult to differentiate into a more specific subtype or cell of origin. New immunohistochemical methods of analysis may help in the future in determination of the primary site in some of these cases.

36a.3   **Answer: (c)**   Both MRI and PET scanning offer the possibility of more accurate determination of primary site in cases of CUP. MRI is particularly useful in evaluation of soft tissues and marrow spaces, whereas PET allows imaging of the entire body in a single study. Both suffer from the limitation of spatial resolution, which prevents detection of very small primary sites.

36a.4   **Answer: (d)**   Comparison between studies of patients with CUP is often difficult because of differences in selection criteria of patients and imaging strategies. If only asymptomatic patients are included, or if only certain types of imaging are done, this drastically alters the results and prevents useful comparison between them.

36a.5   **Answer: (a)**   The skin and subcutaneous tissues are rare sites of presentation of patients with CUP. In one study, lung cancer was the most common primary site ultimately discovered in these cases.

36b.1   **Answer: (d)**   Low-grade astrocytomas, excluding pilocytic astrocytomas, tend to lack enhancement. Glioblastoma multiforme, metastases, and hemangioblastomas should not be included in the differential diagnosis of a nonenhancing lesion.

36b.2   **Answer: (e)**   Cyst formation is often seen in less aggressive lesions. Location is important in tumor differentiation; however, lesions of both high and low grade originate infratentorially. Cytotoxic edema is not generally associated with tumors, aggressive or benign. Rather, vasogenic edema is associated with neoplasms. Gray matter involvement can be seen independent of grade; whereas tumor extension is most often along white matter tracks, a minority of tumors (ie, pleiomorphic xanthoastrocytoma and ganglioglioma) often involve gray matter.

36b.3   **Answer: (c)**   Meningioma is the most common extra-axial lesion.

36b.4   **Answer: (a)**   von Hippel-Lindau disease is associated with multiple hemangioblastomas. These lesions can be solid, cystic, or mixed.

36b.5   **Answer: (c)**   The thyroid gland descends normally from the foramen cecum to its expected location. Thyroglossal duct cysts occur along the path of this descent, that is, anterior and midline.

36c.1   **Answer: (a)**   Although multimodality evaluation is typically used to comprehensively evaluate the anatomic extent of the primary tumor, MRI is particularly useful in the evaluation of patients with superior sulcus tumors. MRI is used to determine the absence or presence and extent of tumor involvement of the brachial plexus as well as extension into the adjacent intervertebral neural canal. Accurate determination of the anatomic extent can influence surgical management in resectable tumors, that is, the decision whether resection is performed by cardiothoracic surgeons alone or a combined approach involving cardiothoracic and neurosurgeons. PET imaging has poor inherent resolution and, although useful in detecting occult metastases, is usually not used to evaluate the local extent of the primary tumor. Radionuclide bone scanning can indicate involvement of ribs and vertebral bodies but offers little additional information that influences management. Radiographic assessment can identify gross invasion of the brachial plexus, ribs, and vertebral bodies but is inaccurate in evaluation of subtle tumor invasion of these structures.

36c.2   **Answer: (e)**   CT is the primary modality used to diagnosis and characterize intra-abdominal lesions, and frequently a confident diagnosis of benignity or malignancy is possible. For instance, if an adrenal mass contains fat or has an attenuation value of < 10 HU on a noncontrast CT scan, the mass can be considered benign without the need for MRI or biopsy. Whole body imaging with FDG-PET is being used to improve the accuracy of staging. FDG-PET has a higher sensitivity and specificity than does CT in detecting metastases to the adrenal glands, bones, and lymph nodes. Whole body PET permits staging of intra- and extrathoracic disease with a single study, reveals occult extrathoracic metastases in patients selected for curative resection, and alters management in up to 40% of patients. Radionuclide bone scanning infrequently reveals occult skeletal metastases; therefore, bone radiography, technetium Tc 99m–labeled methylene diphosphonate bone scintigraphy, and MRI are usually only performed if the patient has focal bone pain or an elevated alkaline phosphatase level.

36c.3   **Answer: (a)**   Although it has been advocated by some that the TNM system be used, SCLC is generally staged as limited disease (malignancy confined to a hemithorax and regional lymph nodes) or extensive disease (malignancy with noncontiguous metastases to the contralateral lung or distant metastases). There is no consensus regarding the imaging studies that should be performed in the staging evaluation of SCLC. Unlike nonsmall cell lung cancer, central nervous system metastases are common at presentation in patients with SCLC. Because most of these patients are asymptomatic, CT or MRI of the brain is often routinely performed in patients with SCLC. For similar reasons, routine CT or MRI of the abdomen is typically performed. Although patients with SCLC and bone and bone marrow metastases are often asymptomatic, isolated bone and bone marrow metastases are uncommon. Consequently, bone scintigraphy and MR imaging are usually performed only if the patient has other findings of extensive disease. Although it has been reported that whole body FDG-PET imaging may be useful in improving and simplifying staging, PET has not been extensively used or evaluated in patients with SCLC.

36c.4   **Answer: (b)**   Although CT provides the requisite information in most patients with mediastinal abnormalities, MRI is especially useful in the evaluation of vascular structures when iodinated contrast-enhanced CT is contraindicated. Normal blood vessels on MRI are typically devoid of intravascular signal and can be differentiated from adjacent soft tissue without contrast administration. Contrast resolution with MRI is superior to CT; thus, MRI can be useful in delineating mediastinal anatomy and demonstrating soft tissue invasion. Because of the similarity in composition of thymomas and lymphomas, CT and MRI cannot differentiate these tumors with certainty. After treatment of mediastinal lymphomas, residual masses are common and distinction of a fibrotic mass from persistent or recurrent tumor can be difficult by CT imaging. MRI can be a useful adjunct to gallium-67 scanning in these cases to monitor and evaluate response to therapy, differentiate fibrosis from residual tumor, and detect recurrent lymphoma. MRI is also the preferred modality for evaluating neurogenic tumors within the mediastinum as it can simultaneously assess intraspinal extension, spinal cord abnormalities, longitudinal extent of tumor, and extradural extension.

36d.1   **Answer: (b)**   MRI is superior to CT and ultrasonography because of its excellent soft tissue resolution and ability to visualize the zonal anatomy. When it is completed by the dynamic contrast scan, it has the highest accuracy in the detection of small tumors and evaluation of depth of stromal and myometrial involvement. Cervical tumors can be accurately identified in 91% of invasive lesions.

36d.2   **Answer: (c)**   The majority of adrenal cortical adenomas are lipid rich. On in-phased images, the adrenal cortical adenomas are iso- to hyperintense, and the signal intensity decreases significantly on out-of-phase images owing to abundant intracellular lipid. This is the same technique that is used to evaluate fatty liver. Usefulness of CT can be comparable to that of MRI by using unenhanced images with the threshold value of < 10 Hounsfield units (HU) and a 60% decrease in HU on enhanced images obtained at 15 minutes after administration of contrast. These enhanced images also help to detect lipid-poor adrenal adenomas.

36d.3   **Answer: (b)**   Multiphasic CT primarily is used to evaluate hypervascular liver lesions, such as hepatocellular carcinoma (HCC) and metastases, to improve the lesions' detectability. Hypervascular tumors have a rapid and brief uptake of contrast during the early arterial phase. This characteristic pattern of enhancement provides key information for the diagnosis. It has been reported that one-third of carcinoid tumors were more conspicuous on arterial phase images, and one-sixth of these lesions were seen only on arterial phase images. Similarly, in HCC, additional lesions can be detected on arterial phase images.

36d.4   **Answer: (c)**

36e.1   **Answer: (b)**   Radiography remains the primary mode of initial evaluation of bone lesions. It is from radiographs that the aggressive or nonaggressive nature of a lesion is best evaluated. MRI is useful in evaluating the extent of a lesion and in assessment of a soft tissue mass, but its results may be misleading in the determination of benign versus malignant lesions. CT scanning is usually not necessary to fully define the osseous characteristics of a lesion and, because of its expense and greater radiation dose, is only used in selected cases to supplement findings on radiographs. Ultrasonography is not particularly useful for primary osseous lesions that do not have a significant soft tissue component. PET imaging has limited usefulness in primary musculoskeletal tumors; currently its primary purpose is identification of distant metastases.

36e.2   **Answer: (e)**   Any of these imaging modalities may be used to guide percutaneous sampling of musculoskeletal tumors. Each has its own advantages and disadvantages. Cost can be an issue—fluoroscopy is often less expensive, but it also provides less anatomic detail. Biopsy with MR guidance requires special equipment because of the magnetic field; therefore, it is often more expensive than other modalities.

36e.3   **Answer: (e)**   CT and radiography are the most useful modalities in the assessment of the character of tumor mineralization. Mineralization causes artifacts on MRI scans because of the effects on the surrounding magnetic field. These artifacts make characterization of the morphology of the mineralization difficult, if not impossible. On ultrasonographs mineralization may act to block sound waves and therefore be detectable as echogenic foci; however, the characterization of morphology of mineralization with ultrasonography is not as straightforward as it is with radiography or CT.

36e.4   **Answer: (d)**   It is best to consult with the treating physician or surgeon before performing a biopsy of a primary musculoskeletal tumor (predominantly sarcomas) as the biopsy tract may need to be resected or included in the area of treatment. It is not true that a definitive diagnosis cannot be made from an FNA biopsy; some tumors may be definitively diagnosed on the basis of imaging characteristics, clinical presentation, and the results of an FNA biopsy. The goal of a biopsy is usually to violate as few anatomic compartments as possible and to avoid contamination of unaffected compartments, which could potentially alter therapy.

36e.5   **Answer: (c)**   Lipomas have a characteristic appearance on MRI that allows them to be definitively diagnosed without the need for biopsy. Many other tumors have a nonspecific high T2, intermediate, or low T1 signal appearance that does not permit a definitive diagnosis. However, other factors such as patient age, location of the tumor, and effect on adjacent structures may allow a narrow differential to be proposed even in these cases.

36f.1   **Answer: (a)**   Diagnostic mammography, also called *consultative* or *problem-solving* mammography, is performed when there are clinical findings, such as a lump or an abnormal screening mammography. A radiopaque *BB* is placed over the palpable mass, so that the interpreting physician can correlate any imaging findings with the clinical abnormality. A radiologist should be present during the examination to supervise the work-up plan and to explain findings and management recommendations to the patient. The procedure is not indicated for screening of asymptomatic high-risk women as they can be properly evaluated by a screening examination.

36f.2   **Answer: (b)**   BI-RADS was developed to improve the communication of results and recommendations for mammography. The breast tissue composition varies from totally fatty to extremely dense, and the sensitivity of mammography is directly related to density (highest sensitivity in the fatty breast and lowest in the extremely dense breast). "Incomplete assessment" after a screening means that additional imaging needs to be performed before arriving at a final assessment for the case. "Suspicious abnormality" indicates a probability of malignancy that warrants a biopsy, and "highly suggestive of malignancy" indicates the findings are classic for cancer. In contrast, "benign findings" means that there are findings, but that they are classic for benign and the recommendation is routine screenings. Generally, this means screening annually. A 6-month follow-up is reserved for an abnormality that is almost certainly benign, with a likelihood of malignancy of < 2%, and can safely be managed with a 6-month screening follow-up.

36f.3   **Answer: (c)**   There are several categories of abnormal findings on a mammogram. These include masses, calcifications, asymmetries, and architectural distortions. Calcifications run the gamut from typically benign, such as vascular or milk of calcium, to suspicious, including pleomorphic and fine linear branching calcifications. The distribution of calcifications is another predictive feature, with a segmental distribution being suspicious for malignancy. Architectural distortion, defined as spicules without a mass, can represent cancer, but can also be because of a radial scar or previous surgery. Masses are described as to shape, margins, and density. Of these, margins are the most predictive of benign versus malignant, and density is the least reliable.

36f.4   **Answer: (d)**   Breast ultrasound images reflect the relative echogenicity of breast structures. For example, the breast fat is less echogenic (hypoechoic) than the fibroglandular tissue (hyperechoic). Simple cysts have no internal echoes (anechoic), a finding so definitive that further work-up is not necessary. Recent studies have focused on features that might differentiate benign from malignant masses. For example, fibroadenomas are typically oval or gently lobular, wider than tall, and have circumscribed margins. If there is any question, an ultrasound-guided biopsy is performed. Ultrasound-guided biopsy is an excellent method for biopsy because it is accurate, done under real-time imaging, and comfortable for the patient, who can lie supine. Cancers typically have an irregular shape, indistinct margins, and are less echogenic (hypoechoic) than surrounding tissue. In contrast, hyperechoic masses are characteristically benign.

36f.5   **Answer: (a)**   Breast core needle biopsy can be guided by ultrasound or stereotactic mammography. The method used depends on the location of the abnormality, the experience of the physician performing the biopsy, and the type of abnormality. For example, calcifications are usually visualized only on mammography; therefore, stereotactic biopsy is generally used to biopsy calcifications. Core needle biopsy has several advantages over open biopsy, including no visible scar, no change in future mammograms, and lower cost. However, the cost-effectiveness of mammography depends on appropriate selection of cases for biopsy. An excessive number of false-positive biopsies (biopsy results are benign) can eliminate the cost savings of the procedure. The positive predictive value (PPV), or positive biopsy rate, indicates the number of cancers diagnosed divided by the number of biopsies performed. In the radiology literature, the desirable range for PPV is 25 to 40%. A range as low as 10% suggests that too many biopsies are being performed for benign findings.

36g.1   **Answer: (e)**   Microbubble contrast agents are not optimally imaged with power and color Doppler imaging when significant artifact from motion and blooming hampers visualization. Rather, the microbubbles are optimally studied with specialized imaging techniques, which selectively detect the signal from the microbubbles with suppression of the signal from the background tissue. This includes both harmonic and pulse inversion imaging.

36g.2   **Answer: (d)**   Detection of a tumor on a liver examination requires a difference between the contrast of the lesion and the background liver. If the two tissues have similar echogenicity, the lesion may not be appreciated, regardless of its size or location.

36g.3   **Answer: (b)**   Identification of additional and unsuspected lesions results in modification and often cancellation of planned surgical procedures in patients with metastatic disease.

36h.1   **Answer: (c)**   Breast, lung, and prostate cancers commonly spread to bone. Women with stage I or II disease have a very low likelihood of having metastatic involvement of the skeleton. Men with PSA levels < 10 are unlikely to have bone involvement. Women with cervical cancer and patients with head and neck cancer are unlikely to have metastatic bone disease until they have extensive metastatic disease.

36h.2   **Answer: (d)**   Medicare has policies that cover lung cancer, colorectal cancer, melanoma, lymphoma, head and neck cancers, esophageal cancer, and breast cancer.

36h.3   **Answer: (b)**   PET is very accurate in the evaluation of the indeterminate pulmonary nodule, with a sensitivity of 97% and a specificity of 78%. The primary cause of false-positive results is granulomatous infections. PET is more accurate than CT in staging the mediastinum, but because the sensitivity is about 80%, most patients still need mediastinoscopy.

36i.1   **Answer: (c)**   PET with ^{18}FDG may be characterized as one of the first molecular imaging techniques validated by basic cancer research and used in clinical settings today. Noncontrast CT provides excellent anatomic detail of disease but no biochemical information. Although perfusion imaging with ^{201}Tl and Gd-DTPA-enhanced MRI generate signals from specific molecules, the signal content reports relatively nonspecific bulk physicochemical information pertaining to blood flow, perfusion, and extracellular space; thus, they do not fulfill the goals of molecular imaging.

36i.2   **Answer: (d)**   All of these represent examples of reporter genes that can be imaged in vivo by PET, single-photon emission computed tomography, or bioluminescence. Additional reporter genes matched with substrates that can be imaged can be detected with MRI and near infrared fluorescence instruments. Clinical gene therapy may someday be monitored noninvasively with molecular imaging of reporter genes that are engineered into the therapeutic vectors.

THERAPEUTIC MODALITIES

DIRECTIONS: Numbering for questions and answers reflects the corresponding chapter in *Cancer Medicine-6*.
Each question contains suggested responses.
Select the best response to each question.
Answers for Therapeutic Modalities begin on page 60.

SURGICAL ONCOLOGY

38.1   Concerning the discipline of surgical oncology, which of the following is true?
a.   Training does not include principles of chemotherapy or radiation oncology.
b.   Surgical oncology is more a technical than a cognitive discipline.
c.   Surgical oncology is more a cognitive than a technical discipline.
d.   Fellowship training is usually of 1 year's duration.
e.   Subspecialty board certification is available through the American Board of Surgery.

38.2   Which of the following is true concerning needle biopsy?
a.   Core needle biopsy and fine-needle aspiration are equally accurate in diagnosing solid tumors.
b.   Recurrences in the biopsy tract are sufficiently frequent to be an important determinant of the selection of needle biopsy as opposed to an open biopsy approach.
c.   Core needle biopsy is best for large tumors, whereas fine-needle aspiration is optimal for small tumors.
d.   Fine-needle aspiration is best performed with radiologic image guidance.
e.   Nuclear pleomorphism is a more important diagnostic feature in fine-needle aspiration than in core needle biopsy.

38.3   Concerning staging systems, which of the following is true?
a.   The American Joint Committee on Cancer (AJCC) sanctioned staging system factors include only T, N, and M (tumor, lymph node, metastasis).
b.   The AJCC, International Union against Cancer (UICC), and World Health Organization (WHO) staging systems are now unified for most common malignancies.
c.   T1N0M tumors are small tumors that have spread to regional lymph nodes.
d.   There are four chronologic classifications designated by a lowercase letter: c (clinical), p (pathologic), r (re-treatment), and a (autopsy).
e.   The r classification requires biopsy proof of recurrence as the criterion of applicability.

RADIATION ONCOLOGY

39.1   Intensity-modulated radiotherapy (IMRT)
a.   Allows for normal tissue sparing
b.   Allows for dose escalation
c.   Has been demonstrated to be effective in randomized trials
d.   Allows for normal tissue sparing and dose escalation
e.   Does none of the above

39.2   Which of the following are gene therapy approaches currently under investigation in combination with radiotherapy?
a.   Radioinducible gene therapy
b.   Prodrug therapy
c.   Radioinducible gene therapy and prodrug therapy
d.   None of the above

39.3   Which of the following is *not* proposed as a limiting factor in radiocurability?
a.   Tumor size
b.   Hypoxic tumor cells
c.   Intrinsic water density of tumors
d.   Intrinsic deoxyribonucleic acid (DNA) repair/sensitivity of tumor cells

39.4   Which of the following is (are) true of Rad51 protein?
a.   It mediates recombination in a complex with other proteins.
b.   It is involved in the end joining pathway.
c.   It is homologous to the bacterial protein RecA.
d.   It phosphorylates CHK 2.
e.   It mediates recombination in a complex with other proteins and is homologous to the bacterial protein RecA.
f.   It mediates recombination in a complex with other proteins and is involved in the end joining pathway.
g.   All of the above are true.

39.5   The interaction of radiation with cells
a.   Is random
b.   Produces hydroxyl radicals

    c.   Mediates DNA double-stranded breaks

    d.   Does all of the above

    e.   Does none of the above

40.1   **Which of the following statements regarding photodynamic therapy (PDT) is *not* true?**

    a.   PDT involves the activation of dyes that are localized in target tissue.

    b.   The most studied light-activated dye or sensitizer is Photofrin.

    c.   The major side effect of PDT is cutaneous photosensitization.

    d.   Photofrin is not recommended in patients who have liver failure.

    e.   All of the above are true.

40.2   **An 81-year-old man is referred to the hospital with dehydration secondary to progressive dysphagia. He first developed dysphagia 18 months before admission. Evaluation at that time included an upper endoscopy that revealed a distal esophageal mass. Biopsy of the mass revealed squamous cell carcinoma. A computed tomography (CT) scan revealed hepatic and mediastinal metastases. The patient subsequently underwent two courses of chemotherapy with some improvement in dysphagia. During the 4 months before admission, the patient's dysphagia worsened, and he underwent several esophageal dilations. Each dilation provided relief of symptoms for no more than 7 days. Radiotherapy was attempted, but the patient refused further therapy because nausea and generalized debility ensued. On admission to the hospital, he was dehydrated, cachectic, and slightly icteric. Admission laboratory test results were notable for blood urea nitrogen, 35 mg/dL; creatinine, 1.3 mg/dL; total bilirubin, 4.4 mg/dL; and AST, 75 U/L. An esophagogastroduodenoscopy was performed, and the patient was found to have nearly complete obstruction of the esophageal lumen by tumor. The use of PDT with porfimer sodium (Photofrin) is considered. Which of the following is a correct statement?**

    a.   The patient's jaundice precludes the use of PTD with porfimer sodium.

    b.   Age greater than 80 years is a contraindication for treatment with PDT with porfimer sodium.

    c.   Total obstruction of the esophagus makes PDT impossible.

    d.   The previous history of chemotherapy is a contraindication to PDT.

    e.   The history of radiotherapy is a contraindication to PDT.

41.1   **Which of the following is known to sensitize cells to killing by hyperthermia?**

    a.   Thermotolerance

    b.   Methotrexate

    c.   Vincristine

    d.   Acidosis

    e.   Synchronization of cells in G_0/G_1 phase of the cell cycle

41.2   **The most likely target that leads to cell death by hyperthermia is**

    a.   Mitochondria

    b.   DNA

    c.   Protein

    d.   Endoplasmic reticulum

    e.   Proton pumps

41.3   **The thermal enhancement ratio (TER) is**

    a.   A method to assess the efficacy of techniques to increase thermal killing in vivo

    b.   Defined as the ratio of doses of radiation to achieve an isoeffect without versus with hyperthermia

    c.   A method that compares the degree of damage to tumor versus normal tissue after hyperthermic treatment

    d.   The degree of visual enhancement of a tumor using a range of different diagnostic tools, after exposure to hyperthermia

41.4   **Which of the following statements about 100 MHz radiofrequency heating is true?**

    a.   The depth of penetration of power is limited to a few centimeters with single antennas placed on the body surface, but by using arrays of antennas that are driven in phase, it is possible to achieve significant power deposition deep within the body.

    b.   Using capacitive coupling, it is possible to heat to great depths, and steering of power can be achieved by varying the size of the coupling electrodes.

    c.   Heating of superficial fat layers is a limitation.

    d.   The method is limited by reflection of radiofrequency fields from air pockets and absorption by bone.

    e.   When driving antennas in phase, the energy cancels out, leading to less power deposition at depth.

41.5   **Phase III clinical trials comparing radiation therapy alone to radiation therapy plus hyperthermia have shown significant improvement in local/regional tumor control and/or a survival advantage in all of the following tumor types except one. Which type has *not* shown a therapeutic advantage?**

    a.   Glioblastoma multiforme

    b.   Cervical tumor

c. Melanoma
d. Esophageal tumor
e. Bladder tumor

MEDICAL ONCOLOGY

42.1 The strategy of adjuvant chemotherapy is increasingly influenced by our understanding of the cellular and molecular biology of metastases. With the understanding that much of this knowledge derives from experimental models, which one of the following is true?
a. A long period of lack of growth (latent period) could result from sustained expression of tumor angiogenesis factors.
b. A failure of growth would necessarily be associated with a marked decrease in the proliferation rate of tumor cells.
c. Except for the lungs, the distribution of metastases is determined primarily by the magnitude of the blood supply to the various organs.
d. The relationship between adhesion molecules on the surface of circulating tumor cells and the endothelium and basement membrane of the organ is the major determinant of the distribution of metastases.
e. Although primary tumors are clonal, metastases are not.

CHEMOTHERAPY

43.1 The original model of tumor growth (also known as the *log-kill model*), which describes tumor growth as exponential, is known as the
a. Delbruck-Luria model
b. Goldie-Coldman model
c. Gompertzian model
d. Skipper-Schabel-Wilcox model
e. Speer-Retsky model

43.2 The model of tumor kinetics based on nonexponential growth of tumors was originally developed by
a. Gompertz
b. Norton
c. Simon
d. Retsky
e. Luria

43.3 After a cell divides, it can either enter the G_1 phase to prepare for another division, die, or
a. Directly proceed to the G_2 phase
b. Enter the S phase
c. Enter a nonproliferative state
d. Directly enter the M phase

44.1 Specificity of a ligand for a molecular target is mainly determined by
a. The vascularity of the tumor
b. The ligand
c. The microenvironment of the tumor
d. The target
e. The lipid (membrane) solubility of the ligand

44.2 Of the following, which may *not* be affected by the dose of a cytotoxic antitumor agent?
a. Cytochrome P-450
b. Kidney function
c. The plasma half-time of the agent
d. Liver function

44.3 The most important factor in the adjuvant treatment of breast cancer is
a. The use of the most active single agent
b. The duration of administration
c. The use of agents emphasizing dose intensity
d. The use of agents in combination
e. The schedule of administration

44.4 The combination of antiestrogen therapy and chemotherapy generally indicates which of the following in the adjuvant treatment of breast cancer? (More than one may be true.)
a. Antagonism $(1 + 1 < 2)$
b. Synergy $(1 + 1 > 2)$
c. Additive effect $(1 + 1 = 2)$
d. Increased toxicity
e. Increased duration of effect

44.5 Neoadjuvant treatment of breast cancer indicates that
a. Chemotherapy may be highly effective in primary breast cancer
b. Contrary to previous indications, the organ of Zuckerkandl is commonly involved in breast cancer
c. When employed in patients with large primaries ($> 3 - 6$ cm), the survival rate has been favorably affected as opposed to the survival rate in patients who receive standard adjuvant chemotherapy
d. Complete responses, pathologically confirmed, do not occur

45.1 Which of the following methods of dose escalation in a phase I trial has *not* been shown to save patients from receiving ineffective dose levels of a new agent?
a. Doubling method
b. Modified Fibonacchi method
c. Pharmacologically guided dose escalation
d. Continual reassessment
e. Geometric mean + extended factor of 2

45.2 The relationship used in toxicology studies to describe how doses in animals relate to doses in humans is best described as
a. Absent—there is no relationship
b. The same on a milligram per kilogram basis
c. Different for each animal
d. The same on a milligram per squared meter basis
e. Different for each pharmacologic class of new agents

45.3 You are talking with a patient about participation in a phase I trial. Which of the following statements best describes how you should present the study to the patient and what knowledge you should impart?
a. "We are obviously in a difficult situation without any real options for you except this phase I trial with a new agent. Phase I trials are not dangerous, and the new drug might help you."
b. "The chances that you will have serious toxicities or even death from the new drug are greater than the chance of your having benefit from the new drug, but it is a reasonable option for you."
c. "The reason we are offering this new drug to you is because there is a chance that the drug will work for you and you will not be at great risk. In general phase I trials are fairly safe, and it is a reasonable option for you."
d. "By participating in this study, you will be helping other patients after you, but there is very little chance that the new agent will help you by shrinking your tumor. However, I suggest you give it a try because it is your only option."

45.4 Which of the following statements best describes the ability of animal models to predict for the antitumor activity of a new agent?
a. Animal tumor models are not at all predictive of anticancer agent activity in patients.
b. Animal leukemia models are predictive of clinical activity, but animal solid tumor models are not.
c. The animal tumor models are reasonable predictors (although not tumor-specific predictors) of activity in the clinic.
d. The animal tumor models are excellent predictors of tumor-specific activity in the clinic.
e. If one uses the appropriate end points, the animal tumor models are very predictive of anticancer activity in the clinic.

45.5 Which of the following statements best describes a pharmacodynamic end point?
a. Serum half-life of the new agent
b. Area under the concentration-time curve for a new agent
c. Effect of the new agent on a particular target
d. Mean residence time for a new agent
e. Dose-limiting toxicity for a new agent

45.6 Which of the following statements best describes what the National Cancer Institute's COMPARE computer program demonstrates?
a. The program indicates whether a new agent will have activity in the clinic.
b. The program is used to detect compounds that have similar patterns of activity in a cell line screen and, therefore, similar mechanisms of action.
c. The program can determine which toxicities in animals are predictive of toxicities in patients.

d. The program determines which agent in an in vivo animal model will have antitumor activity in the clinic.
e. The program is used to compare the pharmacology of a new agent in animal systems versus that in patients.

46.1 Which of these antitumor compounds requires metabolism or chemical change before it has biologic activity?
a. Cisplatin
b. Irinotecan
c. Methotrexate
d. Gemcitabine
e. All of the above

46.2 Nucleoside analogues may inhibit DNA repair via
a. Irreversible alkylation of the DNA
b. Mechanism-based blocking of repair patch excision
c. Insertion into the resynthesized DNA patch
d. Inhibition of topoisomerase I–mediated relaxation of condensed DNA

46.3 Which of the following may be the basis for interpatient variability in the pharmacokinetics of anticancer agents?
a. Abnormalities in drug absorption
b. Variability in drug distribution
c. Heterogeneity in drug elimination
d. Differences in protein binding
e. All of the above

46.4 Pharmacodynamics is the study of dose-response relationships. Which of the following can be characterized as a pharmacodynamic study?
a. The effect of increasing incorporation of gemcitabine into the DNA synthesis in MCF-7 cells in vitro on the clonogenic survival of the cells
b. An investigation in tumor-bearing mice that seeks to relate the systemic exposure of capecitabine to the increase in survival
c. A clinical study that relates renal clearance of carboplatin to the degree of thrombocytopenia
d. All of the above
e. None of the above

47.1 Regional antineoplastic drug delivery has become a standard management option in which clinical setting?
a. Intraperitoneal therapy of recurrent endometrial cancer
b. Intra-arterial therapy of meningioma
c. Intravesical therapy of superficial bladder cancer
d. Intrathecal therapy of meningeal carcinomatosis from melanoma

47.2 Advantages associated with regional antineoplastic drug delivery include all of the following *except*
a. Reduced systemic toxicity
b. Higher peak concentrations of drug directly in contact with tumor
c. Prolonged exposure of drug to tumor within a body compartment
d. Enhanced delivery of drug to tumor via the systemic compartment

47.3 The depth of penetration of cytotoxic agents *directly* into tumor tissue following regional drug delivery is approximately
a. 1 to 2 mm
b. 5 to 8 mm
c. 1 to 1.5 cm
d. 2 to 3 cm

48.1 P-Glycoprotein causes resistance to multiple different classes of chemotherapeutic agents primarily by
a. Increasing the metabolic breakdown of cancer drugs
b. Enhancing the systemic clearance of cancer drugs
c. Blocking the entry of water-soluble cancer drugs into cancer cells
d. Pumping lipid-soluble cancer drugs out of cancer cells

48.2 Which of the following statements about glutathione S-transferases (GSTs) and drug resistance is *not* true?
a. GSTs are classified as phase II drug detoxifying enzymes.
b. GSTs can make some anticancer drugs more polar and, therefore, result in the trapping of these drugs inside of cancer cells.
c. GSTs are directly involved in the detoxification of doxorubicin.
d. Increased GST activity is implicated in cellular resistance to alkylating agents such as chlorambucil and melphalan.

48.3 Which one of the following statements regarding resistance to drugs that target topoisomerase II is *not* true?
   a. Topoisomerase II inhibitors work by destabilizing deoxyribonucleic acid (DNA)-topoisomerase complexes (cleavable complexes).
   b. Drugs subject to cellular resistance owing to changes in topoisomerase II may also be subject to P-glycoprotein-mediated resistance.
   c. Drugs that target topoisomerase II include agents from anthracyline and epidophylotoxin classes of anticancer drugs.
   d. Topoisomerase II inhibitors are generally not effective against solid tumors where there is a large population of quiescent cells.

48.4 Cellular resistance to methotrexate can be obtained by all of the following mechanisms *except*
   a. Increased levels of the target enzyme dihydrofolate reductase
   b. Increased expression of the reduced folate carrier
   c. Decreased polyglutamylation of methotrexate
   d. Increased expression of multidrug resistance–associated proteins (MRPs)

CHEMOTHERAPEUTIC AGENTS

49.1 Since the initial demonstrations of the usefulness of folate antagonists in the treatment of cancer, methotrexate has earned a role in the curative regimens used in the treatment of a wide range of neoplastic diseases. For which of the following malignancies has methotrexate historically shown significant activity?
   a. Osteosarcoma
   b. Non-Hodgkin's lymphoma (NHL)
   c. Acute lymphoblastic leukemia (ALL)
   d. Choriocarcinoma
   e. Osteosarcoma and ALL
   f. All of the above

49.2 As with many other antineoplastic agents, methotrexate causes toxicity to self-renewing tissues, producing mucositis and myelo-suppression after most dosing schedules, similar to that seen with other agents. However, depending on the dose and schedule, methotrexate can also cause end-organ damage in tissues not undergoing frequent cell division. Which of the following toxicities are described after methotrexate administration?
   a. Nephrotoxicity: impaired renal function both as a result of direct tubular damage and as a result of precipitation of methotrexate and its metabolite 7-hydroxymethotrexate
   b. Cardiotoxicity: decreased myocardial contractility proportional to the total cumulative dose of methotrexate received
   c. Neurotoxicity: from irritability and headache to cranial nerve palsies, seizures, and coma, resulting from a biochemical folate deficiency in the central nervous system (CNS)
   d. Nephrotoxicity and cardiotoxicity
   e. Nephrotoxicity and neurotoxicity
   f. All of the above

49.3 All of the following have been described as mechanisms of methotrexate resistance in experimental tumors *except*
   a. Amplification of the target enzyme
   b. Mutation of the target enzyme
   c. Decreased drug uptake
   d. Decreased intracellular drug metabolism
   e. Increased expression of P-glycoprotein

49.4 Understanding the molecular basis of normal folate physiology, of methotrexate cytotoxicity, and of methotrexate resistance is allowing and guiding the rational design of new folate antagonists and strategies to selectively target resistant cells. Although a number of later-generation antifolates are in clinical trial, only two, ralitrexed and trimetrexate, currently have approved indications. Which of the following mechanisms is *not* a mechanism used by newer antifolates to circumvent methotrexate resistance?
   a. Increased affinity for and inhibition of ribonucleotide reductase
   b. Decreased dependence on the reduced folate carrier for transport into the cell
   c. Increased retention within the cell as a result of more efficient polyglutamylation
   d. Increased inhibition of thymidylate synthetase
   e. Increased inhibition of enzymes necessary for purine synthesis (eg, glycinamide ribonucleotide transformylase)

50.1 A patient develops life-threatening toxicity following the administration of a chemotherapy regimen containing 5-fluorouracil and leucovorin. Which of the following is the most likely explanation?
   a. 5-Fluorouracil was administered too rapidly as a bolus.
   b. The leucovorin dose was miscalculated.
   c. The 5-fluorouracil dose was miscalculated.
   d. Genetic susceptibility was present owing to a low level of the enzyme catabolizing 5-fluorouracil.
   e. Genetic susceptibility was present owing to a high level of the enzyme anabolizing 5-fluorouracil.

50.2 **Which of the following is *not* a mechanism of resistance with the cancer chemotherapy drug cytarabine?**
a. Decreased activity of the carrier for cytarabine transport
b. Decreased activity of cytoplasmic deoxycytidine kinase
c. Increased catabolism of cytarabine through the action of dihydropyrimidine dehydrogenase
d. Increased catabolism of cytarabine through the action of cytidine deaminase
e. Decreased activity of deoxycytidine monophosphate (dCMP) deaminase

50.3 **Capecitabine represents a new orally active prodrug of 5-fluorouracil approved for the treatment of metastatic breast cancer and for advanced colorectal cancer. The enzymes required for its activation are**
a. Thymidylate synthase
b. Cytosine deaminase
c. Cytidine deaminase and thymidine phosphorylase
d. Carboxylesterase
e. Carboxylesterase, cytidine deaminase, and thymidine and uridine phosphorylases

50.4 **By mistake a cancer patient receives a dose of 5-fluorouracil of 5,000 mg/m^2 rather then 500 mg/m^2. Within minutes of the bolus infusion of 5-fluorouracil, the patient's care provider realizes the error. How could he/she intervene?**
a. Rapid administration of thymidine
b. Rapid administration of uridine
c. Administration of leucovorin
d. Delayed (6 h) administration of uridine
e. Delayed (6 h) administration of thymidine

51.1 **The alkylating agent busulfan is extensively used**
a. For treatment of sarcomas
b. As a component of chemotherapy preparation for bone marrow transplantation
c. For treatment of acute lymphocytic leukemia

51.2 **An alkylating antitumor agent that can cause cystitis and serious hematuria and whose use calls for adequate hydration of the patient is**
a. Carboplatin
b. Melphalan
c. Chlorambucil
d. Cyclophosphamide

51.3 **A new deoxyribonucleic acid–methylating agent that is proving useful in the treatment of a number of tumors, including brain tumors, is**
a. Dacarbazine
b. Lomustine
c. Hepsulfam
d. Temozolomide

51.4 **The use of alkylating agents, including cyclophosphamide, should be avoided at what stage of pregnancy to prevent damage to the fetus?**
a. First trimester
b. Second trimester
c. Third trimester

51.5 **The platinum-based antitumor agent most associated with renal toxicity is**
a. Carboplatin
b. Iproplatin
c. Cisplatin

52.1 **Topotecan destroys cancer cells by which of the following mechanisms?**
a. Induction of protein-linked breaks in the deoxyribonucleic acid (DNA) backbone
b. Inhibition of the DNA unwinding activity of topoisomerases
c. Intercalation (insertion into the DNA double helix by stacking between bases)
d. Inhibition of ribonucleotide reductase
e. Incorporation into the growing DNA strand

52.2 **Cellular events occurring after exposure to camptothecins include all of the following *except***
   a. Arrest in mitosis because of impaired microtubule formation
   b. Formation of double-strand breaks in DNA owing to collision of replication forks with topoisomerase I–linked single-strand breaks
   c. Activation of DNA repair pathways, such as transcription-coupled DNA repair
   d. Illegitimate DNA recombination
   e. Ubiquitination of topoisomerase I

52.3 **All of the following may confer resistance to doxorubicin *except***
   a. Amplification of the dihydrofolate reductase gene
   b. Down-regulation of topoisomerase IIα protein levels
   c. Point mutations in topoisomerase IIα
   d. Increased expression of *MDR1*
   e. Increased expression of *MRP1*

52.4 **Which of the following statements regarding cardiac toxicities associated with anthracyclines is *not* true?**
   a. Cardiac damage may result from drug-induced formation of reactive oxygen species.
   b. The likelihood of doxorubicin-induced congestive heart failure cannot be predicted from the cumulative dose that a patient has received.
   c. Administered prophylactically, dexrazoxane (Zinecard) can reduce the incidence of doxorubicin-induced cardiomyopathy.
   d. Patients with a pretreatment left ventricular ejection fraction of < 50% are at increased risk of doxorubicin-induced cardiomyopathy.
   e. Cardiac toxicity is more common with doxorubicin than with epirubicin.

52.5 **For which of the following drugs are topoisomerases *not* implicated as a target?**
   a. Gemcitabine
   b. Daunorubicin
   c. Mitoxantrone
   d. Fluorouracil
   e. Irinotecan

53.1 **Under which situation(s) should dose modifications be considered when prescribing either paclitaxel or docetaxel?**
   a. Moderate renal dysfunction (creatinine clearance 20–40 mL/min)
   b. Severe renal dysfunction (creatinine clearance < 20 mL/min)
   c. Both moderate and severe renal dysfunction
   d. Moderate hepatic excretory dysfunction
   e. Moderate transaminitis

53.2 **Which statement(s) is (are) true regarding the neurotoxicity of antimicrotubule agents?**
   a. Diabetes and alcholism are risk factors for taxane-induced peripheral neuropathy.
   b. Antecedent neurologic disorders are risk factors for vinca alkaloid–induced neurotoxicity.
   c. Cranial nerve deficits can be observed following administration of both taxanes and vinca alkaloids.
   d. Diabetes and alcholism are risk factors for taxane-induced peripheral neuropathy, and antecedent neurologic disorders are risk factors for vinca alkaloid–induced neurotoxicity.
   e. All of the above are true.

53.3 **In preclinical studies, resistance to both taxanes and vinca alkaloids has been related to which of the following?**
   a. Multidrug resistance owing to overexpression of P-glycoprotein
   b. Structural mutations in tubulin
   c. Multidrug resistance owing to overexpression of multidrug resistance–associated protein (MRP)
   d. Multidrug resistance owing to overexpression of P-glycoprotein and structural mutations in tubulin
   e. All of the above

54.1 **Monotherapy with a tyrosine kinase inhibitor is most likely to be effective in cancers in which**
   a. The targeted kinase is known to be expressed
   b. The targeted kinase is known to be critical to the pathogenesis of the tumor
   c. The patient has advanced-stage disease
   d. Other pathways not targeted by the kinase inhibitor are also known to be involved in the pathogenesis of the tumor

54.2 **Which of the following is (are) true about *KIT* and gastrointestinal stromal tumors (GISTs)?**
   a. The majority of GISTs express *KIT*.
   b. *KIT* mutations can be identified in the majority of GISTs.

  c. Patients whose tumors express *KIT* mutations are more likely to respond to imatinib than patients whose tumors express the normal *KIT* allele.
  d. All of the above are true.
  e. None of the above are true.

54.3 **Which of the following is (are) a possible reason(s) for lack of efficacy of a tyrosine kinase inhibitor in a clinical trial using standard response criteria?**
  a. The target is not expressed in the tumor.
  b. The target is not critical to the growth or survival of the cancer.
  c. The target is not completely inhibited in the tumor.
  d. The target is in only one of several pathways that are critical for the growth and survival of the cancer.
  e. All of the above are possible reasons.

54.4 **Besides chronic myelogenous leukemia (CML) and GIST, imatinib has also been shown to be effective in which of the following tumors? (More than one may be correct.)**
  a. Chronic myelomonocytic leukemia (CMML)
  b. Dermatofibrosarcoma protuberans (DFSP)
  c. Systemic mastocytosis
  d. Seminoma

BIOTHERAPEUTICS

55.1 **Which asparaginase preparation has the longest circulating half-life?**
  a. *Escherichia coli*
  b. *Erwinia*
  c. Polyethylene glycol (PEG) asparaginase

55.2 **Your patient experiences hives and bronchospasm 30 minutes after an intramuscular (IM) dose of L-asparaginase (Elspar). Her protocol calls for continued asparaginase therapy for 10 more weeks in consolidation. Which treatment plan is correct?**
  a. Abandon all asparaginase therapy for the duration of the treatment protocol.
  b. Substitute *Erwinia* asparaginase.
  c. Premedicate the patient with diphenhydramine (Benadryl) prior to the next dose of L-asparaginase.
  d. Substitute PEG asparaginase.
  e. Substitute either *Erwinia* asparaginase or PEG asparaginase.

55.3 **Your patient develops acute pancreatitis with clinical symptoms and markedly elevated amylase and lipase after 3 weeks of induction therapy for acute lymphoblastic leukemia. The regimen included L-asparaginase (Elspar) IM three times per week for 9 doses. Additional asparaginase therapy is scheduled during consolidation. You should**
  a. Discontinue all asparaginase therapy for the duration of this patient's therapy
  b. Change from L-asparaginase to *Erwinia*
  c. Change from L-asparaginase to PEG asparaginase
  d. Wait until the pancreatitis resolves and resume therapy with L-asparaginase

55.4 **Your patient has experienced a previous clinical hypersensitivity to native *E. coli* L-asparaginase. You are now planning to substitute PEG asparaginase. The planned regimen called for weekly IM *E. coli* asparaginase at a dose of 25,000 IU/m^2. To achieve similar pharmacokinetics, PEG should be given at what dose and dosing interval?**
  a. 1,000 IU weekly
  b. 2,500 IU weekly
  c. 2,500 IU every other week
  d. 2,500 IU every month

55.5 ***Silent hypersensitivity* refers to a phenomenon best described as**
  a. Neutralization of asparaginase activity by antiasparaginase antibodies without accompanying clinical symptoms
  b. Mild clinical reactions after asparaginase administration that can be suppressed by premedication with antihistamines and/or steroids
  c. Anaphylaxis after asparaginase administration
  d. None of the above

56.1 **How many human interferons (IFNs) are there?**
  a. 1
  b. 2

    c.   15

    d.   33

    e.   600

56.2   What cellular signal transduction mechanism mediates the effects of IFNs?

    a.   *Ras* pathways

    b.   Signal transducers and activators of transcription (STATs)

    c.   Cyclic adenosine monophosphate (AMP)

    d.   Retinoid receptor α (RXRα)

    e.   None of the above

56.3   IFNs as single agents have been almost as effective as or more effective than the best chemotherapeutic agents for all of the following metastatic malignancies *except*

    a.   Follicular lymphomas

    b.   Renal carcinomas

    c.   Melanomas

    d.   Colorectal carcinomas

56.4   How many genes are induced in cells after IFNs bind to their receptor?

    a.   None

    b.   1

    c.   3

    d.   60

    e.   > 200

57.1   Which interleukin (IL) was first approved by the US Food and Drug Administration (FDA) and used in a clinical trial?

    a.   IL-1

    b.   IL-2

    c.   IL-6

    d.   IL-10

    e.   IL-12

57.2   Which IL is known as major immunosuppressive cytokine?

    a.   IL-4

    b.   IL-6

    c.   IL-10

    d.   IL-12

    e.   IL-24

57.3   What is the main rationale for the use of immunostimulatory cytokines in patients for cancer treatment?

    a.   To strengthen immunosuppressive effects of cytokines

    b.   To decrease the effect of specific immune reactions

    c.   To increase blood flow to the tumor site

    d.   To suppress antitumor response

    e.   To initiate/augment/stimulate a weak or nonexistent antitumor immune response

58.1   Routine use of granulocyte colony–stimulating factor (G-CSF) should be considered in all of the following settings *except*

    a.   A 58-year-old woman undergoing her first round of chemotherapy for breast cancer

    b.   A 45-year-old woman undergoing her second round of chemotherapy for breast cancer who had become severely neutropenic and septic after her first round of chemotherapy

    c.   A 60-year-old man who is neutropenic, febrile, and hypotensive several days after chemotherapy for a solid tumor

    d.   An 18-year-old patient undergoing allogeneic bone marrow transplantation

58.2   Which of the following is *incorrect*?

    a.   Erythropoietin (EPO) is manufactured by the kidney and the liver.

    b.   EPO receptors are expressed on neural cells.

    c.   Many cancer patients have a relative EPO deficiency despite their high levels of endogenous EPO.

    d.   A patient with anemia due to renal failure has a transferrin saturation of 15% but a high ferritin level. Iron repletion is not necessary because ferritin levels are a more accurate reflection of iron stores.

    e.   Functional iron deficiency, which complicates EPO therapy, is best treated with parenteral rather than oral supplementation.

58.3 **Most growth factors are both pleiotropic and redundant. Which of the following growth factors is nonredundant for lymphoid development in that it cannot be compensated for by the presence of other factors and, hence, leads to a profound defect in lymphocyte development?**
a. Interleukin (IL)-6
b. IL-7
c. IL-8
d. IL-13
e. Thrombopoietin

58.4 **Which of the following is *not* true?**
a. Serum IL-6 levels are an independent prognostic factor for diffuse large cell lymphomas, with higher levels correlating with a poorer outcome.
b. Serum IL-10 levels are an independent prognostic factor for diffuse large cell lymphomas if the assay detects both human and viral IL-10 but not if the assay detects only human IL-10. High levels correlate with a poor outcome.
c. Levels of IL-1 and/or IL-1 receptor antagonist (IL-1RA) may be important prognostic factors in various inflammatory and autoimmune disorders and in certain types of leukemia.
d. Serum levels of EPO tend to be inversely related to the hematocrit.
e. Serum levels of stem-cell factor are very high in patients with aplastic anemia.

58.5 **Which of the following is *not* true?**
a. Viral IL-10 is encoded by the open reading frame *BCRF1* of the Epstein-Barr virus.
b. IL-2 is homologous to an open reading frame of the human immunodeficiency virus (HIV).
c. IL-8 receptor is homologous to a gene encoded by human herpesvirus 8.
d. IL-17 is homologous to an open reading frame of *Herpesvirus saimiri.*

59.1 **Which form of irradiation is least effective for targeted radioimmunotherapy?**
a. α emission
b. β emission
c. γ emission
d. Auger electrons

59.2 **Anti-idiotypic antibodies can inhibit lymphoma growth by several mechanisms including**
a. Antibody-dependent cell-mediated cytotoxicity
b. Complement-dependent cytotoxicity
c. Apoptosis induced by cross-linking B-cell receptors
d. All of the above
e. None of the above

59.3 **Which of the following statements regarding rituximab (Rituxan) is *not* true?**
a. Rituximab reacts with CD20 on the surface of B-cell lymphomas and chronic lymphocytic leukemia cells.
b. A decrease in levels of normal B lymphocytes is associated with a substantial risk of infection.
c. The combination of rituximab with CHOP (cyclophosphamide, doxorubicin [hydroxydaunomycin], vincristine [Oncovin], prednisone) chemotherapy has produced greater event-free and overall survival than did CHOP alone in patients with diffuse large cell lymphoma.
d. Effective treatment of chronic lymphocytic leukemia with rituximab requires higher doses of the antibody and more frequent treatment to neutralize the "antigenic sink" produced by shedding of CD20 from leukemia cells.

59.4 **Which of the following accurately describes the cardiotoxicity associated with trastuzumab (Herceptin)?**
a. Cardiotoxicity is observed when trastuzumab is combined with doxorubicin but not with paclitaxel.
b. Cardiotoxicity relates to the increased expression of *HER2* on cardiac myocytes.
c. Cardiotoxicity is generally reversible if trastuzumab and chemotherapy are discontinued.
d. All of the above are true.
e. None of the above are true.

59.5 **To date, none of the targeted toxins has been approved for clinical use by the US Food and Drug Administration: True/False**

60.1 **Which of the following best describes oncofetal and tissue-specific antigens as vaccine targets?**
a. When used as vaccines, they may theoretically induce autoimmune states.
b. When used as vaccines, they are ineffective because of tolerance.
c. They are expressed only in the fetus.
d. All of the above are true.

60.2   **Problems associated with the development of tumor vaccines include**
   a.   The lack of relevant preclinical models with slow-growing tumors
   b.   The use of screening for efficacy of vaccines in patients with large tumor volumes
   c.   The long time course for clinical end points in patients treated in the adjuvant setting
   d.   All of the above

60.3   **Which of the following is the best strategy of overcoming tumor-cell antigenic heterogeneity in tumor vaccine development?**
   a.   Using multiple vectors
   b.   Simultaneous targeting of multiple antigens
   c.   Treating patients with minimal disease
   d.   Using combination therapy (ie, adding chemotherapy)
   e.   Intratumoral injection

60.4   **Which of the following statements is *not* true regarding vaccine clinical trials in melanoma?**
   a.   Interferon and interleukin-2 (IL-2) have both shown clinical responses in melanoma.
   b.   Melanoma lesions are easily accessible.
   c.   Melanoma lesions can be grown in culture.
   d.   Numerous melanoma-associated antigens have been identified.
   e.   Of all solid tumors, the least potent in vitro responses have been directed against melanoma-associated antigens.

60.5   **Which of the following is an advantage of using poxviruses as a vector? (More than one may be correct.)**
   a.   Efficient post-translational processing of the inserted gene
   b.   Wide host range
   c.   Stable recombinants
   d.   Replication in the cytoplasm
   e.   All of the above

ENDOCRINE THERAPY

61.1   **A 60-year-old man with newly diagnosed metastatic prostate cancer is referred to you for medical treatment of his malignancy. He has no evidence of spinal cord compression, but he has increasing pain in his back and ribs. Results of a neurologic examination are normal. Prostate-specific antigen (PSA) is 200 ng/mL, and a bone scan shows hot areas in the cervical spine, lumbar spine, and pelvis. A magnetic resonance imaging (MRI) scan of the spine does not show extension of these lesions into the spinal canal. The patient has chronic active hepatitis B and has declined surgical castration. What medical treatment would you recommend?**
   a.   Single-agent diethylstilbestrol (DES)
   b.   Monotherapy with a luteinizing hormone–releasing hormone (LH-RH) agonist
   c.   Monotherapy with a LH-RH antagonist
   d.   Chemotherapy
   e.   A nonsteroidal antiandrogen such as flutamide as a single therapy

61.2   **Chronic administration of LH-RH agonists is being used to induce the regression of endocrine-dependent malignant neoplasms, especially prostate and breast cancers. Which of the following are the side effects most likely to be associated with chronic treatment with LH-RH agonists?**
   a.   Myocardial infarction and venous thrombosis
   b.   Permanently elevated LH and follicle-stimulating hormone (FSH) levels
   c.   Impotence or loss of libido in men and hot flashes or climacteric-like vasomotor phenomena and osteopenia in both sexes
   d.   Fetal harm when administered to a pregnant woman
   e.   Hepatic injury

61.3   **A 59-year-old man is referred to you by his family doctor for a second opinion regarding the treatment for a large poorly differentiated and locally advanced prostate cancer (stage T3b). His PSA was 20 ng/mL at the time of screening for prostate cancer, and in the past week it has risen to 28 ng/mL. Findings from a bone scan, chest radiography, and computed tomography and MRI scans of the abdomen and pelvis performed this week are normal. What is the most appropriate treatment for this patient?**
   a.   Radical prostatectomy
   b.   External beam radiation therapy alone
   c.   External beam radiation therapy combined with chronic administration of an agonistic analogue of LH-RH
   d.   Chronic administration of an agonist of growth hormone–releasing hormone (GH-RH)

61.4 A 47-year-old woman has recently been treated surgically for a node-positive estrogen receptor– and progesterone receptor–positive breast cancer. Her oncologist has recommended she undergo chemotherapy, but she has elected not to have this modality of treatment. She comes to your office for advice on hormonal therapy for her breast cancer. What is the appropriate management of this patient at this time?
   a. Treatment with raloxifene hydrochloride
   b. Estrogen replacement
   c. Withhold hormonal treatment because the likelihood of benefit is low
   d. Treatment with an LH-RH antagonist
   e. Combined treatment with an LH-RH agonist and tamoxifen

61.5 Which of the following statements concerning the oncologic applications for somatostatin analogues is *not* true?
   a. Somatostatin analogues are much less toxic than adjuvant chemotherapy.
   b. Somatostatin analogues inhibit the growth of a variety of tumors in animals and various endocrine tumors in patients.
   c. Oncologic applications of somatostatin analogues are based on multiple effects, and several mechanisms of action are likely.
   d. Chronic administration of somatostatin analogues can produce medical castration.
   e. The presence of somatostatin receptors in neuroendocrine and in non-neuroendocrine tumors permits localization of primary tumors and metastases by scintigraphy with radiolabeled somatostatin analogues.

62.1 Increased adrenocorticotropic hormone (ACTH) production in the anterior pituitary is *least* likely to result in
   a. Adrenocortical hypertrophy
   b. Hyperglycemia
   c. Hyperaldosteronism
   d. Increased production of pregnenolone

62.2 Although the combination therapy MOPP (mechlorethamine, vincristine [Oncovin], procarbazine, prednisone) is still considered a highly effective treatment for Hodgkin's lymphoma, a newer regimen now favored as first-line therapy because of its efficacy with improved toxicity profile is
   a. ABVD (doxorubicin [Adriamycin], bleomycin, vinblastine, decarbazine)
   b. NOVP (mitoxantrone [Novantrone], vincristine, vinblastine, prednisone)
   c. CMF (cyclophosphamide, methotrexate, 5-fluorouracil)
   d. VAD (vincristine, doxorubicin (Adriamycin), dexamethasone)

62.3 The cellular effects of glucocorticoids are mediated by the glucocorticoid receptor (GR), which is
   a. A homotrimeric protein
   b. A G-protein coupled receptor
   c. A ligand-dependent deoxyribonucleic acid (DNA)-binding transcription factor
   d. A constitutively nuclear receptor

62.4 Glucocorticoids are not an effective treatment, alone or in combination, for which of the following?
   a. Acute myeloid leukemia
   b. Acute lymphoblastic leukemia
   c. Peritumoral edema in central nervous system tumors
   d. Symptomatic relief of critically ill patients

62.5 Glucocorticoid-mediated apoptosis of lymphoid tissue
   a. Occurs at physiologic levels of glucocorticoid in humans
   b. Is not involved in thymic involution in rodents
   c. Is largely responsible for acute immune suppression in humans treated with pharmacologic doses of glucocorticoids
   d. Occurs in acute lymphocytic leukemias and other malignancies in humans

63.1 Which of the following statements best describes the effect of tamoxifen on breast cancer cells?
   a. Tamoxifen binds irreversibly to the estrogen receptor (ER).
   b. Tamoxifen works equally well in ER-positive and ER-negative patients.
   c. Tamoxifen competitively inhibits the binding of estradiol to the estrogen receptor.
   d. Tamoxifen directly inhibits the production of several kinds of proteins important for breast cancer cell proliferation.
   e. Tamoxifen is a pure estrogen antagonist.

64.1 Which of the following statements best describes the biologic action of the aromatase enzyme system?
   a. It catalyzes the conversion of estrone to estradiol.
   b. It converts dihydrotestosterone to testosterone.
   c. It converts androgens to estrogens within the adrenal gland.

d.   It is the final enzymatic step in the biosynthesis of estrogens.

e.   It is active in surrounding fat tissue but not in breast tumors.

64.2   A 65-year-old woman, status postmodified radical mastectomy for stage II estrogen receptor (ER)-positive breast cancer, was treated with tamoxifen adjuvant therapy for 5 years. Four months after completing this therapy, she developed deep venous thrombophlebitis (DVT) of the left leg and required anticoagulation therapy. She is now admitted 1 month later to the hospital for evaluation of congestive heart failure thought to be secondary to long-standing hypertension. During the course of this evaluation, she was noted to have several subcutaneous nodules around the site of the previous mastectomy. Biopsy of one of the skin nodules reveals adenocarcinoma that is positive for estrogen and progesterone receptor by immunohistochemical staining. A bone scan shows several lesions that are consistent with metastatic disease, although the patient has no bone pain. Which of the following would be the most appropriate management of her breast cancer at this time?

a.   Resume tamoxifen 20 mg PO daily

b.   Megestrol acetate 40 mg PO qid

c.   Anastrozole 1 mg PO daily

d.   Letrozole 5 mg PO daily

e.   Cyclophosphamide (500 mg/m^2), Adriamycin (doxorubicin) (50 mg/m^2), and 5-fluorouracil (500 mg/m^2 q3wk)

64.3   A 37-year-old woman, with a strong family history of breast cancer, underwent a modified radical mastectomy for stage II breast cancer 2 years ago. She refused adjuvant therapy. She now has a malignant pleural effusion, scattered bilateral lung nodules, and chest wall nodules consistent with metastatic breast cancer. Biopsy of a skin metastasis confirms the presence of breast carcinoma. The tumor is ER positive, progesterone receptor negative, and *HER2/neu* 3+ positive. She adamantly refuses chemotherapy but is willing to consider other forms of treatment. Which of the following would be *inappropriate* treatment for this patient?

a.   Herceptin

b.   Bilateral oophorectomy

c.   Tamoxifen

d.   Zoladex (luteinizing hormone–releasing hormone [LH-RH] analogue) and tamoxifen

e.   An aromatase inhibitor

64.4   In separate phase III trials comparing anastrozole or letrozole to megestrol acetate, the data show that

a.   The aromatase inhibitor was less effective

b.   Megestrol acetate was associated with greater weight gain

c.   Responders to letrozole had a response duration similar to that for responders to megestrol acetate

d.   Anastrozole was associated with a higher frequency of thrombophlebitis

e.   The aromatase inhibitors were associated with a high incidence of skin rash

64.5   Which of the following statements best describes the properties of the particular aromatase inhibitor?

a.   Aminoglutethimide is a selective inhibitor of aromatase.

b.   Letrozole is a nonsteroidal competitive inhibitor of aromatase.

c.   Exemestane is a nonsteroidal reversible inhibitor of aromatase.

d.   Anastrozole is a less potent aromatase inhibitor than aminoglutethimide.

e.   In standard doses, all aromatase inhibitors suppress intratumoral estrogen synthesis to the same extent.

65.1   **Progesterone receptor (PR) observed in target tissues**

a.   Is sufficient to predict response to progesterone

b.   Is only the first phase of a complex series of events involved in the regulatory mechanisms that determine the response to this hormone

c.   Is a protein that is only expressed in malignancies

d.   Can be used to select the specific treatment that will produce tumor regression

65.2   **Which of the following statements is true regarding proliferation of breast epithelium?**

a.   It is the result of estrogens, which cause increased mitosis in the follicular phase of the menstrual cycle.

b.   It is greatest in the luteal phase of the menstrual cycle and appears to be stimulated by progesterone after estrogen priming.

c.   It is not influenced by ovarian or adrenal hormones.

d.   It can be completely inhibited by physiologic progesterone.

65.3   **PR is increased as a result of**

a.   Progesterone exposure

b.   Stimulation of the target cell by mifepristone (RU-486)

c.   Exposure to physiologic estrogens or estrogenic agonists

d.   Androgen exposure

65.4   Heat shock proteins (hsp-90, hsp-27) affect PR by
a.   Functioning as a chaperone protein for the PR prior to ligand binding
b.   Altering interaction with coactivator proteins
c.   Binding to the receptor in the absence of ligand and effecting an inactive state for the receptor
d.   All of the above methods

65.5   Administration of progestins is associated with
a.   Support of the products of conception
b.   Proliferation and differentiation of the endometrium and promotion of secretion in the endometrium
c.   Maturation and cornification of the vaginal mucosal epithelium
d.   All of the above

66.1   Which of the following therapies would *not* be recommended as adequate first-line hormonal monotherapy for recurrent prostate cancer?
a.   Orchiectomy
b.   Polyestradiol phosphate (160 mg IM qmo)
c.   Flutamide (250 mg tid)
d.   Goserelin acetate (10.8 mg SQ q12wk)
e.   Any of these choices would be appropriate

66.2   Which of the following is *not* a toxicity effect of LH-RH agonist therapy?
a.   Hair loss
b.   Loss of libido
c.   Impotence
d.   Anemia
e.   Osteoporosis

66.3   Antiandrogen withdrawal responses have *not* been observed with which of the following agents?
a.   Flutamide
b.   Megestrol acetate
c.   Nilutamide
d.   Abarelix
e.   DES

66.4   Based on available data, which of the following patients would be the *least* likely to benefit from early initiation of androgen deprivation therapy?
a.   60-year-old presenting with multiple asymptomatic bony metastases
b.   68-year-old with Gleason grade 9 cancer, with prostate-specific antigen (PSA)-only recurrence 3 years after prostatectomy
c.   65-year-old with Gleason grade 7 cancer and node-positive disease
d.   72-year-old with Gleason grade 6 cancer, with PSA-only recurrence 3.5 years after prostatectomy, and a PSA doubling time of > 10 months
e.   70-year-old with Gleason grade 7 cancer, with PSA-only recurrence 8 months after prostatectomy, and a PSA doubling time of < 10 months

66.5   Which two of the following statements concerning androgens and androgen receptors are true?
a.   Androgen independence occurs because androgen-independent prostate cancer cells no longer express androgen receptors.
b.   Testosterone is inactivated intracellularly by conversion to dihydrotestosterone (DHT).
c.   Antiandrogen withdrawal responses may be secondary to mutations in the androgen receptors in a subset of prostate cancer cells.
d.   Besides blocking the binding to androgen receptors intracellularly, the binding of "pure" antiandrogens such as flutamide to androgen receptors in the hypothalamus and pituitary leads to a decrease in serum testosterone.
e.   Although the glandular cells within the normal prostate are androgen dependent and are eliminated following castration, the stem cells within the basal cell compartment are not eliminated following castration.

GENE THERAPY

67.1   Random insertional mutagenesis is a major concern of which of the following viral vectors used in cancer gene therapy?
a.   Retrovirus
b.   Adenovirus
c.   Herpes simplex virus 1 (HSV-1)
d.   Adeno-associated virus (AAV)
e.   None of the above

67.2 Which of the following oncolytic viral platforms uses a wild-type virus, with no mutations engineered into the viral genome?
a. Adenovirus
b. HSV-1
c. Reovirus
d. All of the above
e. None of the above

67.3 Gene expression can be regulated at either the transcriptional or translational level. Which of the following gene therapy strategies targets transcription?
a. Antisense
b. Triple-helix formation
c. Ribozyme
d. Ribonucleic acid interference (RNAi)

67.4 Tumor-selective replication of the oncolytic virus *dl*1520 (Onyx-015) has been reported to be dependent on the deletion or inactivation all of the following genes *except*
a. *P53*
b. *MDM2*
c. *P14^{ARF}*
d. *E1B*

67.5 The therapeutic index of virus-directed enzyme/prodrug therapy ("suicide gene therapy") is enhanced by
a. Systemic delivery of a relatively nontoxic prodrug
b. A "bystander effect"
c. Use of nonmammalian prodrug-converting enzymes
d. High local tumor drug concentrations
e. All of the above

BONE MARROW TRANSPLANTATION

69.1 Which of the following is the most frequent complication of allogeneic hematopoietic transplantation from a human leukocyte antigen–matched sibling donor for treatment of leukemia?
a. Graft rejection
b. Graft-versus-host disease (GVHD)
c. Tuberculosis infection
d. Epstein-Barr virus–related lymphoproliferative disease

69.2 Acute GVHD is primarily caused by which of the following cell types?
a. T lymphocytes
b. B lymphocytes
c. Macrophages
d. Natural killer cells

69.3 Which of the following viral infections occurs most frequently after allogeneic hematopoietic transplantation?
a. Cytomegalovirus
b. Adenovirus
c. Respiratory syncytial virus
d. Epstein-Barr virus

69.4 Which of the following tissues is directly affected by GVHD?
a. Brain
b. Liver
c. Heart
d. Kidney

ANSWERS

SURGICAL ONCOLOGY

38.1   **Answer: (c)**   Other than a small number of special operations such as hemipelvectomy for soft tissue sarcomas of the pelvis, most surgical procedures performed by surgical oncologists are also performed by general surgeons. Fellowship training is 2 to 3 years' duration and focuses on learning multidisciplinary oncology management; it usually includes rotations on medical oncology and radiation oncology services. There is currently no board certification process in surgical oncology.

38.2   **Answer: (e)**   Fine-needle aspiration suctions cells from within a tumor, thereby disrupting tumor architecture in the biopsy specimen. In contrast, core needle biopsy delivers an intact core of tumor tissue. Consequently, the diagnosis of malignancy using fine-needle aspiration is less accurate than with core needle biopsy and depends on abnormal cytologic features such as nuclear pleomorphism. Biopsy tract recurrences are infrequent with either needle approach, and the selection of open biopsy is usually driven by local pathology diagnostic expertise. Either technique may be suitable for a given tumor regardless of tumor size, and radiologic guidance should be used whenever a tumor is not easily palpated.

38.3   **Answer: (d)**   The AJCC staging system includes T, N, and M designators as well as b (for grade) in some tumors. Almost all tumors are staged the same way in the AJCC and UICC systems—there is no WHO staging system. If a tumor has spread to lymph nodes, the designation is N1. Likewise, if a tumor has spread to non-nodal distant sites, it is designated M1. The four chronologic classifications are c, p, r, and a. The r designation applies to either clinical or pathologic determinants of tumor recurrence, and therefore does not require biopsy proof of recurrence.

RADIATION ONCOLOGY

39.1   **Answer: (d)**   There are as yet no randomized trials demonstrating the superiority of IMRT over three-dimensional or conventional treatment planning.

39.2   **Answer: (c)**

39.3   **Answer: (c)**

39.4   **Answer: (e)**   Rad51 mediates genetic recombination and recombination repair and is homologous to the bacterial protein RecA.

39.5   **Answer: (d)**

40.1   **Answer: (e)**   Photodynamic therapy involves light activation of certain dyes that have been previously localized in target issues. The most explored dyes are the porphyrins, particularly Photofrin. Side effects are infrequent. However, prolonged phototoxicity may occur and last up to 4 to 6 weeks. Because Photofrin is metabolized and excreted via the liver, its use in patients who have compromised hepatic function is not recommended. A number of new non-Photofrin photosensitizers have been developed, including mono-L-aspartyl chlorine, zinc phthalocyanine, and the porphycenes. There are currently more than 30 photosensitizers. Clinical trials have revealed promising results in patients who have a variety of cutaneous tumors, including breast cancers on the chest wall, basal and squamous cell skin cancer, melanoma, mycosis fungoides, and Kaposi's sarcoma.

40.2   **Answer: (a)**   A bilirubin level greater than 4.0 mg/dL or an AST level greater than three times normal is generally considered a contraindication to the use of porfimer sodium. However, advanced age alone is generally not a contraindication to the use of PDT, nor is prior chemotherapy and/or radiotherapy. An advantage of PDT is that it is capable of treating tumors that completely obstruct the esophagus. An interstitial fiber is available that can be inserted directly into the tumor under endoscopic guidance.

41.1   **Answer: (d)**   Thermotolerance is an acquired resistance to killing by hyperthermia. Two types of chemotherapeutic agents that do not work synergistically with hyperthermia are the vinca alkaloids and methotrexate. Alternatively, alkylating agents and nitrosoureas interact synergistically with hyperthermia via a variety of mechanisms, including increased intracellular uptake, inhibition of deoxyribonucleic acid (DNA) damage repair, and inhibition of drug-resistance mechanisms. Cells in G_0 are most resistant to killing by hyperthermia, whereas cells in S phase are most sensitive. Acidosis sensitizes cells to killing by hyperthermia.

41.2   **Answer: (c)**   The primary evidence for protein being the target is threefold. First, heat of inactivation, as derived from Arrhenius' analysis, is in the range of 130 to 170 kcal/mol, which is in the range of energies required for protein inactivation. Second, the process of thermotolerance, which produces heat shock proteins, results in stabilization and/or refolding of denatured proteins and protection against heat-induced cell killing. Third, the cytoskeletal effects are attributable to dissolution of microtubules, which are made of protein.

41.3 **Answer: (b)** If hyperthermia is effective in achieving radiosensitization, then a lesser radiation dose is needed to achieve the isoeffect and the ratio is > 1.0. Ratios > 1.0 have been found for many tumor types, both in preclinical and even clinical data. Importantly, the TER values for normal tissues are less than those for tumor, thereby strongly suggesting that therapeutic gain is achievable with this combination therapy. Option (c) refers to the ratio of TER values for tumor versus normal tissue. This ratio is commonly given the moniker of "therapeutic gain factor" (TGF) or "therapeutic ratio" (TR).

41.4 **Answer: (a)** Options (b) and (c) refer to capacitive radiofrequency heating and are not applicable to phased array devices. Reflection of power off of air cavities and absorption by bone are limitations of ultrasonography. When the antennas are driven in phase, one achieves phase addition at depth, thereby allowing for more power deposition at such locations.

41.5 **Answer: (e)** Positive phase III trials have been reported for all of the other tumors listed. The positive results for cervical tumors were found in a subset analysis of part of a larger phase III trial for advanced pelvic tumors. Two additional tumor types in this study did not show therapeutic benefit for hyperthermia: bladder and colorectal cancers. Other positive phase III trials that have been conducted include retreatment of chest wall recurrences of breast cancer and head and neck cancer.

MEDICAL ONCOLOGY

42.1 **Answer: (d)** A long latent period could indeed result from failed, not sustained, activation and expression of tumor angiogenesis factor genes. Tumors up to 0.5 mm in diameter can survive by diffusion of oxygen and metabolites, but growth beyond this requires angiogenesis. A long latent period might indeed be associated with G_0 (resting) cells, but at least some experimental models, including the aforementioned angiogenesis model, suggest that cytokinetic activity may be prominent in small microscopic tumors and that growth does not occur because cell death and cell differentiation are in equilibrium with cell proliferation. Metastases require the ability of cancer cells to break through the basement membrane, travel through lymphatics or blood vessels, and bind to a distant organ, presumably via adhesion molecules. Metastases may exhibit clonal evolution compared with the primary but are not polyclonal.

CHEMOTHERAPY

43.1 **Answer: (d)** The Skipper-Schabel-Wilcox model is a model of tumor growth developed by researchers at the Southern Research Institute. It is based on the observation that leukemia cells in mice grow exponentially with a constant doubling time. This model presumes that the doubling time of tumor cells is fixed. Although this model is not consistent with the growth pattern of all clinically observable tumors, it remains of great importance in the field of cancer biology.

43.2 **Answer: (a)** The Gompertzian model of tumor growth, developed in 1825, describes a pattern whereby the doubling time increases as the tumor size increases. The etiology of this occurrence has not been clearly explained, although it might be related to autocrine and paracrine growth factors. Several subsequent kinetic models such as the Speer-Retsky model and the Norton-Simon model are based on the Gompertzian concept.

43.3 **Answer: (c)** The cell cycle proceeds from G_1 to the S phase (deoxyribonucleic acid [DNA] synthesis), then the G_2 phases (the gap between DNA synthesis and cell division), then the M phase (mitosis). The G_1 phase is the gap between cell division and DNA synthesis. G_0 refers to those cells that are not in a proliferative state. Some cells are in a temporary G_0, from which they subsequently proliferate if recruited, whereas others are thought to be permanently nonproliferative. Tumor stem cells may have long G_0 phases during which time susceptibility to therapy may be reduced.

44.1 **Answer: (d)**

44.2 **Answer: (c)**

44.3 **Answer: (d)** When determining which of these factors is *most* important, Dr. Frei employed a ranking scale of 1 to 10. The use of agents in combination ranked highest with an 8. The use of the most active single agent was a 6, the use of agents emphasizing dose intensity was a 3, the schedule of administration was a 5, and the duration of administration was a 5.

44.4 **Answer: (b) and (c)** The combination usually indicates at least an additive effect, if not a synergistic effect.

44.5 **Answer: (a)** Chemotherapy may be highly effective in primary breast cancer. The studies have not yet definitively proven that the survival rate would be favorably affected by the neoadjuvant treatment.

45.1 **Answer: (b)** The modified Fibonacchi method of dose escalation is the original method for performing dose escalation in a phase I setting. With this method the initial dose is doubled, but after that there is a tapering off of a percent dose escalation at each level, which leads to just 33% increases in dose at each level. This results in many patients receiving ineffective doses of a new agent. All other above choices represent more aggressive dose escalation schemes, which result in fewer patients receiving ineffective doses of a new agent.

45.2   **Answer: (d)**   The way to best describe the relationship between doses in animals and doses in humans is on a milligram per squared meter basis. This reliable method was described by Freireich and colleagues.

45.3   **Answer: (c)**   This is the most proper approach to explaining participation in a phase I trial because there is a small but a real chance the patient will respond, and phase I trials are fairly safe; it is a reasonable option for patients. Statement (a) is not proper because it says that there are not any real options for the patient. There are always other options for patients including giving optimal supportive care only. Statement (b) is not correct because, in general, phase I trials are safe, and death from a phase I agent is an extremely uncommon event. Finally, statement (d) is not appropriate because there is a chance that a patient will have a response to a new agent in a phase I setting and, as noted above, the patient always has other options (such as supportive care only).

45.4   **Answer: (c)**   There are multiple studies to indicate that, although certainly not perfect, animal tumor models do predict, in general, anti-tumor activity in the clinic. That predictive ability is not tumor-specific (ie, if a new agent has antitumor activity in an animal breast cancer model, it does not mean that the new agent will have clinical activity against breast cancer).

45.5   **Answer: (c)**   A pharmacodynamic end point is the effect the new agent has on a particular target. For example, if a new agent has been shown to affect the target farnesyl transferase, a pharmacodynamic end point would be the measurement of farnesyl transferase in the patient's tumor both before and after treatment with the new agent (in relationship to dose of the new agent).

45.6   **Answer: (b)**   Paull and colleagues developed the COMPARE program to evaluate new compounds as they were screened in the institute's 60 cell line screening panel. Using this method, a new compound is evaluated in the 60 cell line screen, and the program is used to compare the pattern of activity of the new compound with the pattern of activity of other compounds (which have already been evaluated in the screen) to determine if the new compound has similar activity to any other compounds. It has been shown that a significant correlation coefficient between the new compound and other agents indicates a similar mechanism of action. A poor correlation coefficient indicates that the new compound probably has a new mechanism of action, which makes the new compound highly interesting.

46.1   **Answer: (e)**   The requirement of metabolism or chemical transformation is common for the majority of anticancer drugs. For instance, cisplatin undergoes aquation to lose two chloride molecules. Irinotecan is hydrolyzed to the active metabolite SN-38. Methotrexate binding to the target enzyme dihydrofolate reductase is much greater after several glutamic acid moieties are added. Gemcitabine, like many other deoxyribonucleic acid (DNA)-directed nucleoside analogues, must be phosphorylated in three separate reactions to become a substrate for DNA polymerases.

46.2   **Answer: (c)**   Damaged DNA is repaired by several defined processes that are triggered by the particular type of adduct or alteration of DNA. Several of these, collectively termed excision DNA repair processes, remove as few as one or as many as 1,000 nucleotides that are either actually damaged or are adjacent to the damage. These processes require replacement of the excised nucleotides by resynthesis of DNA. This provides an opportunity for insertion of nucleotide analogues into the repair patch. If these fraudulent nucleotides inhibit the repair process, signals for cell death may be generated. Thus, activation of nucleotide excision repair processes may enable nucleotide analogues to have a DNA-directed activity in tumor cells that are not replicating their DNA.

46.3   **Answer: (e)**   Differences in all of the parameters noted among patients give rise to the large variability seen in plasma pharmacokinetics among patients. Absorption is influenced by the incidence of vomiting and gut motility. Prior surgery can have an effect as can radiation therapy and chemotherapy. Drug distribution is affected by obesity. Also, changes in weight may affect the distribution of lipophilic drugs. Both hepatic and renal dysfunction can affect drug elimination, as can concomitant medications. Finally, hypoalbuminemia as well as concomitant medications can result in variability in protein binding and therefore the effective bioavailability of the agent.

46.4   **Answer: (d)**   All of these are examples of investigations of the pharmacodynamic relationship of the indicated drugs. Regardless of whether the setting is in cells in culture, in an experimental model, or in the context of a clinical trial, all of these examples relate a dose response of each drug on some aspect of the biology involved in the experimental design. Thus, it is clear that incorporation of gemcitabine nucleotide into DNA is critical for the inhibition of DNA synthesis and subsequently cell death. Extension of the survival of tumor-bearing mice is the classic experimental therapy model for the pharmacodynamics of agents in development. Finally, renal function is a dominant determinant of systemic exposure to carboplatin and is related to the extent of thrombocytopenia, the dose-limiting toxicity. This pharmacodynamic relationship is the basis for prediction of tolerable carboplatin doses knowing creatinine clearance.

47.1   **Answer: (c)**   A number of antineoplastic agents, including thiotepa, mitomycin-C, and bacillus Calmette-Guérin have been documented to produce objective and long-lasting responses and to prevent progression to invasive disease when instilled directly into the bladder as treatment of superficial bladder cancer.

47.2   **Answer: (d)**   Following regional antineoplastic drug delivery, there will likely be *less* exposure of the systemic compartment to the active agent compared with systemic treatment. The aim of regional drug delivery is to increase exposure of a tumor within a body compartment to the antineoplastic agent, while reducing systemic drug delivery.

47.3   **Answer: (a)**   Experimental observations demonstrate that chemotherapeutic agents are able to penetrate to a maximum of 1 to 2 mm into tumor or normal tissue following direct delivery into a body compartment. This explains why regional antineoplastic drug delivery is a rational management strategy only into those settings where microscopic or very-small-volume macroscopic disease is present within the compartment being treated.

48.1   **Answer: (d)**   P-Glycoprotein is a drug-efflux pump. Drugs associated with the multidrug-resistant phenotype are lipid-soluble drugs freely permeable across the cell membrane.

48.2   **Answer: (c)**   GSTs play a role in the detoxification of chlorambucil and melphalan but not the anthracycline doxorubicin. GSTs are phase II enzymes. Conjugation of drugs with glutathione may make these drugs less toxic, but the conjugated drug may be more polar than the parent drug and may therefore decrease cell membrane permeability and lead to increased cellular retention.

48.3   **Answer: (a)**   Topoisomerase II drugs stabilize the DNA-topoisomerase complex, resulting in production of lethal DNA strand breaks. Topisomerase II drugs may also be P-glycoprotein substrates. Since topoisomerase drugs require cell division for toxicity, tumors with a large number of quiescent cells are resistant to topoisomerase II drugs. Anthracyclines and epidophylotoxins are topoisomerase II poisons.

48.4   **Answer: (b)**   Resistance to methotrexate is caused by the down-regulation of the reduced folate carrier, which results in decreased intra-cellular accumulation of methotrexate. Increased dihydrofolate reductase, decreased polyglutamylation, and increased expression of *MRP* genes are all proven mechanisms of methotrexate resistance.

CHEMOTHERAPEUTIC AGENTS

49.1   **Answer: (f)**   Although several folate antagonists have been developed, and several are now in clinical trial, methotrexate is the antifol with the most extensive history and widest spectrum of use. Despite a single-agent response rate of only 20%, randomized trials of pre- and post-definitive treatment have demonstrated the beneficial effect of chemotherapy that includes high-dose methotrexate with leucovorin rescue. Based on experimental studies showing that methotrexate and cytarabine produce additive and possibly synergistic effects, this combination has also been used in regimens to treat NHL. Methotrexate is used as part of all combination regimens to treat ALL, especially as treatment during remission, and as intrathecal administration for prophylaxis of meningeal leukemia. Choriocarcinoma is unique in that single-drug treatment with methotrexate produces a substantial number of cures.

49.2   **Answer: (e)**   Both conventional- and high-dose methotrexate regimens are reported to cause renal toxicity. This toxicity is believed to be owing to precipitation of methotrexate and its less soluble metabolite 7-hydroxymethotrexate in the tubules, as well as to a possible direct effect of this drug on the renal tubule. The use of vigorous hydration, often with osmotic diuresis and alkalinization of urine to increase solubility of methotrexate and 7-hydroxymethotrexate, has markedly ameliorated this problem.

Possible mechanisms of methotrexate neurotoxicity include increases in cerebral spinal fluid levels of adenosine, a potent autocoid in the CNS, and alterations in and elevations of homocysteine (an excitatory amino acid, active at the *N*-methyl-D-aspartate receptor).

49.3   **Answer: (e)**   Methotrexate inhibits the enzyme dihydrofolate reductase (DHFR), which is responsible for regenerating the reduced folates necessary for thymidylate synthesis. Inhibition of DHFR therefore leads to shutdown of pyrimidine synthesis and rapid cell death. Gene amplification of DHFR (often associated with double-minute or centromereless chromosomes) and mutations in DHFR leading to decreased affinity for methotrexate can both produce methotrexate resistance. Polyglutamylation of methotrexate by the enzyme folylpolyglutamate synthetase (FPGS) results in increased affinity of methotrexate for target enzymes, as well as prolonged intracellular retention. Reductions in FPGS activity and elevations in the activity of the enzyme γ-glutamyl hydrolase, which removes glutamyl residues, have both been linked to methotrexate resistance. Impaired ability to transport methotrexate into cells through the reduced folate carrier also can cause intrinsic resistance. Decreased transport has been shown to be a common mechanism of acquired resistance to methotrexate in leukemic blasts from patients with relapsed ALL, for example. Methotrexate is not one of the chemotherapeutic agents known to be a substrate for the multidrug-resistance molecule GP170.

49.4   **Answer: (a)**   The nonclassic antifolates, trimetrexate and piritrexim, are lipophilic and cross the cell membrane by passive or facilitative diffusion rather than by the reduced-folate transport carrier. Other new antifols, such as 10-ethyldeazaaminopterin were chosen for clinical trial after detailed structure activity studies demonstrated that hydrophobic substitutions at the N10 position of aminopterin resulted in improved uptake and retention (polyglutamylation) by tumor cells compared with normal cells. During recent years, other targets for the development of folate antagonists have been identified, including TS, GAR, and AICAR transformylase, and methionine synthetase. Potent inhibitors of TS and GAR transformylase have been synthesized and are now under active investigation.

50.1   **Answer: (d)**   Deficiency of the enzyme dihydropyrimidine dehydrogenase, which is the critical rate-limiting step in the catabolism of 5-fluorouracil, can result in an excess of 5-fluorouracil being available to be anabolized. The clinical picture is similar to what occurs when an overdose of 5-fluorouracil is mistakenly administered. This pharmacogenetic syndrome occurs in approximately 3% of the US population and has been associated with severe toxicity including death in its most severe form.

50.2   **Answer: (c)**   Cells can become resistant to cytarabine because of decreased activities of the carrier for cytarabine transport and of cytoplasmic deoxycytidine kinase; increased catabolism of cytarabine through the action of cytidine deaminase; increased formation of deoxycytidine triphosphate (dCTP) by ribonucleotide reductase and nucleoside diphosphate kinase; or decreased activity of dCMP deaminase, which could lead to increased competition by dCTP with ara-CTP for incorporation into deoxyribonucleic acid (DNA). An increased activity of 3' to 5' exonuclease, which could remove cytarabine-CMP from the DNA-chain terminus, has also been suggested. Cytarabine is not metabolized by dihydropyrimidine dehydrogenase.

50.3   **Answer: (e)**   Capecitabine is a carbamate prodrug that requires an initial hydrolysis of the *N*-pentyl carbamate chain by hepatic carboxylesterase to form 5'-deoxy-5-fluorocytidine, subsequently deaminated to 5'-deoxy-5-fluorouridine by cytidine deaminase. In the final step, both thymidine and uridine phosphorylases hydrolyze 5'-deoxy-5-fluorouridine to produce 5-fluorouracil.

50.4   **Answer: (d)**   A delayed administration of uridine would provide the only rescue regimen to overcome both DNA- and ribonucleic acid–related toxicities. The immediate administration of either uridine or thymidine would actually saturate the same catabolic enzymes used in the degradation of 5-fluorouracil, thereby prolonging the tissue exposure to fluoropyrimidine and increasing the fraction of the antineoplastic agent that would be converted to its fluoronucleotide forms.

51.1   **Answer: (b)**   Although an old agent, busulfan is still a component, usually in combination with cyclophosphamide, of allogeneic bone marrow transplantation regimens. In the past 5 years, the importance of monitoring busulfan concentrations to reduce hepatic damage has been recognized.

51.2   **Answer: (d)**   These toxic side effects appear to be caused by the metabolite acrolein and can rarely be fatal. Use of the agent mesna may reduce hemorrhagic cystitis, but adequate hydration of the patient is still necessary to reduce the incidence of these complications.

51.3   **Answer: (d)**   Temozolomide appears to be more effective and less toxic than is dacarbazine, and it is now being used in the treament of a number of tumors including sarcomas.

51.4   **Answer: (a)**   Many patients have been successful treated in the second and third trimesters of pregnancy without damage to the fetus, but abnormalities of the fetus have occurred following treatment during the first trimester. Therefore, treatment of lymphoma with CHOP (cyclophosphamide, doxorubicin [hydroxydaunomycin], vincristine [Oncovin], prednisone) and other alkylating agent–containing regimens should be delayed until at least the second trimester.

51.5   **Answer: (c)**   The later generations of platinum compounds are less toxic to the renal system than is cisplatin; careful attention to renal status and hydration must be made when using cisplatin.

52.1   **Answer: (a)**   Topotecan does not bind DNA by itself but binds to topoisomerase I–DNA covalent complexes ("cleavable complexes") that represent a reaction intermediate in the topoisomerase I catalytic cycle. Drug binding to this complex prevents religation of the DNA by topoisomerase I, resulting in the formation of protein-linked DNA double-strand breaks, which subsequently result in cell death. Thus, the cytotoxicity of topotecan is mediated by "poisoning" rather than by simply inhibiting the unwinding activity of topoisomerase I. This important distinction is also exemplified by the finding that cells resistant to topotecan typically have reduced rather than increased levels of topoisomerase I.

52.2   **Answer: (a)**   Mitotic arrest owing to altered microtubule function is caused by microtubule-targeting drugs such as the taxanes, not camptothecins. Camptothecins stabilize a normally transient topoisomerase I–DNA complex, resulting in the formation of enzyme-linked single-strand DNA breaks, which are subsequently converted to double-strand breaks by collision with replication forks. Certain DNA repair pathways are known to be involved in processing camptothecin-induced DNA damage, including transcription-coupled repair. Camptothecins and topoisomerase II inhibitors have been shown to cause illegitimate DNA recombination, which may induce secondary neoplasias. Also, topoisomerase I has recently been shown to be ubiquitinated after cells are treated with camptothecins; this response is likely a mechanism to minimize the DNA damage caused by these drugs.

52.3   **Answer: (a)**   Amplification of the dihydrofolate reductase gene is associated with resistance to methotrexate. Doxorubicin destroys cells by stabilizing a normally transient reaction intermediate involving a covalent linkage of topoisomerase II with DNA. Thus, either decreased topoisomerase II protein levels or mutations that impair formation of the drug-enzyme-DNA ternary complex may confer resistance. Increased expression of certain drug efflux proteins, such as the *MDR1* and *MRP1* gene products, may also confer drug resistance by decreasing cellular accumulation of doxorubicin.

52.4   **Answer: (b)**   The incidence of anthracycline-induced cardiomyopathy is related to both the cumulative dose and schedule of administration and is increased in patients with underlying cardiac failure. When doxorubicin is given at doses of 40 to 75 mg/m^2 q3wk, the incidence of congestive heart failure is < 1% for a cumulative dose of 350 mg/m^2, but 30% for a cumulative dose of 700 mg/m^2. The mechanism of anthracycline-induced cardiomyopathy probably involves the formation of reactive oxygen species via metabolism of anthracyclines to quinones. Certain free radical scavenging drugs such as dexrazoxane have been shown to decrease the incidence of anthracycline cardiomyopathy. In addition, cardiomyopathy occurs less frequently with administration of epirubicin and idarubicin than with doxorubicin.

52.5 **Answer: (d)** Fluorouracil inhibits thymidylate synthase and does not target topoisomerases. Although structurally distinct, daunorubicin and dactinomycin are DNA intercalators that impair (poison) the topoisomerase II catalytic cycle by stabilizing a normally transient reaction intermediate in which topoisomerase II is covalently linked to DNA. Irinotecan is not a DNA intercalator but targets topoisomerase I, resulting in the formation of topoisomerase I–linked DNA strand breaks. Incorporation of gemcitabine in DNA induces DNA structural changes that result in topoisomerase I poisoning and consequent topoisomerase I–linked DNA breaks.

53.1 **Answer: (d)** Hepatic disposition is the predominant disposition mechanism for both paclitaxel and docetaxel. These agents are metabolized, albeit not completely, and both parent compound and metabolites are excreted into the bile and feces. Dose modifications are not required in renal dysfunction but must be considered when there is evidence of hepatic excretory dysfunction (eg, hyperbilirubinemia).

53.2 **Answer: (d)** Diabetes and alcoholism are known to predispose patients to taxane-induced neurotoxicity, whereas antecedent neurologic disorders (particularly Charcot-Marie-Tooth disease, hereditary and sensory neuropathy type I, Guillain-Barré syndrome, and childhood poliomyelitis) are known to predispose patients to vinca alkaloid–induced neurotoxicity. Cranial nerve deficits have been reported in patients following treatment with the vinca alkaloids but are not associated with taxane treatment.

53.3 **Answer: (d)** Resistance to both the taxanes and vinca alkaloids has been related to overexpression of P-glycoprotein, as well as structural mutations in tubulin. However, overexpression of MRP has been related to vinca alkaloid resistance but not taxane resistance.

54.1 **Answer: (b)** Although expression of a kinase is an important criterion for the use of an agent that targets that kinase, expression does not necessarily equate with a critical role for that kinase in the growth or survival of a tumor. However, if a kinase has been shown to be critical to the pathogenesis of a tumor, an agent that targets that kinase would be predicted to be effective. The effectiveness may depend, in part, on how many other pathways are also critical to the growth and survival of the tumor and the likelihood that the number of pathways required increases with more advanced disease.

54.2 **Answer: (d)** More than 90% of patients with GISTs express *KIT*, and 86% have *KIT* mutations. Response rates in patients with the most common *KIT*-activating mutation in exon 11 were 72% compared with a response rate of 9% in patients whose tumors had no detectable mutations.

54.3 **Answer: (e)** All answers listed are possible reasons that a kinase inhibitor may not result in objective responses. Carefully designed clinical trials that include target modulation as an end point may be able to distinguish between some of these possibilities. For example, if the target is found to be expressed and inhibited in the cancer by the kinase inhibitor, either the target is not critical to the growth or survival of the cancer or there are several pathways that are critical for the growth and survival of the cancer.

54.4 **Answer: (a) and (b)** Imatinib is an inhibitor of the ABL, platelet-derived growth factor receptor (PDGFR), and KIT tyrosine kinases. It has been shown to be effective in the subset of CMML patient that expresses TEL-PDGFR, the product of a (5;12) chromosomal translocation. Imatinib also has activity in DFSP. These tumors are characterized by a (17;22) translocation involving the *COL1A1* and *PDGFB* genes, which results in overproduction of fusion COL1A1-PDGF-BB ligand and consequent hyperactivation of PDGFR. Although many cases of systemic mastocytosis are caused by a KIT-activating mutation and 10% of seminomas also have KIT-activating mutations, these mutations are biochemically resistant to imatinib.

BIOTHERAPEUTICS

55.1 **Answer: (c)**

55.2 **Answer: (e)**

55.3 **Answer: (a)**

55.4 **Answer: (b)**

55.5 **Answer: (a)**

56.1 **Answer: (c)** IFNs are a family of proteins, each residing at a specific genetic locus. Three major classes of IFNs (α, β, γ) were initially defined on the basis of chemical, antigenic, and biologic differences. These have now been confirmed to result from significant differences in primary amino acid sequence. With advances in molecular biology and sequencing technology, complete sequences for 15 expressed human proteins were defined. Human IFN-α and IFN-β are structurally similar and located on chromosome 9. Both IFN-α and IFN-β are 166 amino acids in length with an additional 20–amino acid secretory peptide present on the amino-terminal end. Comparison of the sequences of IFN-α and IFN-β has defined approximately 45% homology of nucleotides and 29% homology of amino acids. Each of the nonallelic human IFN-α genes differs by approximately 10% in nucleotide sequences and 15 to 25% in amino acid sequence. IFN-γ is 143 amino acids in length, is located on chromosome 12, and also contains 20–amino acid secretory peptide. IFN-γ has only minimal sequence homology with IFN-α or IFN-β. A fourth human IFN class, omega, has subsequently been defined. All IFNs have the defining biologic effect of induction of cellular resistance to replication of both ribonucleic acid (RNA) and deoxyribonucleic acid (DNA) viruses.

56.2 **Answer: (b)** After receptor binding by IFN-α or IFN-β, specific tyrosine kinases known as tyk2, which are not actually part of the receptor structure, together with one or more additional tyrosine kinases, such as JAK-1 and JAK-2, are phosphorylated. These activated tyrosine kinases activate signal-transducing peptides and induce the formation of complex protein subunits (ISGF-3α) consisting of STAT 1α or STAT 1β and STAT 2. The proteins STAT 1α and STAT 1β are alternatively spliced products of the same gene. The STAT 1α protein contains at its carboxyl end 39 additional amino acids. The phosphorylated ISGF-3α complex is translocated to the nucleus and forms (with the addition of a fourth subunit, *P48* or *IRF9*) a DNA-binding complex specific for the IFN-stimulated response element, ISRE, and results in activation of IFN-specific genes. IFN-γ receptor binding results in a similar sequence of events, although the gene-activation complex consists of a homodimer of STAT 1, which binds to DNA elements termed γ-activated sites. Other signaling cascades are also activated by IFNs, including phosphatidylinositol-3-kinase and the mitogen-activated protein kinase cascade.

56.3 **Answer: (d)** INFs exceed the effectiveness of the best chemotherapeutic agents for renal carcinomas and chronic myelogenous leukemia. For follicular lymphomas and melanoma, IFNs have equivalent activity. However, in colorectal carcinoma, even when combined with 5-fluorouracil, IFNs to date have had no therapeutic effectiveness.

56.4 **Answer: (e)** IFNs regulate gene expression, modulate expression of proteins on the cell surface, and include synthesis of new enzymes. Alterations in gene expression result in modulation of levels of receptors for other cytokines, concentration of regulatory proteins on the surface of immune effector cells, and enzyme activities that modulate cellular growth and function. On a cellular basis, these effects translate into alterations of the state of differentiation, rate of proliferation and cell death, and functional activity of many cell types. A problem in attributing the effects of IFNs to specific gene products has been the evidence that they induce many hundreds of genes. This has been confirmed by determining mRNA profiles from IFN-α, IFN-β, or IFN-γ, treatments of the human fibrosarcoma cell line, HT1080, using oligonucleotide arrays. Until overexpression or deletion can manipulate these genes, delineation of their specific role in cellular response to IFNs can only be speculative. However, a number of genes induced by type I IFNs are involved in apoptosis, including *PKR, PML, RAP46/BAG1*, phospholipid scramblase, and hypoxia inducible factor-1α. Consequently, it is likely that the antitumor effects of IFNs in vivo can be augmented by combination with apoptosis-inducing agents.

57.1 **Answer: (b)** IL-2 (aldesleukin [Proleukin]) was the first IL approved by the FDA and by regulatory authorities in Canada and the European community for the treatment of patients with metastatic renal cell carcinoma or melanoma.

57.2 **Answer: (c)** IL-10 is an important immunoregulatory cytokine whose principal biologic function appears to involve the suppression of cytokine synthesis in the Th1 subset of CD4 T helper cells. The suppression by IL-10 of IL-2 and interferon-γ production by Th1 CD4 cells and of IL-1, tumor necrosis factor (TNF), IL-6, IL-8, and colony-stimulating factors by monocytes, coupled with IL-10's ability to stimulate B-cell growth and immunoglobulin production, suggest that IL-10 may be of therapeutic use in sepsis and a number of autoimmune diseases that are associated with inflammation. The suppressive effects of IL-10 on cell-mediated immunity suggest that it might play a role in transplant rejection or the treatment of graft-versus-host disease.

57.3 **Answer: (e)** Various immunostimulatory cytokines, particularly ILs, are currently administered to patients in an attempt to initiate/augment/stimulate a weak or previously nonexistent antitumor immune response. In addition to immune response stimulation, some ILs have been used to stimulate the growth and differentiation of various subpopulations of blood cells after chemotherapy or bone marrow transplantation in a restorative role.

58.1 **Answer: (a)** Based on published studies, the American Society of Clinical Oncology (ASCO) committee guidelines recommend that routine use of G-CSF is not necessary in primary prophylaxis of patients with a risk of febrile neutropenia less than 40%. Use of G-CSF appears reasonable after induction therapy of acute myelogenous leukemia in patients over 55 years old, in complicated febrile neutropenia, in secondary prophylaxis of patients who have experienced a prior episode of febrile neutropenia, and in the transplant setting.

58.2 **Answer: (d)** EPO is produced predominantly by the kidneys and to a lesser extent by the liver. Many anemic cancer patients have high EPO levels, but their levels are not as high as they would be in a well patient who has that degree of anemia. Therefore, there is a relative deficiency of endogenous EPO. Functional iron deficiency (despite normal or high iron stores) has been found to be a significant problem in patients receiving EPO therapy for anemia of renal failure. In patients with a transferrin saturation of < 20%, parenteral iron repletion significantly improves response. Interestingly, EPO receptors are found on neural cells. Many other hematopoietic growth factors also are found in and affect the central nervous system.

58.3 **Answer: (b)** Although IL-4, IL-6, and IL-7 all affect the lymphoid system, only IL-7 is considered nonredundant. Ablation of IL-7 or parts of the IL-7 receptor in gene knockout mice leads to a profound defect in lymphopoiesis. IL-8 is considered mainly a chemotactic factor and thrombopoietin a platelet growth factor.

58.4 **Answer: (e)** Both IL-6 and IL-10 have been reported to be important independent prognostic factors for diffuse large cell lymphoma in multivariate analysis. In the case of IL-10, however, this correlation appears only if the assay measures both viral and human IL-10. Both IL-1 and IL-1RA levels have been found to correlate with prognosis in some myeloid leukemias, although whether these levels are independent variables is not clear. In general, endogenous EPO levels correlate inversely with the hematocrit. Stem-cell factor levels are, however, not elevated in patients with aplastic anemia. The latter finding has been one of the triggers that first led to the currently ongoing clinical trials of this molecule in patients with aplastic anemia.

58.5   **Answer: (b)**   A relationship between several cytokines, cytokine receptors, and viruses is emerging. The viral cytokine genes may represent ancestral-captured cellular genes, a situation similar to that observed with oncogenes. The function of these proteins, as produced by the virus, may play an important role in their ability to produce disease. Even so, there is no relationship between IL-2 and HIV.

59.1   **Answer: (c)**   The path length of γ emission is too great for effective targeting.

59.2   **Answer: (d)**

59.3   **Answer: (b)**   Despite low levels of normal B lymphocytes, infections are observed in only 2% of recipients during 1 year of follow-up.

59.4   **Answer: (c)**   Cardiotoxicity is generally reversible. It is observed when trastuzumab is combined with either doxorubicin or paclitaxel, although it is less frequently observed with the latter combination. *HER2* is only sparsely expressed on cardiac myocytes.

59.5   **Answer: False**   Denileukin diftitox (Ontak), a fusion protein that contains interleukin-2 and diphtheria toxin, has been approved for treatment of cutaneous T-cell leukemia.

60.1   **Answer: (a)**   Since many oncofetal antigens (eg, carcinoembryonic antigen) and tissue-specific antigens (eg, melanoma and melanocyte antigens) are also expressed to some extent on normal adult tissue, one must always be concerned with the induction of autoimmunity.

60.2   **Answer: (d)**

60.3   **Answer: (b)**   Two possible solutions to this problem are (1) developing vaccines that target two or more antigens and (2) using biologic modifiers (ie, cytokines) to up-regulate tumor-associated and human leukocyte antigens.

60.4   **Answer: (e)**   The vast majority of vaccine clinical trials to date have been conducted in patients with melanoma. All of the above, except choice (e), are reasons for this occurrence. Choice (e) is incorrect because it should state that perhaps the *most* potent in vitro immune responses have been directed against melanoma-associated antigens. It should also be pointed out that previous adoptive transfer clinical studies with TILs have demonstrated that immune T cells directed against melanoma-associated antigens, in the presence of IL-2, can kill melanoma cells in situ.

60.5   **Answer: (e)**   The advantages of using poxviruses include its ability to insert large amounts of deoxyribonucleic acid and high immunogenicity, as well as all of the choices listed above.

ENDOCRINE THERAPY

61.1   **Answer: (c)**   This patient with chronic active hepatitis and symptomatic disseminated prostate carcinoma who has declined surgical castration may benefit from appropriate hormonal treatment. The aim of endocrine therapy is to improve the quality of life and prolong survival. Approximately 80% of such patients can benefit from endocrine treatment with improvement in bone pain, decreases in tumor markers such as PSA and acid phosphatase, and objective evidence of tumor regression. These beneficial effects can last an average of 2.5 years; most patients with advanced prostate carcinoma relapse and finally die, apparently of androgen-independent prostate cancer. The estrogen DES is contraindicated for this man who has chronic active hepatitis. DES is rarely used now because it is associated with serious cardiovascular, hepatic, and mammotropic side effects. Treatment with an LH-RH antagonist appears to be the best choice for this patient with advanced prostate carcinoma and metastases to the spine because it involves no risk of tumor flare-up, which occurs during the first few weeks of therapy in about 10% of patients treated with LH-RH agonists alone. Recent work with the LH-RH antagonist cetrorelix in patients with advanced prostate cancer and paraplegia owing to metastatic invasion of spinal cord suggests that LH-RH antagonists may be indicated for patients with extensive metastases in whom the LH-RH agonists cannot be used as single agents because of the possibility of flare-up. Chemotherapy for prostate cancer shows poor response rates and significant toxicity. Nonsteroidal antiandrogens are less effective than orchiectomy or LH-RH analogues and are contraindicated in patients with severe hepatic impairment. Administration of antiandrogens such as flutamide, nilutamide, and bicalutamide prior to and during early therapy with agonists can prevent disease flare-up in prostate cancer patients treated with LH-RH agonists.

61.2   **Answer: (c)**   The administration of DES was once commonly used for the treatment of prostate cancer, but it is associated with cardiovascular side effects such as myocardial infarction and venous thrombosis. Surgical castration causes chronically elevated levels of LH and FSH. The main side effects caused by chronic administration of LH-RH agonists are those that can be attributed to sex-hormone deficiency. These consist of impotence and loss of libido in men and hot flashes or climacteric-like vasomotor phenomena and osteopenia in both sexes. Episodes of temporary flare-up in disease that are manifested by an increase in bone pain during the first week of administration have been reported in 5 to 10% of patients with prostate cancer. None of the patients with prostate cancer treated with LH-RH analogues have developed thromboembolic episodes, which have occurred with DES treatment, or hepatic injury, which has been reported with flutamide.

Flutamide is indicated for use in combination with LH-RH agonists for the treatment of metastatic prostatic carcinoma (stage D2). LH-RH agonists may cause fetal harm when administered to a pregnant woman. Hepatic injury has been described during flutamide treatment. Approximately half of the reported cases occurred within the initial 3 months of the administration of flutamide. The hepatic injury was reversible after discontinuation of therapy in some patients. Serum transaminase levels should be measured prior to starting treatment with flutamide, then monthly for the first 4 months and periodically thereafter.

61.3   **Answer: (c)**   Radical prostatectomy alone is not the best choice for clinical stage T3 disease, especially for those patients with high-grade tumors. In addition, a complete tumor removal in patients with locally advanced prostate cancer is frequently not possible, and evidence suggests that radiotherapy alone does not provide long-term control of prostate cancer. Patients with stage T3 disease, especially those with poorly differentiated tumors, should be treated with adjuvant hormonal therapy combined with surgery or nonsurgical modalities. Recently, it has been demonstrated that adjuvant therapy with LH-RH agonists, started at the beginning of external irradiation treatment and continued for 3 years, can improve the 5-year overall survival of patients with locally advanced prostate cancer. GH-RH agonists should not be confused with gonadotropin-releasing hormone agonists (an LH-RH), which is also called Gn-RH. Today agonists of LH-RH alone or with an antiandrogen are used for the treatment of all stages of prostate cancer. Agonistic analogues of GH-RH have been used in clinical trials for the treatment of children with short stature owing to growth hormone deficiency. Because agonists of GH-RH release growth hormone and stimulate hepatic secretion of insulin-like growth factor I (IGF-I), this class of compounds should be avoided in patients with malignancies, including prostate cancer.

61.4   **Answer: (e)**   Raloxifene hydrochloride is a selective estrogen receptor modulator (SERM) that has not been adequately studied in women with a prior history of breast cancer. Raloxifene is indicated for the treatment and prevention of osteoporosis in postmenopausal women. This patient has an estrogen receptor–positive tumor, and she should not receive estrogen replacement therapy because it could stimulate residual cancer cells. LH-RH antagonists have not been evaluated in patients with breast cancer. About 30% of unselected premenopausal patients with breast cancer have estrogen-dependent tumors and can be treated with hormonal manipulations. Clinical trials conducted since 1982 with Decapeptyl, buserelin, goserelin acetate (Zoladex), or leuprolide in women with metastic breast cancer revealed frequent objective responses in premenopausal patients with estrogen receptor–positive tumors. The antiestrogen tamoxifen has been proven a useful therapy in premenopausal women with advanced breast cancer, particularly those with estrogen receptor–positive tumors. The combination of an LH-RH analogue with an antiestrogen in the treatment of breast cancer might provide complete "estrogen blockade." Recently Klijn and colleagues demonstrated that the combination of the LH-RH agonist buserelin with tamoxifen was more effective and resulted in longer overall survival in premenopausal patients with advanced breast cancer than did treatment with either drug alone.

61.5   **Answer: (d)**   Somatostatin analogues are much less toxic than adjuvant chemotherapy. Oncologic applications of somatostatin analogues are based on multiple effects, and several mechanisms of action are likely. It is probable that somatostatin analogues, by virtue of having a wide spectrum of activities (which include the suppression of the secretions of the pituitary, pancreas, stomach, and gut; interference with growth factors; and direct antiproliferative effects on some tissues), inhibit various tumors through multiple mechanisms. Administration of somatostatin analogues inhibits the levels of growth hormone, IGF-I, insulin, glucagon, and other gastrointestinal hormones but not the secretion of LH, FSH, and sex steroids. The presence of somatostatin receptors may permit the localization of some tumors and metastases using scanning techniques. Radiolabeled analogues of somatostatin, such as indium In 111 pentetreotide (OctreoScan) and (^{123}I-Tyr^3)-octreotide, have been used clinically for the localization of tumors containing receptors for somatostatin. Technetium Tc-99m labeled RC-160 or ^{111}In-DTPA-RC-160 could be also used. Scintigraphy with the radiolabeled somatostatin analogue octreotide has been used with success for detection of both neuroendocrine and non-neuroendocrine tumors. Non-neuroendocrine tumors that contained somatostatin receptors and that could be localized in vivo with the radiolabeled somatostatin analogue octreotide included nonsmall cell lung cancer, meningiomas, breast cancer, and astrocytomas, but not exocrine pancreatic tumors. Other radiolabeled somatostatin analogues such as RC-160 have yet to be evaluated clinically.

62.1   **Answer: (c)**   The zona glomerulosa of the adrenal cortex, where aldosterone is produced, is relatively unaffected by ACTH; therefore, aldosterone levels change very little in response to ACTH exposure.

62.2   **Answer: (a)**   ABVD is preferred because, among other reasons, it does not contain a glucocorticoid and therefore obviates the glucocorticoid-related toxicities. CMF does not contain a steroid, but it is a breast cancer therapy. NOVP and VAD both contain steroids.

62.3   **Answer: (c)**   GR is a cytoplasmic protein that translocates to the nucleus in response to ligand binding, binds DNA as a homodimer, and activates gene transcription. It is not a G-protein coupled receptor.

62.4   **Answer: (a)**   There is little evidence for the efficacy of glucocorticoids in treating acute myeloid leukemia. Glucocorticoids are used successfully for the other three conditions listed and are, in fact, highly useful in palliative care and edema relief as described in options (d) and (c), respectively.

62.5   **Answer: (d)**   Although at physiologic doses of glucocorticoids, human lymphoid tissue does not respond as rodent tissue does with apoptotic events, human lymphoid malignancies do undergo apoptosis. Acute glucocorticoid immune suppression in humans appears to result from lymphocyte sequestration, not apoptosis; therefore, answer (c) is incorrect.

63.1 **Answer: (c)**   Tamoxifen competitively inhibits the binding of estradiol, which is required for the proliferation of ER-positive breast cancer cells, to the ER. Estrogens cause an increase in stimulatory growth factors such as tumor growth factor alpha (TGF-α) and a decrease in inhibitory growth factors such as TGF-β; antiestrogens, such as tamoxifen, interrupt these estrogen stimulatory effects, thereby causing the cell to be held in the G_1 phase.

The dose schedule of choice is 10 mg bid. Tamoxifen is a partial agonist as well as being a competitive antagonist, thereby producing weak estrogen-like effects in postmenopausal women. Tamoxifen is generally prescribed (1) to treat metastatic breast cancer in those who have ER tumors or primary bony disease and (2) as adjuvant therapy for older patients and/or those who have ER-positive tumors.

64.1 **Answer: (d)**   The aromatase enzyme complex system catalyzes the conversion of androstenedione and testosterone to estrone via three hydroxylation steps. The resulting saturation of the A-ring of the steroid molecule creates an aromatic compound, hence the name of the enzyme system. This enzyme pathway is the final step in the synthesis of estrone starting with cholesterol, and its activity accounts for the greatest source of estrogen in postmenopausal women. Aromatase enzyme is most abundant in adipose tissue, but approximately two-thirds of human breast tumors express aromatase activity, and this may be an important source of estrogen autocrine growth stimulation. Estrone is converted to estradiol through the action of the enzyme 17-β steroid dehydrogenase, not aromatase. Conversion of dihydrotestosterone to testosterone is mediated by 5-α reductase.

64.2 **Answer: (c)**   This clinical situation is an excellent one for the use of aromatase inhibitors as palliative management in advanced hormone-dependent breast cancer, especially in elderly patients. Letrozole could also be used, but the approved dose is 2.5 mg. Resumption of tamoxifen might be considered but is usually recommended for patients who have not been treated with this agent for 12 months or longer. Clinical studies have reported responses to aromatase inhibitors in patients with disease refractory to tamoxifen. Megestrol acetate would be a less optimal choice in this patient with a history of DVT and heart failure. Randomized trials have shown a reduced incidence of cardiovascular and thromboembolic side effects associated with aromatase inhibitors when compared with megestrol acetate. Hormonal therapy in general would be a better choice than chemotherapy in this elderly patient with comorbidities, and Adriamycin (doxorubicin) would be contraindicated in view of her history of heart failure.

64.3 **Answer: (e)**   Aromatase inhibitors are currently indicated only in the management of postmenopausal patients. Older agents have not been sufficiently potent to inhibit ovarian aromatase. Furthermore, any lowering of estrogen production by the intact ovary would lead to a reflex increased secretion of gonadotropins, which would stimulate further aromatase production in the ovary. The newer more potent compounds could possibly overcome this problem but have not been adequately tested and, in theory, could induce a clinical problem of polycystic changes in the ovary. Either of the other options could be employed, but bilateral oophorectomy would be the classic approach. Tamoxifen is active in metastatic cancer of premenopausal women but does not produce the endocrinologic equivalent of castration. Recent evidence suggests that an LH-RH analogue combined with tamoxifen might be superior to either agent used alone. Since this patient's tumor is *HER2/neu* positive, her disease might respond to treatment with Herceptin (trastuzumab). However, the single-agent activity of Herceptin is considerably lower than that of hormonal therapy in this setting. Nevertheless, this treatment, although expensive, is relatively free of side effects, which this patient wishes to avoid.

64.4 **Answer: (b)**   In five very large phase III clinical trials comparing aromatase inhibitors (anastrozole, letrozole, vorozole, and exemestane) with megestrol acetate, it was observed that the patients receiving the progestin reported a much higher incidence of undesired weight gain, which they considered a toxicity. In this same generation of trials, the aromatase inhibitor was either equivalent to or associated with greater efficacy than megestrol acetate and with fewer side effects such as thrombophlebitis and cardiovascular events. Unlike with aminoglutethimide, the incidence of skin rash from the newer aromatase inhibitors was very low.

64.5 **Answer: (b)**   Letrozole and anastrozole are both nonsteroidal competitive inhibitors of aromatase. These types of inhibitors compete with the substrate on a molar basis for the enzyme. Aminoglutethimide can inhibit a number of cholesterol side-chain cleavage enzymes, in addition to aromatase, and is thus not a specific inhibitor. Exemestane is a steroidal compound that is a structural analogue of androstenedione. It functions predominantly as a mechanism base or suicide inhibitor of the enzyme by forming an irreversible inactivating complex with the enzyme. Enzymatic blockade by this type of inhibitor would only be overcome by the synthesis of new enzyme. Third-generation inhibitors, such as anastrozole and letrozole, are considerably more potent than first-generation inhibitors, such as aminoglutethimide, and this may explain their greater clinical efficacy. Preclinical in vivo and in vitro studies show that third-generation inhibitors, particularly letrozole, significantly reduce estrogen synthesis by inhibiting intratumoral aromatase.

65.1 **Answer: (b)**   Progesterone interaction with its receptor is only the first phase of a complex series of events involved in the regulatory mechanisms that determine the response to this hormone. In addition to the sequence of events in the assembly of a preinitiation complex of ribonucleic acid (RNA) polymerase II and general transcription factors, a series of proteins serve to modulate the response to progestins in target issues in health and disease. These proteins that modulate transcriptional activity are referred to as coregulators (coactivators, corepressors, and cointegrators) and produce a series of protein–deoxyribonucleic acid (DNA), protein-RNA, and protein-protein interactions to either enhance or repress gene transcription. This complex interaction of PR with bound progestin and coregulator proteins provides potential selectivity. It is requisite, but not sufficient, to predict response to progesterone. The PR is expressed in normal target tissue. The demonstration of PRs in tissues does not serve to predict the specific type of endocrine treatment that will be effective; it only serves to identify a tumor that has the potential for being responsive to endocrine manipulation.

65.2 **Answer: (b)** Breast epithelial proliferation is associated with progesterone and is most pronounced in the luteal phase of the menstrual cycle. Although estrogen appears to be required for priming the cells for progesterone response, estrogen by itself is not associated with breast proliferation. In the uterus, however, estrogen is dominant in the follicular phase of the cycle when uterine endometrial proliferation is maximized, whereas progesterone inhibits proliferation in the endometrium.

Clearly, ovarian and adrenal hormones, progestins, and estrogens influence proliferation; estrogens do this by priming for progestin stimulation. Although high levels of progestins appear to inhibit breast epithelial proliferations, physiologic levels do not.

65.3 **Answer: (c)** PR should be considered a target gene for estrogen response in that a functional estrogen receptor and estrogen exposure are required to up-regulate the synthesis of PR. Progesterone has the effect of down-regulating its own receptor, whereas the antiprogestin RU-486 does not appear to alter synthesis of PR. Androgen exposure also appears to act similarly to progestins in reducing PR.

65.4 **Answer: (d)** Progesterone functions in RNA transcription regulation through a complex series of interactions initiated by binding the hormone to its cognate receptor. When the ligand is bound, hsp-90, hsp-70, and hsp-27 are released. In the absence of progesterone, the PR is functionally inactive and is associated with chaperone protein hsp-90. The chaperone function of the hsp-90 is intimately associated with inactivity of the steroid receptor. The activation of the PR directly involves its binding to its conserved activation function (AF-2) at the carboxyl end of the PR. This interaction modifies the molecular constraints, including the release of the hsp-90. The modifications, which involve the release of the chaperone protein(s) and corepressor proteins, as well as binding of coactivator proteins, permit enhanced access to the DNA binding domain. The results from the laboratory of D.R. Ciocca suggest that in human breast cancers hsp-27 may be involved in cell growth, arrest, and enhanced differentiation. Hsp-70 also appears to be involved in cell proliferation. In the absence of progesterone, the PR is functionally inactive. The function of the heat shock protein has also been associated with cell death or apoptosis as well as differentiation. The synthesis of hsp-27 is modulated in the endometrium during different phases of the menstrual cycle. The synthesis of hsp-90, which stabilizes the inactive form of the receptor, is modulated by environmental or other stress, resulting in increased cellular concentrations. Higher concentrations of the hsp-90 appear to suppress sex steroid receptor–dependent transcription in general.

65.5 **Answer: (d)** All of the effects noted are seen with progestins. The support of products of conception and the differentiation of the endometrium to a secretory pattern require progestins. The maturations and cornification of the vaginal mucosal epithelium may be achieved with either estrogen, estrogen plus progestin, or appropriate doses of progestin.

66.1 **Answer: (c)** The Veterans Administration Cooperative Urological Research Group studies demonstrated that orchiectomy is equivalent in response rates and survival to diethylstilbestrol (DES). Several studies have documented that the effectiveness of luteinizing hormone–releasing hormone (LH-RH) agonists such as goserelin acetate is also equivalent to both orchiectomy and/or DES. Flutamide was found to be inferior to DES in terms of overall survival in at least one study.

66.2 **Answer: (a)** The toxicity of the LH-RH agonists is related to gonadal suppression of testosterone production. These side effects include loss of libido, impotence, and muscle wasting. Longer androgen deprivation is associated with mild anemia, and the development of osteoporosis has been reported in one study. Hair loss is not a side effect.

66.3 **Answer: (d)** Antiandrogen withdrawal responses have been observed with all three nonsteroidal antiandrogens (flutamide, bicalutamide, nilutamide), megestrol acetate, and DES. Abarelix is not an antiandrogen but is an LH-RH antagonist.

66.4 **Answer: (d)** Although the optimal timing of androgen deprivation remains controversial, results of the MRC study show a benefit of early initiation in patients with metastatic disease. Messing and colleagues have performed a randomized study comparing early versus delayed hormonal therapy in patients with node-positive disease following prostatectomy and reported a survival advantage in patients receiving early therapy. Pound and colleagues recently analyzed the time course of disease progression in 1,997 men with biochemical recurrence after radical prostatectomy. This study identified Gleason score, time to PSA recurrence, and PSA doubling time as effective prognostic factors. Patients with a Gleason score of 5 to 7, a PSA recurrence of > 2 years, and a PSA doubling time of > 10 months had the highest probability of disease-free survival at 3, 5, and 7 years. In this instance, based on the algorithm presented in Pound and colleagues' report, the patient in answer (d) has all three positive indicators and would have an 82% probability of remaining disease free at 7 years. The patient in answer (e), with a shorter time to recurrence, would have a 59% chance, and the patient in answer (b), with Gleason score of 9 would have a 47% probability of remaining metastases free at 7 years. Although it is not known if these latter two patients would benefit from early initiation of androgen deprivation therapy, the patient in answer (d), with a very low probability of early recurrence, would be least likely to benefit.

66.5 **Answer: (c) and (e)** Prostate cancer cells taken from metastatic sites in "hormone-refractory" patients continue to express the androgen receptors; therefore, answer (a) is a false statement. Pure antiandrogens (ie, flutamide, bicalutamide, and nilutamide) bind to androgen receptors in prostate cancer cells and to androgen receptors in the hypothalamus and pituitary. This receptor binding blocks the negative feedback of androgens at the hypothalamic-pituitary level, leading to an eventual increase in LH released into the circulation. This leads to an increase, rather than a decrease, in serum testosterone; thus, answer (d) is false. Testosterone is converted to DHT by 5α-reductase. DHT is the active intracellular androgen that binds to androgen receptors stimulating cell growth and inhibiting cell death of androgen-dependent cells.

GENE THERAPY

67.1   **Answer: (a)**   Adenovirus and HSV-1 are both double-stranded deoxyribonucleic acid (DNA) viruses that are form episomes in the infected cell. AAV does integrate into the cellular genome, but this insertion is not random. It integrates into the long arm of chromosome 19 (q19.3–q-ter). Retroviruses, however, integrate in a random fashion into the cellular genome, which can result in insertional mutagenesis and the expression of oncogenes or repression of tumor suppressor genes.

67.2   **Answer: (c)**   Wild-type HSV-1 is a neurotropic virus with the ability to cause herpes encephalitis. Replication-competent HSV-1 is therefore neuroattenuated by deletion of one or more viral genes. Although infection with wild-type adenovirus is not associated with fatal infections, all oncolytic adenoviral vectors to date have deletions in one or more genes to restrict viral replication to tumor cells. Reovirus infection was dubbed an "orphan virus" because no disease process was associated with it. Wild-type reovirus replication is also reported to be dependent on an active *ras* pathway. Because tumor cells frequently have activating mutations in *ras,* wild-type reovirus is reported to replicate selectively in tumors.

67.3   **Answer: (b)**   Antisense molecules, ribozymes, and RNAi are all strategies to target messenger RNA specifically and block translation of transcribed genes. Triple-helix forming oligonucleotides, however, block transcription of the target gene by binding to duplex DNA.

67.4   **Answer: (b)**   The adenoviral mutant *dl*1520 (Onyx-015) contains a deletion in the *E1B* gene affecting the 55 kDa E1B protein. The paradigm to date with this virus is that it selectively replicates in cells with inactivation of the P53 protein. This can occur with mutations in the pathway affecting *P53* stability. Inactivating mutations in *P53* and *P14^{ARF}* or activating mutations in *MDM2* all have the net result of blocking *P53* activity.

67.5   **Answer: (e)**   Virus-directed enzyme/prodrug therapy has several advantages. The prodrug is relatively nontoxic and therefore can be delivered systemically in higher concentrations than active drugs (ie, chemotherapies). Viral delivery of specific prodrug-converting enzymes to the tumor bed restricts the conversion of the prodrug to its active metabolite. The use of viral or bacterial converting enzymes provides further restriction because these enzymes do not exist endogenously. Further advantages include the ability of active metabolites to diffuse to surrounding cells that have not been transfected with the converting enzyme "bystander effect." Certain active metabolites are also radiosensitizers (eg, 5-fluorouracil) and can be combined with radiotherapy to enhance the therapeutic index.

BONE MARROW TRANSPLANTATION

69.1   **Answer: (b)**

69.2   **Answer: (a)**

69.3   **Answer: (a)**

69.4   **Answer: (b)**

MULTIDISCIPLINARY

MANAGEMENT

DIRECTIONS: Numbering for questions and answers reflects the corresponding chapter in *Cancer Medicine-6*. Each question contains suggested responses. Select the best response to each question. Answers for Multidisciplinary Management begin on page 80.

PSYCHO-ONCOLOGY

70.1   The best regimen for managing a confused agitated patient who has a delirium owing to an underlying medical problem that cannot be eliminated is
    a.   A benzodiazepine
    b.   An antidepressant
    c.   An antipsychotic
    d.   An antipsychotic plus a benzodiazepine

70.2   What is the most useful psychotropic drug for a patient who has somnolence and low energy owing to side effects of narcotics given for pain?
    a.   A tricyclic antidepressant
    b.   A serotonin and norepinephrine reuptake inhibitor
    c.   A psychostimulant
    d.   A mood stabilizer

70.3   What is (are) the most common offender(s) in producing medication-induced depression?
    a.   Corticosteroids
    b.   Interferon and interleukin-2
    c.   Tamoxifen
    d.   Narcotic analgesics
    e.   All of the above

ONCOLOGY NURSING

71.1   To be eligible for certification as an oncology certified nurse (OCN), a nurse must have which of the following?
    a.   A master's degree in oncology nursing
    b.   A minimum of 1,000 hours of oncology nursing practice within 2.5 years of application and a bachelor's degree or higher in nursing
    c.   Current registered nurse (RN) licensure only
    d.   Current RN licensure and a minimum of 1,000 hours of oncology nursing practice within 2.5 years of application

71.2   Oncology nurses are most likely to be found practicing in all of the following settings *except*
    a.   Ambulatory care clinics
    b.   Home health care agencies
    c.   Hospital/multihospital settings
    d.   Private oncologists' offices

71.3   Which of the following most accurately represents the multiple facets of the role of the oncology nurse?
    a.   Direct patient care, patient assessment, patient education, and symptom management
    b.   Direct patient care, coordination of care, symptom management, and administration
    c.   Coordination of care, nursing research, health policy advocacy, and patient assessment
    d.   Symptom management, nursing research, nursing education, and health policy advocacy

71.4   Which of the following four traditional advanced practice nursing roles are most commonly seen in the oncology setting?
    a.   Nurse midwife and nurse anesthetist
    b.   Nurse practitioner and clinical nurse specialist
    c.   Nurse practitioner and nurse anesthetist
    d.   Clinical nurse specialist and nurse midwife

71.5   Which of the following best represents the reasons underlying a predicted nursing shortage of over 400,000 nurses by 2020?
    a.   An expected increase in elderly persons being diagnosed with cancer, an increase in younger women and men choosing nursing as a career, and a younger nursing workforce
    b.   An aging nursing workforce, increasing numbers of young men and women choosing nursing as a career, and maintenance of the status quo in professional collaborative relationships
    c.   An expected increase in the elderly population and corresponding cases of cancer, an aging nursing workforce that is expected to retire, and a lack of young men and women choosing nursing as a career
    d.   A workplace environment that respects the contributions of nurses, an aging nursing workforce, and an expected decrease in the number of persons diagnosed with cancer

CANCER REHABILITATION MEDICINE

72.1   **In a patient with neurologically complete thoracic paraplegia due to metastatic disease of the spine, the primary functional goal is to**
a.   Obtain spinal stability by application of a thoracolumbar sacral orthosis
b.   Provide electrical stimulation of the spinal cord to encourage neural regeneration
c.   Restore neurologic function by prompt surgical decompression
d.   Obtain independence in the activities of daily living by an interdisciplinary rehabilitation approach
e.   Provide personal assistance at home or at a nursing facility as early as possible in order to reduce the length of stay and cost of care

72.2   **In metastatic disease of the femur, the person *least* likely to suffer a pathologic fracture would be an individual who**
a.   Has a cortical bone lesion that affects 25% of the bony circumference as seen on an imaging study
b.   Has a large single lytic lesion in the proximal femur
c.   Is a woman
d.   Has persisting or increasing pain
e.   Has metastatic disease in other bones and organs

72.3   **Successful prosthetic use following above-the-knee amputation for a sarcoma in the distal femur depends on all of the following factors *except***
a.   Surgical techniques
b.   Preoperative counseling
c.   Length and shape of residual limb
d.   Absence of phantom pain
e.   Emotional adjustment

MULTIDISCIPLINARY MANAGEMENT

74.1   **Systemic chemotherapy during pregnancy is associated with fetal malformation risks. These risks are greatest**
a.   When the mother has multiple comorbid conditions
b.   When the chemotherapy includes anthracyclines and corticosteroids
c.   When the chemotherapy is given during the third trimester close to the time of delivery
d.   When the chemotherapy includes antimetabolites during the first trimester
e.   When the chemotherapy includes taxanes and platinum compounds during the second trimester

74.2   **Staging and assessing extent and location of malignant disease most often include diagnostic imaging techniques. Which of the following increases the risk of fetal abnormalities?**
a.   Magnetic resonance imaging of the thoracic and lumbar spine during the second trimester of pregnancy
b.   Computed tomography of the abdomen and pelvis during the first trimester of pregnancy
c.   Mammography during the first trimester of pregnancy
d.   Chest radiography during the second trimester of pregnancy
e.   Ultrasonography of the liver any time during the pregnancy

74.3   **The most frequent cancers occurring concurrent with pregnancy include *all but* which one of the following?**
a.   Cervical cancer
b.   Thyroid cancer
c.   Hodgkin's disease
d.   Breast cancer
e.   Small cell lung cancer

74.4   **From the available data, which of the following statements about treatment of leukemia during pregnancy is true?**
a.   Acute promyelocytic leukemia cannot be treated with all-*trans* retinoic acid because retinoids are known teratogens.
b.   Imatinib is the most beneficial first treatment for chronic myeloid leukemia.
c.   Delaying treatment of acute myeloid leukemia (AML) until after delivery gives the mother and fetus the best chance for survival.
d.   Chemotherapy for AML begun at time of diagnosis offers the best chance for a favorable outcome for mother and fetus.
e.   Acute lymphocytic leukemia is frequently associated with transplacental transmission of leukemia to the fetus.

74.5   **Issues that might impact on the treatment decision for the pregnant patient with cancer include effects of treatment for the patient and fetus. Which of the following also can influence the treatment planning process?**
a.   Termination of pregnancy
b.   The risk of fetal death due to cancer treatment

c. Type and relevance of diagnostic procedures used to assess disease
d. Placental metastasis and transplacental malignancy risks
e. The patient's ethical/moral value system
f. All of the above
g. None of the above

75.1 What percentage of all cancers occurs in patients ≥ age 65 years?
a. 20%
b. 40%
c. 60%
d. 80%
e. 100%

75.2 All of the following physiologic changes occur with aging *except*
a. Decreased response to catecholamines
b. Decreased response to hypoxemia
c. Decreased antibody response
d. Decreased high-frequency hearing
e. Decreased bone marrow fat

75.3 All of the following characteristics are used to describe a frail patient *except*
a. Age > 75 years
b. Dependence in activities of daily living
c. Dementia
d. Urinary or fecal incontinence
e. Failure to thrive

75.4 A comprehensive geriatric assessment includes an evaluation of which of the following?
a. Functional status
b. Comorbid medical conditions
c. Cognition
d. Nutritional status
e. All of the above

75.5 Which of the following physiologic changes with aging contribute(s) to changes in the volume of distribution of medications?
a. Increase in body fat
b. Increase in total body water
c. Increase in lean body mass
d. Increase in serum albumin
e. Increase in hemoglobin

75.6 Which of the following renal and hepatic changes occur with aging?
a. Decrease in glomerular filtration rate
b. Decrease in phase I hepatic reactions
c. Decrease in phase II hepatic reactions
d. Decrease in glomerular filtration rate and phase I hepatic reactions
e. Decrease in glomerular filtration rate and phase II hepatic reactions

76.1 All of the following interventions are supported by evidence from randomized trials *except*
a. Massage to reduce anxiety
b. Music therapy for mild depression
c. Acupuncture for chemotherapy nausea
d. Hypnosis for acute pain related to cancer treatment
e. Herbal medicine for hot flashes related to hormone therapy

76.2 Use of which of the following is acceptable?
a. St John's wort to treat depression and fatigue associated with chemotherapy
b. Reishi mushroom, said to activate immunity and fight cancer, in place of chemotherapy
c. High-dose vitamins C and E to reduce side effects of radiotherapy
d. "Fuzheng Baozhen Decoction," a Chinese patent herbal medicine, to treat cancer before surgery
e. Reishi mushroom after completion of chemotherapy

76.3 Which of the following alternative cancer therapies, promoted as prolonging survival from cancer, actually has been disproved and shown not to extend survival?
a. High-dose vitamin C
b. European mistletoe (Iscador)
c. Psychotherapy and support groups
d. All of the above
e. None of the above

76.4 Which of the following botanicals has been shown to extend survival as an adjunct to chemotherapy after colectomy?
a. MGN-3 (derived from rice bran)
b. Essiac
c. Mushroom extracts
d. Garlic
e. Ginseng

PAIN AND PALLIATION

77.1 A patient verbalized to the physician and his nurse his wish not to be resuscitated in the event of a cardiac or pulmonary arrest. Discussion was documented and the do not resuscitate (DNR) order was written in the chart. When the patient lost capacity to direct medical care, his wife requested that the DNR order be canceled. What would be the appropriate response?
a. The wife is the next of kin and has a right to represent her husband in making decisions about his care. The DNR order should be revoked.
b. Should the wife be the health care proxy, the DNR order should be revoked based on her wish.
c. The institution's ethics committee should be asked to validate the DNR order.
d. The DNR should not be revoked. Supportive counseling and education should be provided.

77.2 You are called to evaluate a patient well known to you. He is a 68-year-old man with metastatic melanoma and intractable diffuse skin pain of the chest wall caused by diffuse skin metastases. In spite of the ongoing attempt to control the patient's pain with different opioids and adjuvant analgesic medication, including steroids, the pain remains poorly controlled. The patient reports feeling "out of agony" only when he is asleep. He is requesting that you increase the dose of the sedating medications so that he does not have to wake up and experience the pain again. What is the appropriate response?
a. Increase the sedating medications immediately as per the patient's request
b. Refuse to increase the sedating medications, explaining that you cannot participate in euthanasia or physician-assisted suicide
c. Call an interdisciplinary meeting with the patient's medical caregivers and family to involve them in the discussion about sedating the patient
d. Call the hospital lawyer

77.3 Which conditions satisfy the doctrine of double effect?
a. The act should be good or morally neutral.
b. The intent of the health care provider must be good. Although the good effect and not the bad effect is intended, the bad effect can be foreseen, tolerated, and permitted.
c. Death must not be the means to the good effect, which is relief of suffering.
d. The good effect must exceed or balance the bad effect.
e. All of the above.

78.1 Barriers to effective pain management include
a. Inadequate assessment
b. Patient reluctance to take opioids
c. Physician reluctance to prescribe opioids
d. Inadequate staff knowledge about pain management
e. All of the above

78.2 The percentage of cancer patients surveyed who reported that severe pain might lead them to consider suicide was in the range of
a. 10–20%
b. 25–50%
c. 60–75%
d. 75–90%
e. 90–100%

78.3 The neospinothalamic pathway
a. Mediates the affective/suffering aspects of pain
b. Mediates the sensory-discriminative aspects of pain

c.   Is responsible for the transmission of position sense and light touch
d.   Is implicated in diseases of the cerebellum
e.   Transduces the signals for both visceral and neuropathic pain

78.4   Which of the following is true about fentanyl?
a.   It is available only in an intravenous and transdermal preparation.
b.   It is on the World Health Organization (WHO) Step 2 list of opioids for the management of cancer pain.
c.   It is now available in a transmucosal preparation for the management of breakthrough pain.
d.   It is named by the WHO as the drug of choice for the management of cancer pain.
e.   It is 20 times more potent than morphine.

78.5   Advantages of using methadone in cancer pain include
a.   85% bioavailability
b.   Lack of active metabolites
c.   Low cost
d.   Long half-life resulting in fewer required daily dosages and improved compliance
e.   All of the above

78.6   Which of the following is true in long-term cancer pain management?
a.   Meperidine is an excellent and safe agent.
b.   Attempt should be made to discontinue opioids regardless of clinical status due to the significant risk of addiction.
c.   Tolerance to the sedating effects of the opioids rarely develops.
d.   Effective symptom control may be achieved in the vast majority of patients.
e.   Nonsteroidal anti-inflammatory drugs are the first choice in the management of severe pain.

78.7   Which of the following is true regarding dose escalation among patients who are taking opioids for cancer pain?
a.   It suggests the onset of addiction.
b.   It most likely indicates progression of disease, which necessitates evaluation.
c.   It represents opioid failure and the need to substitute adjuvant drugs.
d.   It represents opioid failure and the need to rotate to another opioid drug.
e.   None of the above are true.

SOCIETAL ONCOLOGY

79.1   A 16-year-old girl develops a nonmetastatic Ewing's sarcoma of the tibia. She is treated with surgical resection and a year of chemotherapy. At age 19, after a 3-year disease-free interval, she is diagnosed with recurrent disease. She has tumor at the primary site as well as multiple pulmonary nodules. Her parents insist that you not tell her about her metastatic disease. What should you do next?
a.   Decline to provide care for the young woman unless you receive permission to speak frankly with her about her illness
b.   Discuss with her parents that she has attained the age of legal majority and therefore has a legal and ethical right to full and accurate information about her illness and care
c.   Ask her parents to sign a written waiver stating their request that information not be provided to their daughter
d.   Request an ethics consultation

79.2   A 34-year-old woman develops breast cancer. Her mother died of ovarian cancer at age 42 years. She is found to carry a mutation in the *BRCA1* gene. She expresses concern that her two daughters, ages 4 and 7 years, may also carry the mutation, and she requests that they undergo genetic testing. The most appropriate response at this time would be to
a.   Consult your hospital attorney
b.   Order testing for the children after thorough pretest counseling with their parents
c.   Order testing only if the children assent to being tested
d.   Discuss the pros and cons of testing, and ask the mother to take a few months to consider her decision
e.   Decline to provide testing until the girls are old enough to make their own decisions

79.3   A 36-year-old man has poor-risk testicular cancer. He is eligible for a protocol comparing standard-dose BEP (bleomycin, etoposide, cisplatin) with BEP followed by high-dose chemotherapy and stem cell rescue (the experimental arm). After researching the treatment options on the Internet, he requests that you treat him with BEP plus high-dose chemotherapy. What would be the most appropriate next step?
a.   Offer him the choice between randomization and treatment off-protocol with standard BEP
b.   Ask him to accept randomization, but agree to remove him from the protocol and treat him with BEP plus high-dose chemotherapy if he is assigned to the standard arm

    c.   Treat him off-protocol with BEP plus high-dose chemotherapy

    d.   Refer him to a colleague who might be willing to offer treatment with BEP plus high-dose chemotherapy off-protocol

79.4   **A 65-year-old male has had chronic lymphocytic leukemia for 5 years that has been treated with episodic chemotherapy. Because of sustained growth of his lymph nodes and progressive decline in his white and red blood cell counts, it is decided to begin CHOP (cyclophosphamide, doxorubicin [hydroxydaunomycin], vincristine [Oncovin], prednisone) chemotherapy. On day 14 after the second cycle of chemotherapy, the patient suffers a gastrointestinal perforation with hypotension and loss of consciousness. He is resuscitated and placed in the intensive care unit (ICU). After 10 days the patient has not regained consciousness, is still dependent on the ventilator, and requires dialysis. He has no advance-care directive. At a meeting involving the ICU staff, oncologists, and the patient's wife and only daughter, the patient's poor prognosis is delineated and the physicians recommend terminating life-sustaining treatments. His daughter is willing to stop both the ventilator and dialysis, but his wife refuses. After another 7 days with no improvement in the patient's condition, the medical team requests an ethics consultation. After meeting with the ethics consultation service, his wife still refuses to have the ventilator and dialysis stopped, and demands that "everything be done" for the patient. What would be the appropriate next step for the oncologist?**

    a.   Declare treatment with a ventilator and dialysis treatments extraordinary care and withdraw them

    b.   Request the hospital attorney go to court to make the daughter the patient's proxy

    c.   Declare the ventilator and dialysis treatments are futile care and withdraw them

    d.   Recognize the wife as the patient's proxy and accept her decision

79.5   **A 54-year-old woman with extensive bladder cancer that has invaded all her pelvic structures is hospitalized for pain relief. She is bed bound all day, has stopped chemotherapy, and has opted for palliative care. She is admitted because she is in excruciating pain, despite being on 210 mg morphine q3h around the clock. Intravenous morphine is begun at a dose of 20 mg/h without total pain control. Over the following 24 hours, the dose is increased to 40 mg/h, and still the patient is experiencing significant pain. The following day the dose is increased to 80 mg/h. The patient is sedated, with a respiratory rate of 7. Still she grimaces and cries out when she moves in the bed or is moved. A new nurse is assigned to the patient and objects to the order to increase the morphine to 100 mg/h. She claims that increasing the morphine dose to 100 mg/h exceeds the maximal dose, and that this will cause respiratory depression and therefore constitutes attempted euthanasia. Which of the following statements is true?**

    a.   The nurse is correct. Increasing the morphine dose so rapidly despite respiratory depression is euthanasia.

    b.   The nurse is incorrect. Increasing the morphine dose to control pain despite respiratory depression is ethical as long as it is done with the aim of controlling the patient's pain.

    c.   The nurse is incorrect. Increasing the morphine dose so rapidly with respiratory depression is not euthanasia; it is physician-assisted suicide.

    d.   The nurse is incorrect. Increasing the morphine dose to more than 100 mg/h exceeds the maximal dose and therefore constitutes euthanasia.

80.1   **In order for a patient to establish a cause of action for medical malpractice he or she must prove**

    a.   That a duty existed

    b.   That a duty was breached

    c.   That a breach of duty caused an injury

    d.   All of the above

80.2   **The physician-patient relationship, which creates a duty to treat, may be established in which of the following circumstances?**

    a.   Where a physician enters into a managed care contract and the patient is a member of that managed care unit

    b.   Where a physician is on call for an emergency room and is called to treat an emergency

    c.   Where a physician listens to the patient's signs and symptoms and gives medical advice even in a casual setting

    d.   All of the above

80.3   **Which of the following does *not* legally terminate a physician-patient relationship?**

    a.   A mutual agreement between the physician and the patient

    b.   A unilateral decision by the physician to terminate the relationship with either an unstable patient or without giving the patient an opportunity to obtain alternative services

    c.   A unilateral decision by the physician to terminate the relationship with stabilization of the patient and an opportunity for the patient to obtain alternative services

    d.   Failure by the patient, who has been informed of his or her condition, to maintain appointments and/or patient refusal of care

80.4   **Which of the following is *not* necessary when obtaining informed consent from a patient?**

    a.   That the consent be in writing

    b.   That the physician describes the illness from which the patient suffers

    c.   That the physician presents recommendations for treatment and reasonable alternative recommendations

    d.   That the physician describes the substantial risks of the reasonable alternative treatments

80.5 **A physician is *not* responsible for the acts of**
a. The nurses and office staff whom he employees
b. Consultants who are specialists in their own fields and who have been selected appropriately
c. Residents and interns the physician directs, in a detailed manner, with regard to care
d. An individual whom the physician has held out in such a manner that the public reasonably believes that the individual is the agent and/or employee of the physician

81.1 **Through the National Cancer Act of 1971, the director of the National Cancer Institute (NCI) was granted the statutory authority to**
a. Determine all cancer budgets for all National Institutes of Health (NIH) agencies
b. Determine budgets of over all NIH budgets
c. Submit a "bypass budget" to the US president, bypassing the director of the NIH
d. Determine only cancer center budgets
e. Do all of the above

81.2 **Disease-specific research plans are generated by the NCI primarily via**
a. Progress review groups (PRGs)
b. Special programs of research excellence
c. RO1 and PO1 grants
d. Cancer center grants
e. Research contracts

81.3 **Imatinib (Gleevec STI571), approved for the treatment of chronic myelogenous leukemia (CML) in 2001, specifically targets**
a. The *ras* gene
b. The cell membrane
c. Normal cells
d. All tumor cells
e. A molecular defect found in CML cells identified as Bcr-Abl

82.1 **The expected large increase in the number of cases of cancer over the next 20 years is largely explained by which of the following?**
a. An increasing incidence of the common cancers
b. Increasing environmental carcinogens
c. The aging of the population
d. Improved cancer treatments
e. Increasing immigration

82.2 **The failure of managed care to control health care costs over the long term may be explained by all of the following *except***
a. Patient demand for access to the physician of their choice
b. Increasing costs of pharmaceuticals
c. New diagnostic tests
d. Increasing physician reimbursement
e. State legislatures passing "patient rights" legislation

82.3 **The factor *least* likely to improve cancer care over the next decade is**
a. Increasing usage of the National Comprehensive Cancer Network guidelines
b. Improved access to clinical trials at the community level
c. A significant increase in the number of practicing oncologists
d. New molecular-based treatments of cancer

ANSWERS

PSYCHO-ONCOLOGY

70.1 **Answer: (d)** An antipsychotic such as haloperidol, a potent dopamine blocker, in a low dose of 0.5 to 1.0 mg bid reduces confusion. Similarly, risperidone at 1 to 3 mg bid or olanzapine 2.5 to 5.0 mg improves cognition. For the agitation, low doses of lorazepam 0.5 to 1.0 mg bid may be added; however, a benzodiazepine alone may actually increase confusion and lead to more disturbed behavior.

70.2 **Answer: (c)** A common side effect of narcotic analgesics is somnolence, poor energy, and lack of motivation to undertake usual activities. A psychostimulant often increases the patient's level of alertness and energy. Methylphenidate 5.0 mg or dextroamphetamine 5.0 mg is the least expensive and works well. The dose of either may need to be raised. Pemoline 18.75 mg in the morning and at noon is useful and can be taken as a chewable tablet. Newer and effective, although expensive, is modafinil; 100 mg taken in the morning and at noon counters many of the psychomotor slowing effects of narcotics and improves a patient's performance and desire to engage in activities.

70.3 **Answer: (e)** All the medications listed can cause significant depressive symptoms. The most dramatic examples are the cytokine-related agents such as interferon and interleukin-2, which can produce profound depression. The corticosteroids can produce a depressed mood, anhedonia, and withdrawal, and they may incur mild cognitive changes as well. Narcotic analgesics produce depressed mood and depressive symptoms. Tamoxifen is the least frequent offender on the list, but because it is often given at the time of a medical-induced menopause, women need to be monitored for depression. These medication-induced depressive states respond best to the selective serotonin reuptake inhibitors (SSRIs; fluoxetine, paroxetine, sertraline, citalopram) at the usual daily dose. Some centers start an SSRI prophylactically when high-dose interferon or interleukin-2 is to be used.

ONCOLOGY NURSING

71.1 **Answer: (d)** To be eligible to sit for certification as an OCN, a nurse must meet the following criteria: hold a current RN license, have a minimum of 1 year (12 mo) experience as an RN within the 3 years (36 mo) prior to application, and a minimum of 1,000 hours of oncology nursing practice within the 2.5 years (30 mo) prior to application, and completion of a minimum of 10 contact hours of continuing education in the specialty of oncology nursing or an academic elective in oncology nursing within the 3 years prior to application. For basic oncology certification, there are no stipulations on educational preparation. To obtain an advanced oncology nurse certification, a nurse must hold a master's degree or higher.

71.2 **Answer: (c)** Although many nurses who consider themselves oncology nurses may work in home health care or a hospice, only about 3% of nurses who belong to the Oncology Nursing Society (ONS) work in this setting.

71.3 **Answer: (a)** Although all activities listed may be performed by oncology nurses depending on their educational level and practice setting, the majority of ONS members and oncology nurses work in a direct patient care role that includes other key roles of patient assessment, patient education, and symptom management.

71.4 **Answer: (b)** Although each traditional role may include components of oncology practice, the correct answer is nurse practitioner and clinical nurse specialist. In these roles there is emphasis on providing nursing care at an advanced level to patients and families through comprehensive health assessments; the identification of normal and abnormal health characteristics; and treatment of a variety of human responses throughout the cancer care continuum according to practice guidelines, protocols, or standing orders.

71.5 **Answer: (c)** The current and impending nursing shortage is a complex situation that has no single solution. A variety of factors such as an aging nursing workforce and the anticipation of an increasing number of elderly in the United States that may receive a diagnosis of cancer are clearly a collision of demographics. In addition, there are many options open to young men and women today. Few have chosen to enter nursing, which is often viewed as a women's profession and a profession that does not receive full recognition of its contribution to the health care systems. Many medical and nursing professional organizations are working to address different components related to the shortage. Oncologists can play a key role in the fostering of a workplace environment that is respectful of the contributions of oncology nurses and promotes a collaborative working relationship.

CANCER REHABILITAION MEDICINE

72.1 **Answer: (d)** Independence in the activities of daily living is the most important goal. After complete paraplegia, there is no basis to anticipate neural recovery despite the surgery, spine stabilization, or electrical stimulation. Personal assistance is not a satisfactory substitute for independence.

72.2   Answer: (a) Pathologic fractures most often occur with large lesions in weight-bearing bones, more often in women than men, and when widespread metastatic disease is present, more bones are put at risk. Pain, particularly when increasing, may signal impending fracture. A lesion that affects only 25% of cortical bone rarely fractures.

72.3   Answer: (d) Phantom pain does not preclude successful use of a prosthetic limb. Inadequate performance status, emotional adjustment, stamina, motivation, and family support can all compromise successful prosthetic use. The surgical approach should provide an adequately shaped and sized stump.

MULTIDISCIPLINARY MANAGEMENT

74.1   Answer: (d) Doll and colleagues have reviewed chemotherapy effects on fetal malformations. They reported that first trimester exposure had the greatest risk of fetal malformation—19%. Antimetabolites, especially methotrexate, were associated with the highest risk.

74.2   Answer: (b) Computed tomography exposes the patient and fetus to ionizing radiation. Doses of radiation of up to 900 mrad may occur. Exposure at 2 to 8 weeks of pregnancy may result in fetal malformation. Mental retardation may result with radiation exposure of this amount between 8 and 25 weeks of gestation. If there has been > 15 cGy of fetal radiation exposure during the first trimester, the National Commission on Radiation Protection recommends that the pregnancy be terminated.

74.3   Answer: (e) Smith and colleagues reviewed more than three million deliveries over a 5-year period in California. Two thousand two hundred forty-seven cases of primary malignancy were diagnosed in the prenatal time period, at delivery, or within 12 months of delivery. Breast, thyroid, and cervical cancers were most common (1.3, 1.2, and 0.8, respectively, per 1,000 live singleton births). Hodgkin's disease and ovarian cancer occurred with equal frequency (0.5 per 1,000 live singleton births). There have been few case reports of small cell lung cancer concurrent with pregnancy.

74.4   Answer: (d) A Mayo Clinic report noted that outcomes for mother and fetus were best when leukemia was treated during pregnancy. Five of nine patients treated for AML during pregnancy had complete remissions. Only one of four patients who delayed treatment until after delivery survived.

A number of case reports have confirmed the benefit of all-*trans* retinoic acid in pregnant women with acute promyelocytic leukemia. Fetal malformations have not been reported.

There are no case reports or other clinical data on the outcome of pregnancy for women with chronic myeloid leukemia treated with imatinib. There have been no fetal malformations reported with the use of hydroxyurea or interferon-α.

Transplacental transmission of malignancy is a rare complication of cancer with concurrent pregnancy. Acute lymphocyte leukemia cells have been identified in the circulation; however, leukemic cell engraftment has not been seen.

74.5   Answer: (f)

75.1   Answer: (c) Sixty percent of all cancers occurs in people ≥ age 65 years. Cancer is a disease that disproportionately affects older patients. People age 65 years and older have an 11-fold increase in the incidence of cancer and a 15-fold increase in cancer mortality compared with people < age 65 years.

75.2   Answer: (e) Hematopoietic changes with aging include a decrease in bone marrow mass and an increase in bone marrow fat. Despite this, peripheral blood cell concentrations in healthy older patients are similar to those of younger patients. As the cardiovascular system ages, there is a decrease in cardiac output, a decrease in maximal heart rate, and prolonged recovery following exertion. During times of stress, there is a decreased response to catecholamines. As the pulmonary system ages, there is a decreased response to hypoxemia or hypercapnia, a decreased elasticity in the lung tissue, an increased ventilation-perfusion mismatch, and a decreased forced expiratory volume. Endocrine changes with aging include a decrease in certain hormone levels and an increase in others. For example, there is a decrease in insulin-like growth factor, growth hormone, renin, aldosterone, dehydroepiandrosterone, and sex steroids and an increase in insulin, norepinephrine, parathyroid hormone, vasopressin, and atrial natriuretic peptide. Changes to the neurologic system with aging include neuronal loss, decrease in brain weight, decreased vision, loss in high-frequency and low-frequency hearing, and alterations in both taste and smell. Changes in the immune system manifest as a decrease in thymic mass, a decrease in production of thymic hormones, a decrease in naive lymphocytes, and a decrease in antibody response.

75.3   Answer: (a) The following clinical characteristics are often used to describe a frail older person: age > 85 years, dependence in activities of daily living, comorbid (coexisting) medical conditions (including serious cardiovascular, respiratory, or cerebrovascular conditions), and one or more geriatric syndromes (dementia, delirium, urinary or fecal incontinence, history of osteoporotic fractures, failure to thrive, neglect, and abuse).

75.4   Answer: (e) A comprehensive geriatric assessment provides information about an individual's functional status (ability to complete tasks at home and in the community), comorbid medical conditions (other concurrent medical illnesses), cognition, nutritional status, and social support. Each of these variables has individual prognostic implications in terms of risk of mortality and should be considered in the evaluation and determination of the treatment plan in the older patient.

75.5   Answer: (a)   There are significant changes in the volume of distribution with aging, including an increase in body fat (leading to slower metabolism of lipid-soluble drugs), a decrease in total body water (leading to an increase in the plasma level of water-soluble drugs), a decrease in lean body mass, a decrease in serum albumin, and a decrease in hemoglobin.

75.6   Answer: (d)   Renal mass decreases by 25 to 30% over the lifespan, leading to a decreased number of functional nephrons. Consequently there is a decrease in glomerular filtration, tubular secretion, and reabsorption with aging. Renal blood flow decreases by 1% per year after age 50 years, and glomerular filtration decreases by 1 mL/min/yr after age 40 years.

    Hepatic metabolism changes with aging, secondary to decreased liver volume and decreased hepatic blood flow. Phase I hepatic reactions (oxidation, deamination, hydroxylation) decrease with aging. These include reactions mediated via cytochrome P-450, which decrease by approximately 30% in older patients. There is no significant change in phase II hepatic reactions (conjugation: acetylation, glucuronidation, sulfation) with aging.

76.1   Answer: (e)   Options (a) to (d) are all supported by randomized trials. No good-quality evidence suggests that herbal agents can reduce hot flashes in cancer patients.

76.2   Answer: (e)   St John's wort is unacceptable because it may interact metabolically with chemotherapy, reducing blood concentrations to subtherapeutic levels. Herbal remedies in place of proven treatment should be discouraged. Antioxidants may interfere with the activity of radiotherapy against cancer. Radiotherapy acts in part by creating oxidative damage within tumor cells, an effect that can be diminished by antioxidant supplements. The use of herbal medicines with unknown constituents, particularly those imported from developing countries, should be discouraged. Some herbs have anticoagulant effects. It is therefore advisable to stop nonprescription products at least 2 weeks before surgery. Patients wishing to use herbs or other dietary supplements after completing treatment should not be dissuaded unless there are reasons to believe the product may be harmful.

76.3   Answer: (d)   Alternative cancer therapies are often described as "unproved" or said to have "no evidence" to support effectiveness. In fact, many have been investigated and shown to be of no benefit.

76.4   Answer: (c)   Two randomized trials of mushroom extracts in colorectal cancer showed significant differences between groups for disease-free and overall survival.

PAIN AND PALLIATION

77.1   Answer: (d)   A DNR decision cannot be overturned by the next of kin or the health care proxy if the patient, while able to direct his care, stated clearly that his wish was not to be resuscitated. The ethics committee may be consulted as needed.

77.2   Answer: (c)   It is important to distinguish between physician-assisted suicide and sedation in the imminently dying. Although physician-assisted suicide is illegal (except in Oregon), sedation to relieve suffering caused by intractable pain is legal and acceptable. Ethical and moral dilemmas do arise and are best addressed by a discussion involving the caregivers and the patient's family. The informed consent of the patient or the surrogate is mandatory and should be obtained after a discussion of reasons for accepting sedation as a side effect of treatment directed toward intractable symptoms; people other than the patient and the doctor should be present during the discussion.

77.3   Answer: (e)

78.1   Answer: (e)   The undertreatment of pain among patients with cancer remains an alarming clinical problem. The publication of numerous guidelines and dissemination of public information are important tools in ensuring appropriate attention to symptom control.

78.2   Answer: (c)   These data have important implications for the current debate on the legalization of physician-assisted suicide given the well-documented inadequate assessment and undertreatment of pain in the cancer population.

78.3   Answer: (b)   This pathway originates in the spinal cord and terminates in the somatosensory cortex of the parietal lobe. The paleospinothalamic pathway has more diffuse projections and mediates the emotional aspects of pain. The dorsal columns in the spinal cord transmit proprioceptive impulses.

78.4   Answer: (c)   Fentanyl is 80 to 100 times more potent than morphine and is on the WHO Step 3 analgesic ladder.

78.5   Answer: (e)   Although the duration of analgesic effect is 4 to 6 hours, the biologic half-life may range from 15 to 60 hours. Due to potential difficulties with drug accumulation, opioid rotations to methadone should be performed only by experienced clinicians. Although a second-line agent, methadone is a useful alternative for some patients with poorly controlled pain on the usual first-line agents.

78.6   **Answer: (d)**   Meperidine is not recommended in the management of chronic cancer pain due to the potential for accumulation of toxic metabo-lites, especially in the setting of renal failure. The use of opioids in the management of pain due to medical illness rarely results in psychological dependence or addiction. Tolerance typically develops to all side effects of the opioids, except constipation. Opioids are the first-line agents in the management of severe cancer pain. Nonsteroidal anti-inflammatory agents are useful as adjuncts especially in the setting of bone pain.

78.7   **Answer: (b)**   A comprehensive evaluation in the management of cancer pain is critical and frequently results in new diagnoses. New pain complaints in patients already taking opioids should prompt the clinician to initiate a thorough search for additional sites of disease.

SOCIETAL ONCOLOGY

79.1   **Answer: (b)**   Adults who have reached the age of legal majority in the relevant jurisdiction are presumed competent to receive medical information and to make decisions affecting their care. Now that she is 19, the patient's parents may no longer control the information that she receives. As a result, they cannot waive her right to information and their permission is not required to speak with her. Withholding information from the patient would violate her right to be treated as an autonomous human being. She can, however, decline to receive the information and ask that decisions be made by her parents. Such a request, if freely made, would constitute an exercise rather than a waiv-er of her autonomy.

79.2   **Answer: (e)**   Each daughter has a 50% chance of inheriting their mother's *BRCA1* mutation. However, onset of *BRCA1*-related cancers is extremely rare in childhood, and there are no strategies available to reduce an affected child's risk of developing adult-onset cancer. Testing now would take away the girls' opportunity to make their own decisions about whether to be tested when they reach adulthood. Thus, test-ing of the children at this time would be inappropriate.

79.3   **Answer: (a)**   Although this situation is complex and there is no ethical consensus on the best approach, most people would argue that patients should not be treated with the experimental arm of a randomized trial without enrolling in that trial. Thus, if patients are unwilling to accept randomization (and agree to abide by its outcome), they should receive standard treatment. If the patient still refuses standard chemotherapy after you have discussed these issues with him, referral for a second opinion would be a reasonable option. You are not obli-gated to treat him with the experimental chemotherapy, nor to find him a clinician who will provide the experimental treatment.

79.4   **Answer: (d)**   The distinction between extraordinary and ordinary care is imprecise to guide decision making. The use of *futility* to termi-nate medical care despite the wishes of patients and their proxies has been shown to be unhelpful. Futility is not clearly defined, and physi-cians do not consistently apply it. Therefore, neither extraordinary care nor futility should be used to justify decision making. Without a for-mal proxy designation, the wife is the closest relative and, unless she is mentally incompetent in some way, the legal proxy. Trying to switch proxies would not be successful. In this case, with great reluctance, the oncologists must adhere to the wife's wishes. This reinforces the importance of discussing advance-care planning with patients before they become terminally ill and lose the ability to make decision for themselves.

79.5   **Answer: (b)**   Using morphine or another opioid to control pain is both ethical and legal, even if it causes respiratory depression and might result in the patient's death—although this is exceedingly rare because patients become tolerant to the respiratory depressive effects of opi-oids. When controlling pain there is no upper dose limit; hence (d) is incorrect. *Euthanasia* is the administration of medication or other inter-vention with the intention of ending the patient's life. *Physician-assisted suicide* is the provision of a prescription that the patient can take to end his or her own life. Since the medical team is administering the morphine, this cannot be a case of physician-assisted suicide; hence (c) is incorrect.

80.1   **Answer: (d)**   The United States judicial system is consistent in this regard. To establish liability, a plaintiff/patient must demonstrate that the care provider owed them a duty. In other words, a physician-patient relationship existed. There must be a breach of that duty, which gen-erally is described as a breach of the appropriate standard of care, and lastly that breach must have caused an injury.

80.2   **Answer: (d)**   The most common manner in which a physician establishes a doctor-patient relationship is by actually rendering care to the patient, whether or not compensation is received. However, there are other circumstances in which such a relationship may be created. These generally involve contractual agreements, such as managed-care agreements, and/or hospital bylaws requiring that care be rendered. However, they may also involve a circumstance that, although casual in nature, involves the evaluation of symptoms and recommendations for treatment.

80.3   **Answer: (b)**   A physician-patient relationship with regard to a specific illness continues until appropriately terminated. When a physician terminates the relationship inappropriately, he or she may be held liable for abandoning the patient. Obviously, a relationship may be termi-nated by mutual consent of the parties. Similarly, it may be terminated by the physician alone, if the physician is confident that the patient is stable, and the physician has given the patient sufficient time to seek alternative services. Patients who refuse to maintain appointments and/or follow medical advice once the consequences have been made clear to them may also be considered to have terminated the relationship.

80.4   **Answer: (a)**   It is not necessary, unless specifically required by state statute, that a consent agreement between a physician and patient be in writing. However, it is always recommended, as it is the physician's best means to protect against allegations that an informed consent was not obtained.

80.5   **Answer: (b)**   A physician may find himself liable for the acts of others. These most often include his own employees. However, responsibility may be expanded for those whom the physician directs in a detailed manner with regard to care rendered, such as an intern or resident. Additionally, a physician may be liable for the acts of an individual whom he or she holds out to the public as one that is either his agent or employee. In most circumstances, consultants are not the responsibility of the requesting physician as long as their credentials warrant being involved in the case.

81.1   **Answer: (c)**   The National Cancer Act of 1971 significantly expanded the scope and authority of the national cancer program. The most unusual authority granted by the Act was direct access to the president of the United States. The director of NCI submits a bypass budget to the president each year, which defines the "professional needs" of the national cancer program.

81.2   **Answer: (a)**   The NCI convenes panels of experts through the progress review mechanism to analyze the status of research on a specific type of cancer and to determine where gaps and barriers exist to achievement of future progress. PRGs submit their recommendations and plans to the NCI for implementation.

81.3   **Answer: (e)**   The US Food and Drug Administration fast-tracked the approval of imatinib in 2001 for the treatment of CML patients. Leukemia, but not normal, cells from CML patients exhibit the abnormal signaling protein Bcr-Abl, making imatinib a targeted agent that sets the stage for a paradigm shift in the development of future therapeutics for cancer.

82.1   **Answer: (c)**   Over the next 20 years the actual incidence of common cancer is most likely to remain stable or, in the case of lung cancer, decrease. However, the prevalence of cancer will increase dramatically as the number of people over age 65 years increases.

82.2   **Answer: (d)**   Physician reimbursement has not increased significantly over the past 10 years when compared with cost increases in pharmaceuticals and diagnostic tests. Failure of the gatekeeper model has also prevented managed-care companies from better controlling their costs.

82.3   **Answer: (c)**   We are actually likely to face a significant manpower shortage in medical oncology. This is influenced by the predicted significant increase in the number and complexity of cancer cases in the aging American population, a modest and stable number of trainee positions and graduates per year, and the eventual retirement of a large cadre of oncologists trained in the decade since the passage of the National Cancer Act.

CANCER MANAGEMENT

DIRECTIONS: Numbering for questions and answers reflects the
corresponding chapter in *Cancer Medicine-6*.
Each question contains suggested responses.
Select the best response to each question.
Answers for Cancer Management begin on page 122.

CENTRAL NERVOUS SYSTEM

83.1   **Which of the following primary brain tumors has necrosis and microvascular proliferation as its histologic hallmarks?**
   a.   Glioblastoma multiforme (GBM)
   b.   Anaplastic astrocytoma
   c.   Oligodendroglioma
   d.   Medulloblastoma
   e.   Ependymoma

83.2   **Which of the following statements concerning GBM is *false*?**
   a.   Median overall survival is only 11 to 12 months.
   b.   The most significant prognostic factors for GBM are age of the patient at diagnosis and score on Karnofsky performance scale.
   c.   Even an apparent gross total resection on magnetic resonance imaging (MRI) of a GBM lesion leaves residual microscopic tumor cells.
   d.   Typically, a GBM lesion enhances with contrast on T1-weighted MRI images.
   e.   Standard treatment for GBM includes maximal resection, hyperfractionated irradiation, and nitrosourea chemotherapy.

83.3   **Which of the following primary brain tumors has a definitive molecular marker that significantly predicts a response to a specific chemotherapy regimen?**
   a.   Medulloblastoma
   b.   GBM
   c.   Oligodendroglioma
   d.   Meningioma
   e.   Ependymoma

83.4   **Which of the following statements regarding meningioma is *false*?**
   a.   The most consistent karyotypic alteration in meningioma is deletion of the long arm or all of chromosome 22.
   b.   There is a well-known association between meningioma and female gender.
   c.   On MRI, meningiomas are intra-axial in location, enhance homogeneously, and are characterized by the "dural tail" sign.
   d.   Meningioma is a characteristic brain tumor type associated with neurofibromatosis type 2 (NF2).
   e.   The rate of meningioma recurrence is associated with the extent of resection.

84.1   **The most common primary tumor associated with hemorrhagic brain metastases is**
   a.   Lung cancer
   b.   Melanoma
   c.   Thyroid cancer
   d.   Choriocarcinoma

84.2   **Stereotactic radiosurgery should be reserved for brain metastases that**
   a.   Are > 4 cm
   b.   Originate from melanoma
   c.   Are ≤ three lesions
   d.   Are associated with significant edema

84.3   **A patient with known lung cancer develops headache. A magnetic resonance scan shows evidence of multiple metastases. His physician places him on 16 mg of dexamethasone and 300 mg of phenytoin per day. The headaches resolve, but 2 weeks later he develops a diffuse morbilliform rash. What should the next step be?**
   a.   Biopsy the skin lesions
   b.   Discontinue the phenytoin and start another anticonvulsant
   c.   Discontinue the phenytoin and do not start another anticonvulsant
   d.   Discontinue both drugs

84.4   **Evidence-based medicine suggests that the treatment of a single brain metastasis most likely to promote long-term survival is**
   a.   Surgical excision followed by whole brain radiotherapy
   b.   Surgical excision and systemic chemotherapy
   c.   Radiosurgery and whole brain radiation
   d.   Radiosurgery without whole brain radiation

THE EYE

85.1 Which of the following combinations below represents the most common primary malignant intraocular and orbital tumors in children and adults?
  a. Intraocular (children)—rhabdomyosarcoma; orbital (children)—leukemia; intraocular (adults)—uveal melanoma; orbital (adults)—lymphoma
  b. Intraocular (children)—retinoblastoma; orbital (children)—rhabdomyosarcoma; intraocular (adults)—uveal melanoma; orbital (adults)—lymphoma
  c. Intraocular (children)—retinoblastoma; orbital (children)—cavernous hemangioma; intraocular (adults)—choroidal nevus; orbital (adults)—lymphoma
  d. Intraocular (children)—capillary hemangioma; orbital (children)—retinoblastoma; intraocular (adults)—uveal melanoma; orbital (adults)—sinus cancer

85.2 Which of the following statements about retinoblastoma is *false*?
  a. There are 250 to 350 cases/yr in the United States.
  b. Worldwide, the 5-year mortality rate of patients with retinoblastoma is approximately 5%.
  c. The genetic defect responsible for the development of the tumor occurs on the long arm of chromosome 13.
  d. In the United States, the most common presenting sign is leukokoria, followed by strabismus.

85.3 Which of the following is *not* a proven risk factor for progression of a choroidal nevus into a melanoma?
  a. Posterior location
  b. Increasing size
  c. Presence of serous fluid
  d. Presence of drusen
  e. Presence of orange pigment

ENDOCRINE GLANDS

86.1 A 43-year-old woman presents with weight gain. Laboratory testing reveals an elevated urinary-free cortisol. Magnetic resonance imaging (MRI) with and without gadolinium reveals no lesion. The next step in her evaluation should be to
  a. Repeat the MRI in 6 months
  b. Repeat the urinary-free cortisol
  c. Advise her about proper nutrition
  d. Obtain a cavernous sinus sampling study

86.2 A 50-year-old man reports an increasing shoe size over the last couple of years, and you notice the characteristic facial features of acromegaly. He tells you that he is not bothered by the changes in facial features or the growth of his hands and feet. You recommend
  a. No further follow-up in deference to the patient's wishes
  b. Proceeding with an evaluation as a probable elevation in the patient's growth hormone (GH) places him at increased mortality risk
  c. Getting an MRI should the patient change his mind about treatment at some later date
  d. Checking a serum prolactin (PRL) level and, if elevated, proceeding with an MRI

86.3 The patient described in the preceding question consents to undergoing fasting serum GH testing and an MRI. Although his GH is elevated, careful review of the MRI discloses no intrasellar pathology. The next step in the evaluation should be to
  a. Obtain a serum IGF-1 level. If this value is not elevated, then the patient does not have acromegaly
  b. Assume that the GH-secreting pituitary adenoma is simply too small to detect on MRI at this time; obtain a follow-up MRI in 6 months
  c. Assume an ectopic source of GH secretion; initiate a search for a carcinoid tumor
  d. Assume a GH-secreting microadenoma that is too small to visualize on MRI; obtain cavernous sinus sampling to look for elevated GH in the venous drainage of the pituitary

86.4 A patient you have been following with a known PRL-secreting macroadenoma has been asymptomatic on bromocriptine mesylate. He now calls your office to report a sudden bilateral loss of vision. His serum PRL level is stable at > 500 ng/mL. At this point you
  a. Increase his bromocriptine dose and have him schedule an appointment with the neurosurgeon
  b. Arrange for him to be evaluated by the neurosurgeon immediately and administer hydrocortisone for the possibility of sudden hypopituitarism
  c. Realize that his high serum PRL level makes a surgical cure exceedingly unlikely; you arrange for him to be seen by the radiation oncologist immediately
  d. Take the patient off bromocriptine and start him on cabergoline

86.5 **A 60-year-old man presents to your office with decreased libido and a bitemporal hemianopsia. Endocrine evaluation reveals panhypopituitarism. An MRI discloses a pituitary macroadenoma, with invasion into both cavernous sinuses. You recommend**
   a. Referral to the radiation oncologist, with treatment to begin as soon as possible
   b. Starting bromocriptine in an effort to shrink the tumor, with a follow-up MRI scheduled in 2 months
   c. Radiation treatment concurrent with bromocriptine and a follow-up MRI on completion of radiotherapy
   d. Referral to the neurosurgeon for decompression of the optic chiasm, followed by radiation therapy for the residual tumor in the cavernous sinuses

87.1 **The most appropriate diagnostic test to perform on a patient with a solitary 2 cm thyroid nodule is**
   a. Serum thyroglobulin
   b. Ultrasonography of the thyroid
   c. Fine-needle aspiration of the nodule
   d. Ultrasonography-guided fine-needle aspiration of the nodule
   e. Radioiodine thyroid scan

87.2 **A 35-year-old woman presents with a right lateral neck mass that proves by biopsy to be papillary thyroid carcinoma metastatic to a cervical lymph node. On examination she has a 1.5 cm right thyroid lobe nodule. The most appropriate initial therapy should be**
   a. Right hemithyroidectomy, radioactive iodine treatment, and thyroid hormone suppression therapy
   b. Total thyroidectomy, radical neck node dissection, radioactive iodine, and thyroid hormone suppression therapy
   c. Total thyroidectomy, modified radical neck node dissection, radioactive iodine treatment, and thyroid hormone suppression therapy
   d. Total thyroidectomy, external beam radiotherapy, and thyroid hormone suppression
   e. Total thyroidectomy and thyroid hormone suppression

87.3 **A 48-year-old woman, in otherwise good health, presents with a pathologic fracture of the left humerus when she slips on the ice. Her initial physical examination is otherwise unremarkable. Following surgical stabilization of the fracture, pathology of the biopsy of the bone lesion reveals metastatic follicular thyroid carcinoma. Directed examination of the neck reveals no evidence of a primary thyroid lesion. Chest radiography reveals multiple nodules approximately 1 to 2 cm in diameter throughout all lung fields and suggestion of metastasis in an eighth rib is also identified. Appropriate initial therapy would include all of the following *except***
   a. Total thyroidectomy
   b. Doxorubicin 60 mg/m^2 monthly
   c. Radioactive iodine, 150 to 200 mCi
   d. External beam radiotherapy to symptomatic bone lesions
   e. Thyroid hormone suppression therapy

87.4 **Which of the following events is most closely associated with the development of anaplastic thyroid carcinoma?**
   a. A somatic codon 634–inactivating mutation of the *RET* proto-oncogene
   b. History of exposure of the neck to ionizing radiation
   c. History of radioactive iodine treatment for hyperthyroid Graves' disease
   d. Somatic mutation of the *P53* tumor suppressor gene in a differentiated thyroid carcinoma
   e. Inadequate thyroid-stimulating hormone (TSH) suppression therapy during long-term management of differentiated thyroid carcinoma

87.5 **A 19-year-old man presents for a pre-employment physical examination. Family history reveals multiple relatives with thyroid cancer and high serum calcium levels. Further testing in the patient reveals a serum calcitonin of 560 pg/mL (normal less than 15 pg/mL). His *RET* proto-oncogene analysis identifies a codon 634 mutation. Ultrasonography of the neck reveals a 6 mm nodule in the right thyroid lobe and no other abnormalities in the neck. He undergoes a right hemithyroidectomy with pathology demonstrating a medullary thyroid carcinoma. Two months postoperatively, the patient's serum calcitonin remains elevated, 96 pg/mL. Appropriate further management of the patient would include all of the following *except***
   a. Dacarbazine-based chemotherapy
   b. Completion thyroidectomy and central neck node dissection
   c. Lateral neck modified radical dissections if abnormal lymph nodes are identified
   d. Thyroid hormone replacement therapy
   e. Measurement of serum calcium and urinary catecholamine metabolites, vanillylmandelic acid (VMA), and metanephrines

88.1 **Adrenal cortical carcinoma is occasionally seen as part of familial cancer syndromes. Which of the following gene mutations have been associated with these syndromes?**
   a. Insulin-like growth factor II (*IGF-II*)
   b. H19 (unknown function)
   c. c-*myc*
   d. *P53* tumor suppressor gene
   e. *P57^{kip2}* (cyclin-dependent kinase inhibitor)

88.2   **What is the manner in which small nonhormone secreting adrenal cortical carcinomas are usually detected?**
   a.   Local symptoms
   b.   A computed tomography (CT) scan of the abdomen for unrelated complaints
   c.   Urine tests for steroid hormone precursors
   d.   Abdominal positron emission tomography
   e.   Iodocholesterol nuclear scan (δ)

88.3   **What criterion is best to determine prognosis in patients with adrenal cortical carcinoma?**
   a.   Hormone production
   b.   Size of the primary tumor
   c.   Mitotic rate
   d.   Age of the patient
   e.   Duration of symptoms

88.4   **Which is the best approach to the management of patients with cortisol-secreting adrenal cortical carcinomas that do not respond to antitumor chemotherapy?**
   a.   Radiation therapy of the largest lesions
   b.   Blockers of cortisol synthesis
   c.   Tumor debulking
   d.   Hospice care
   e.   Treatment with androgens for their anabolic effects

88.5   **Which therapeutic interventions are most appropriate in patients with stage IV adrenal cortical carcinoma?**
   a.   Debulking surgery alone
   b.   Mitotane
   c.   Combination chemotherapy
   d.   Surgical resection of the primary tumor and metastases
   e.   Debulking surgery plus combination chemotherapy

HEAD AND NECK

90.1   **What is the risk of squamous cell carcinoma of the head and neck (SCCHN) in those currently smoking?**
   a.   < 50% increased risk
   b.   50 to 100% increased risk
   c.   100 to 200% increased risk
   d.   600 to 700% increased risk
   e.   > 1500% increased risk

90.2   **First described by Slaughter in 1953, the theory of field cancerization, or condemned mucosa syndrome, explains why patients with squamous carcinoma of the upper aerodigestive tract (UADT) can be expected to develop metachronous or synchronous primaries at what rate?**
   a.   < 1% per year
   b.   1 to 4% per year
   c.   4 to 7% per year
   d.   7 to 10% per year
   e.   > 10% per year

90.3   **Stages III and IV, and possibly stage II, squamous cell carcinoma of the oral cavity is best managed with which of the following?**
   a.   Surgery alone
   b.   Radiation therapy alone
   c.   Surgery and, if indicated, postoperative radiotherapy
   d.   Combination of chemotherapy and radiotherapy
   e.   Induction chemotherapy followed by surgery and postoperative radiotherapy

90.4   **The sequential use of chemotherapy and radiation therapy in the treatment of SCCHN has been shown to**
   a.   Improve long-term survival of appropriately selected patients
   b.   Improve local control in treated patients
   c.   Improve regional control in treated patients
   d.   Decrease the incidence of distant metastases
   e.   Accomplish all of the above

90.5   In its publication in 1991, the VA Laryngeal Cancer Study Group (VACSP) showed that, for patients with advanced laryngeal cancers in need of total laryngectomy, induction chemotherapy (5-fluorouracil and cis-platinum) followed by definitive radiotherapy
   a.   Was superior to surgery and radiotherapy in terms of long-term survival
   b.   Improved local control better than surgery and postoperative radiotherapy
   c.   Effectively preserved laryngeal function in treated patients
   d.   Was as effective as surgery and postoperative radiotherapy in controlling disease
   e.   Provided no benefit over the then-standard surgery and postoperative radiotherapy

91.1   Which of the following odontogenic tumors is best described by the term *benign aggressive*?
   a.   Complex odontoma
   b.   Ossifying fibroma
   c.   Ameloblastoma
   d.   Adenomatoid odontogenic tumor

91.2   A radiographic pattern of mixed density on plain films would be most likely for which of the following odontogenic tumors?
   a.   Odontogenic fibroma
   b.   Ameloblastoma
   c.   Clear cell odontogenic tumor
   d.   Calcifying epithelial odontogenic tumor

91.3   The malignant ameloblastoma is distinguished from the ameloblastic carcinoma by which of the following characteristics?
   a.   A benign histologic pattern
   b.   Predominance of metastasis to bone
   c.   Systemic hypercalcemia
   d.   A characteristic immunofluorescent pattern

91.4   Among the fibro-osseous lesions, which of the following is considered to be a true tumor?
   a.   Focal cemento-osseous dysplasia
   b.   Cemento-ossifying fibroma
   c.   Periapical cemental dysplasia
   d.   Fibrous dysplasia

91.5   Malignancies metastatic to the jawbones are most likely to present in the posterior mandible. In women the most common index lesion is the breast. Which is the most common for men?
   a.   Lung
   b.   Prostate
   c.   Kidney
   d.   Colon

THE THORAX

92.1   Evaluation of a new 1 cm noncalcified left lower lobe mass could be performed by
   a.   Review of any old films (chest radiographs, computed tomography [CT] scans of the chest)
   b.   Repeat CT scans of the chest after 2 to 3 months
   c.   Positron emission tomography (PET) scans of the chest
   d.   Wedge resection of the nodule
   e.   All of the above

92.2   All of the following tumors can be approached surgically *except*
   a.   A 4.5 cm tumor with focal involvement of the superior vena cava and no nodal involvement
   b.   A 2 cm tumor involving the carina tracheae with no nodal involvement
   c.   A 3 cm peripheral lung cancer with an ipsilateral pleural effusion containing malignant cells
   d.   A 5 cm tumor with rib involvement and N1 nodal positivity

92.3   Which of the following statements is true with regard to lung cancer screening?
   a.   Recent trials with CT screening have established its ability to reduce lung cancer mortality.
   b.   Improved survival seen in the Mayo Clinic lung cancer project was correlated with a reduction in disease-specific mortality.
   c.   CT screening identifies a high proportion of T1 tumors.
   d.   CT screening is highly specific.

92.4 Survival of stage 1 nonsmall cell lung cancer (NSCLC) is higher if patients are treated with surgery than with radiotherapy alone. Which one of the following statements does *not* help to explain this?
   a. Surgically treated patients are also surgically staged, whereas irradiated patients tend to be clinically staged.
   b. Radiation does not kill enough cancer cells without chemotherapy to cure NSCLC.
   c. Surgically treated patients tend to have better performance status than irradiated patients.
   d. Lung tumors tend to move with respiration. Because motion is often not explicitly measured, some irradiated tumors are outside the radiation ports for a portion of their treatment.

93.1 A 72-year-old retired man was admitted for recent dyspnea on exertion. Chest radiographs revealed a right pleural effusion. Physical findings were otherwise unremarkable, and he was afebrile. Thoracentesis yielded 1,200 mL of clear exudate, and cytology was negative for malignant cells. Pleural needle-biopsy showed "reactive fibrosis." He had a 20 pack-year history of cigarette smoking, and he quit smoking 30 years prior. A history-taking revealed that during World War II he worked for 10 months as a pipe-fitter in a naval shipyard. A computed tomographic (CT) scan of the chest showed minimal residual pleural fluid and thickening. Bronchoscopy results were entirely normal. The most appropriate course of action for this patient is
   a. Injection of a sclerosing agent into the pleural cavity
   b. A short trial of oral corticosteroid therapy
   c. Careful follow-up including chest radiography every 3 months
   d. Thoracoscopy
   e. Exploratory thoracotomy

93.2 Exposure to asbestos can lead to the following pleural manifestations *except*
   a. Pleural calcifications
   b. Benign pleural plaques
   c. Benign pleural effusion
   d. Malignant mesothelioma
   e. Benign mesothelioma

93.3 Besides asbestos exposure, other factors incriminated in the etiology of malignant mesothelioma in men include all of the following *except*
   a. Exposure to zeolite fibers (erionite)
   b. Prior history of radiotherapy
   c. Cigarette smoking
   d. A family history of malignant mesothelioma

94.1 The malignant nature of a thymoma is best determined by
   a. The histologic characteristics of epithelial cells
   b. The ratio of epithelial cells to lymphocytes
   c. The presence of myasthenia gravis
   d. The invasive nature of the tumor

94.2 Syndromes associated with thymomas include
   a. Red cell aplasia
   b. Hypogammaglobulinemia
   c. Myasthenia gravis
   d. Hypogammaglobulinemia and myasthenia gravis
   e. Red cell aplasia, hypogammaglobulinemia, and myasthenia gravis

94.3 Which of the following statements regarding thymic carcinomas is *not* true?
   a. At the difference of thymomas, epithelial cells appear cytologically malignant.
   b. Some thymic carcinomas have been linked to Epstein-Barr virus.
   c. Thymic carcinoma includes a small cell type, similar to oat cell lung cancer.
   d. Thymic carcinoma does not include a lymphoepithelioma type.

94.4 A 42-year-old patient underwent surgery for a lymphoepithelial thymoma. In one area the tumor invaded the thymic capsule and mediastinal fat. A complete en bloc surgical resection was performed with pathologically negative margins. What further course of treatment would you recommend?
   a. No further treatment but regular follow-up visits and CT scans
   b. A course of adjuvant chemotherapy with a platinum combination
   c. Radiotherapy to the mediastinum
   d. Treatments in both answers (b) and (c)

95.1 **The most common cardiac tumor is**
a. Lipoma
b. Myxoma
c. Fibroelastoma
d. Angiosarcoma

95.2 **The most common site of cardiac myxoma is the**
a. Right atrium
b. Right ventricle
c. Left atrium
d. Left ventricle

95.3 **Which one of the following manifestations does *not* occur in cardiac myxomas?**
a. Clubbing
b. A characteristic finding at auscultation (tumor plop)
c. Embolic episodes
d. Fever and leukocytosis indicating associated infectious endocarditis

96.1 **A variety of hematologic neoplasms including acute myelomonocytic leukemia and acute megakaryocytic leukemia have been associated with which of the following neoplasms?**
a. Primary mediastinal seminoma
b. Primary mediastinal teratocarcinoma
c. Embryonal carcinoma of the testis
d. Primary retroperitoneal teratocarcinoma
e. All of the above

96.2 **A 25-year-old male is referred from a thoracic surgeon to consider further therapy. This patient had a 5 cm asymptomatic mediastinal mass discovered on a chest radiograph taken during an army entrance physical examination. A chest computed tomography (CT) scan showed a well-circumscribed 5 × 5 cm anterior mediastinal mass; the remainder of the staging work-up was normal. He underwent a mediastinal exploration through a sternal incision, and a well-circumscribed tumor was removed in its entirety. Pathology revealed a mediastinal seminoma. Postoperatively, serum human chorionic gonadotropin (hCG) and α-fetoprotein (AFP) levels are normal. At this point, you would recommend**
a. Close observation with no further treatment
b. Radiation therapy (30 Gy) to the mediastinum
c. Radiation therapy (50 Gy) to the mediastinum
d. Two courses of chemotherapy with cisplatin, etoposide, and bleomycin
e. Three courses of chemotherapy with cisplatin and etoposide

96.3 **A 27-year-old male develops rapidly worsening substernal chest pain as well as swelling of his arms, face, and neck. On physical examination, it is determined that he has superior vena cava syndrome. Chest radiographs reveal a large anterior mediastinal mass. CT scans of the chest/abdomen confirm the presence of a 14 cm anterior mediastinal mass; in addition, three noncalcified lung nodules are seen (two in the right lung, one in the left lung). Routine laboratory evaluation is normal except for a lactate dehydrogenase level of 650 U/L. Serum levels of hCG and AFP are normal. A core needle biopsy of the anterior mediastinal mass reveals a seminoma. Appropriate management includes which of the following?**
a. Open biopsy of the mediastinal mass, via a parasternal incision, to confirm diagnosis
b. Fine-needle aspiration biopsy of one of the lung nodules to confirm the presence of metastatic disease
c. Immediate radiation therapy to relieve superior vena cava syndrome
d. Immediate chemotherapy with cisplatin, etoposide, and bleomycin
e. Immediate therapy with concurrent radiation therapy and carboplatin or etoposide

96.4 **A 30-year-old man presents with cough, substernal chest pain, and increasing dyspnea. He is found to have a 10 cm anterior mediastinal mass as well as a right pleural infusion. Serum tumor markers indicate an AFP level of 8,500 and an hCG level of 450. A needle biopsy of the mediastinal mass reveals nonseminomatous tumors with features of teratocarcinoma mixed with endodermal sinus tumor. After four courses of chemotherapy with cisplatin, etoposide, and bleomycin, restaging reveals a persistent 5 × 4 cm mediastinal mass as the only residual radiographic abnormality. Serum tumor markers are normal. Optimal management of this patient now includes**
a. Surgical resection of the residual anterior mediastinal mass
b. Two additional courses of cisplatin, etoposide, and bleomycin
c. Monthly follow-up with chest radiography and determination of AFP and hCG levels
d. Consideration for further treatment with high-dose ifosfamide, carboplatin, and etoposide and autologous peripheral stem cell support
e. Salvage chemotherapy with vinblastine, ifosfamide, and cisplatin

97.1   What is the probability that a clinically detectable pulmonary nodule is malignant in a patient with *no* history of malignancy?
   a.   < 10%
   b.   10–20%
   c.   20–30%
   d.   30–40%
   e.   40–50%

97.2   Which of the following is *not* a criterion for surgical resection of a malignant pulmonary nodule?
   a.   An absence of extrathoracic metastases
   b.   Control of the primary tumor
   c.   Prior reception of induction chemotherapy
   d.   A > 60-day tumor doubling time (TDT)
   e.   The number of metastases

97.3   Which of the following is *not* true about TDT?
   a.   It can be calculated using chest radiography or computed tomography (CT).
   b.   In patients with multiple metastases, it should be determined on the fastest-growing lesion.
   c.   A TDT of > 500 days generally indicates a benign lesion.
   d.   TDT is not related to the histology of the primary neoplasm.
   e.   It can be used to determine candidates for pulmonary metastasectomy.

97.4   Pulmonary metastasectomy has *not* been shown to improve survival with which of the following tumor types?
   a.   Colorectal carcinoma
   b.   Melanoma
   c.   Osteogenic sarcoma
   d.   Pancreatic carcinoma
   e.   Testicular cancer

97.5   Which of the following is *not* true concerning surgical pulmonary metastasectomy?
   a.   If the primary and metastatic lesions present simultaneously, the primary lesion should be addressed first.
   b.   Patients with bilateral metastases should undergo resection of the most involved side first.
   c.   A margin of 1 to 2 cm is adequate.
   d.   Video-assisted thoracic surgery (VATS) should only be used a diagnostic tool.
   e.   Continuity with the chest wall is not a contraindication for pulmonary metastasectomy.

GASTROINTESTINAL TRACT

98.1   The most common esophageal neoplasm in North America is
   a.   Adenocarcinoma
   b.   Squamous cell carcinoma
   c.   Leiomyoma
   d.   Small cell carcinoma
   e.   A metastatic nodule from another tumor site

98.2   Esophageal cancer patients most commonly present with
   a.   Weight loss
   b.   No symptoms
   c.   Heartburn
   d.   Dysphagia
   e.   Pain

98.3   The most accurate method of assessing tumor depth in nonobtructing esophageal cancer is
   a.   A positron emission tomography scan
   b.   A computed tomography scan
   c.   Barium swallow
   d.   Endoscopic ultrasonography (EUS)
   e.   Clinical symptoms

98.4   Surgery alone is best suited for which stage of esophageal cancer?
   a.   Stage I
   b.   Stage IIA/IIB

c. Stage III
d. Stage IVA
e. All of the above

98.5 **Locoregionally advanced esophageal cancer (stage I–IVA) is often treated with a combined modality approach because of the high rate of failure with surgery alone. Which multimodality approach has shown the *least* promise in this stage of disease compared with surgery alone?**
a. Surgery followed by postoperative radiation
b. Preoperative chemotherapy followed by surgery
c. Preoperative chemoradiation followed by surgery
d. Chemotherapy and radiation with surgery as salvage therapy
e. All of the above

99.1 **Endoscopic mucosal resection (EMR) is suitable for definitive management of which of the following lesions?**
a. T1 lesion, 1.5 cm in diameter with signet ring histology, detected by ultrasonography
b. T1 lesion, 2.5 cm in diameter, Borrmann type IIa, detected by ultrasonography
c. Ultrasound T1 lesion, 1 cm in diameter with central ulcer, detected by ultrasonography
d. Ultrasound T2 lesion, 1 cm in diameter, well differentiated, detected by ultrasonography

99.2 **Among patients in the United States, the 5-year survival rates for resected stage IIIA and IIIB gastric cancer are**
a. 34% and 20%
b. 28% and 20%
c. 20% and 8%
d. 44% and 28%

99.3 **A 54-year-old Hispanic woman presents with abdominal distention, weight loss, and early satiety. On examination she was found to have ascites, a periumbilical nodule, and a right adnexal mass. Biopsy revealed a mucinous adenocarcinoma. Esophagogastroduodenoscopy showed gastritis and prominent gastric folds. Colonoscopy was normal. You recommend**
a. Surgical debulking followed by carboplatin and paclitaxel
b. Jumbo biopsy of the stomach
c. Induction chemotherapy with carboplatin and paclitaxel
d. Cancer antigen (CA) 125 and carcinoembryonic antigen (CEA) tests

100.1 **Treatment of a small hepatoma in a cirrhotic patient includes all of the following *except***
a. Radiofrequency ablation
b. Liver transplantation
c. Chemoembolization
d. Hepatic lobectomy
e. Ethanol ablation

100.2 **Over the past two decades in the United States, incidence and mortality rates have been**
a. Increasing for hepatocellular carcinoma (HCC) and decreasing for cholangiocarcinoma
b. Decreasing for HCC and increasing for cholangiocarcinoma
c. Increasing for both HCC and cholangiocarcinoma
d. Decreasing for both HCC and cholangiocarcinoma

100.3 **The higher incidence rates of HCC seen in men compared with those in women are likely partly explained by**
a. Higher rates of alcoholic cirrhosis in men
b. A protective effect of oral contraceptive use in women
c. More frequent tobacco use in men

101.1 **Which of the following define a high risk of recurrence in patients after resection of liver metastases derived from colorectal cancer? (More than one may be correct.)**
a. Node-positive primary
b. Age
c. Largest tumor > 5 cm
d. Sex

101.2 **The proportion of patients with colorectal cancer and liver metastases at diagnosis is**
a. 5%
b. 15%

    c.   35%

    d.   40%

101.3   **The most appropriate treatment for hepatic metastases (three or less) derived from colorectal carcinoma is**

    a.   Systemic chemotherapy

    b.   Cryosurgery

    c.   Liver resection

    d.   Radiofrequency ablation

101.4   **Factors that prevent a patient from being a candidate for resection are**

    a.   A high number of lesions

    b.   Synchronous disease

    c.   Involvement of both the right and left lobes

    d.   None of the above

101.5   **Treatment with hepatic arterial infusion results in which of the following toxicities? (More than one may be correct.)**

    a.   Nausea and vomiting

    b.   Ulcer disease

    c.   Diarrhea

    d.   Hepatic enzyme elevations

103a.1   **Symptoms of pancreatic cancer include all of the following *except***

    a.   A change in bowel function

    b.   Hyperglycemia

    c.   Abdominal and/or back pain

    d.   Hypertension

    e.   Scleral icterus

103a.2   **Environmental factors may be responsible for what percentage of pancreatic cancers?**

    a.   10%

    b.   20%

    c.   40%

    d.   80%

103a.3   **When pancreatic cancer is suspected, the most useful radiographic study is**

    a.   Transabdominal ultrasonography

    b.   Computed tomography (CT)

    c.   Magnetic resonance imaging (MRI)

    d.   Endoscopic retrograde cholangiopancreatography (ERCP)

    e.   Endoscopic ultrasonography (EUS)

103a.4   **The optimal management of a patient with obstructive jaundice secondary to a presumed pancreatic head cancer is**

    a.   Exploratory laparotomy with surgical biliary bypass

    b.   ERCP with endobiliary stent placement

    c.   Percutaneous transhepatic cholangiography with catheter placement

    d.   Nasobiliary endoscopic decompression

103a.5   **A patient underwent pancreaticoduodenectomy, and the final pathology demonstrated a 2.5 cm adenocarcinoma confined to the pancreatic head with three positive regional lymph nodes. The correct American Joint Committee on Cancer (AJCC) tumor/node/metastasis (TNM) staging for this patient would be**

    a.   Stage IB

    b.   Stage IIA

    c.   Stage IIB

    d.   Stage III

103b.1   **Patients with periampullary neoplasms usually present with**

    a.   Abdominal and/or back pain

    b.   Jaundice

    c.   Weight loss

    d.   Nausea/vomiting

103b.2 Which of the following is *not* true regarding lymph node metastases in a patient with an ampullary carcinoma?
   a.   It is a contraindication to potentially curative surgery.
   b.   It is associated with a less favorable outcome after curative resection.
   c.   It is not as powerful a prognostic factor as it is with pancreatic cancer.
   d.   It is a reason to consider the patient for adjuvant therapies.

103b.3 The overall accuracy of endoscopic ultrasound (EUS) in staging depth of tumor invasion is
   a.   ≤ 50%
   b.   50 to 70%
   c.   71 to 85%
   d.   > 85%

103b.4 Contraindications for local excision of periampullary neoplasms include all of the following *except*
   a.   A high false-negative endoscopic biopsy rate
   b.   The technical difficulty of the operation
   c.   The frequent local recurrence
   d.   The difficulty of determining depth of tumor invasion by EUS

103b.5 Duodenal cancer develops in what percentage of patients with familial adenomatous polyposis (FAP) syndrome?
   a.   ≤ 5%
   b.   10 to 20%
   c.   30 to 50%
   d.   > 75%

104.1 The most common symptomatic benign tumor of the small bowel is
   a.   Lymphangioma
   b.   Adenoma
   c.   Hemangioma
   d.   Lipoma
   e.   Leiomyoma

104.2 All of the following systemic diseases increase the risk of small bowel adenocarcinoma *except*
   a.   Regional enteritis
   b.   Celiac disease
   c.   Nontropical sprue
   d.   Rheumatoid arthritis
   e.   Crohn's disease

104.3 The most common site in the small bowel for carcinoid tumors is the
   a.   Ampulla of Vater
   b.   Duodenum
   c.   Jejunum
   d.   Proximal ileum
   e.   Distal ileum

104.4 Gastrointestinal (GI) stromal tumors express which mutated tyrosine kinase?
   a.   Epidermal growth factor receptor
   b.   *bcr-abl*
   c.   c-*kit*
   d.   *src*
   e.   Platelet-derived growth factor receptor

104.5 The current drug of choice for patients with unresectable or locally advanced GI stromal tumors is
   a.   Doxorubicin
   b.   Ifosfamide
   c.   5-Fluorouracil
   d.   Imatinib mesylate
   e.   Platinum

105.1 The most common tumor of the appendix is
   a.   Adenocarcinoma
   b.   Carcinoid

    c.   Lymphoma

    d.   Cystic borderline neoplasm

    e.   Sarcoma

105.2   **Management of appendiceal carcinoid tumors is based on**

    a.   Grade

    b.   Size

    c.   Degree of differentiation

    d.   Depth of invasion into the appendiceal muscle wall

    e.   Presence or absence of vascular invasion

105.3   **Pseudomyxoma peritonei is most aggressively treated with**

    a.   Systemic chemotherapy

    b.   Radiation therapy

    c.   Surgical debulking plus intraperitoneal chemotherapy

    d.   Surgical resection of the appendix

    e.   Observation

105.4   **The management of adenocarcinoma of the appendix is determined by**

    a.   Size

    b.   Grade

    c.   Depth of wall invasion

    d.   Degree of differentiation

    e.   Vascular invasion

106.1   **Risk factors for colorectal cancer include all of the following *except***

    a.   Peutz-Jeghers syndrome

    b.   Age

    c.   Gender

    d.   Family history of colorectal cancer

    e.   Prior history of adenomas

106.2   **Tumor markers routinely used clinically in the management of colorectal cancer include**

    a.   TP53

    b.   18q deletion

    c.   Microsatellite instability (MSI)

    d.   All of the above

    e.   None of the above

106.3   **Which of the following statements is correct?**

    a.   If the primary tumor is adherent to contiguous organs or structures, en bloc resection is *not* necessary if the patient is planned for postoperative chemotherapy and/or radiation therapy.

    b.   Primary colorectal tumor resection is contraindicated in the presence of hepatic metastases.

    c.   Cytoreductive therapy is routinely performed for carcinomatosis in patients with peritoneal dissemination from colorectal cancer.

    d.   Obstruction and perforation of colorectal cancer have no adverse prognosis in terms of survival.

    e.   Patients with colon adenocarcinoma and metastatic disease do not need to have their primary tumor resected prior to starting systemic therapy.

106.4   **Which of the following statements is *not* true?**

    a.   Preoperative neoadjuvant chemoradiation has not been proven to be more effective than postoperative chemoradiation for stage II and stage III rectal adenocarcinomas.

    b.   Both preoperative radiation therapy and postoperative radiation therapy have been shown to decrease local recurrence rates after the treatment of stage II and III rectal adenocarcinomas.

    c.   The Dutch Mesorectal Trial proved that radiation therapy is not necessary if a total mesorectal excision is performed.

    d.   Obtaining a negative radial margin of resection is important in the management of rectal cancer.

    e.   The expertise of the surgeon performing rectal cancer surgery has been shown to influence prognosis.

106.5   **Adjuvant chemotherapy after curative resection of colon cancer is indicated in which of the following scenarios?**

    a.   Stage I colon cancer

    b.   Stage I colon cancer with lymphovascular invasion

    c.   Stage II colon cancer

d. Stage III colon cancer
e. All of the above

107.1 The most common infectious agent correlated with the development of anal canal cancers is
a. *Chlamydia*
b. Human papillomavirus (HPV)
c. Gonorrhea
d. Human immunodeficiency virus (HIV)
e. *Trichomonas*

107.2 The most common serious toxicity in trials of multimodality therapy for anal carcinoma, using the combination of 5-fluorouracil and mitomycin-C, has been
a. Hematologic
b. Gastrointestinal
c. Renal
d. Pulmonary

107.3 Overall 5-year survival for anal carcinoma with combination 5-fluorouracil/mitomycin-C chemotherapy and radiation therapy in a large number of studies is generally in the range of
a. 35 to 40%
b. 55 to 60%
c. 75 to 80%
d. 95 to 100%

107.4 Which of the following treatments is not an acceptable alternative in the management of positive inguinal lymph nodes?
a. Multimodality therapy *with* an excisional biopsy of the involved node(s)
b. Radiation therapy alone in patients who cannot tolerate chemotherapy
c. Multimodality therapy *without* an excisional biopsy of the involved node(s)
d. Superficial and deep groin dissection

107.5 The prognosis of primary melanoma of the anal canal is primarily related to which of the following?
a. DNA ploidy
b. Percentage of S-phase cells
c. Tumor thickness
d. Tumor grade

GENITOURINARY TRACT

108.1 The gene for von Hippel-Lindau disease is located on chromosome
a. 1
b. 3
c. 8
d. 11
e. 17

108.2 The most common presenting symptom of renal cell carcinoma is
a. Frequency
b. Urgency
c. Hematuria
d. Flank pain
e. Palpable mass

108.3 Imaging of the inferior vena cava is best accomplished by
a. Ultrasonography
b. Computed tomography scan
c. Magnetic resonance imaging
d. Positron emission tomography scan
e. Inferior venacavography

108.4   **The preferred treatment for a 3 cm renal cell carcinoma is**
a.   Enucleation
b.   Partial nephrectomy
c.   Radical nephrectomy
d.   Radiation therapy
e.   Combination immunotherapy and chemotherapy

108.5   **Debulking nephrectomy prior to immunotherapy should be considered in patients with**
a.   Poor performance status
b.   Bilateral renal cell carcinoma
c.   Disease predominant in the kidney
d.   Inferior vena caval involvement
e.   Multiple hepatic metastases

109.1   **Transitional cell carcinoma (TCC) of the renal pelvis is**
a.   More common than bladder cancer
b.   Equal in incidence to bladder cancer
c.   More common in men than women
d.   Often bilateral
e.   Less common than ureteral carcinoma

109.2   **The most common symptom of renal pelvic TCC is**
a.   Flank pain
b.   Hematuria
c.   Urinary frequency
d.   Urinary urgency
e.   Bone pain

109.3   **Staging evaluation for renal pelvic TCC should include all *except***
a.   Chest radiography
b.   Determination of alkaline phosphatase levels
c.   Magnetic resonance imaging
d.   Urinary cytology
e.   Serum multichannel analysis test

109.4   **The preferred management of high-grade TCC of the renal pelvis with a normal contralateral kidney is**
a.   Partial nephrectomy
b.   Radical nephrectomy
c.   Nephroureterectomy with bladder cuff
d.   Radiation therapy
e.   Chemotherapy

109.5   **The preferred chemotherapy for TCC of the renal pelvis is**
a.   M-VAC (methotrexate, vinblastine, doxorubicin [Adriamycin], cisplatin)
b.   Carboplatin
c.   Paclitaxel
d.   Gemcitabine
e.   Cisplatin

110.1   **Which of the following is *not* a known risk factor for bladder cancer?**
a.   Cigarette smoking
b.   Male gender
c.   Black race
d.   Infection with *Schistosoma haematobium*
e.   Exposure to aromatic amines

110.2   **Which of the following intravesical agents has *not* been shown to reduce the risk of recurrence of Ta (noninvasive) bladder tumors?**
a.   Bacille Calmette-Guérin (BCG)
b.   Mitomycin-C
c.   Doxorubicin

d.   Thiotepa
e.   5-Fluorouracil

110.3   A patient undergoes a radical cystectomy for a muscle-invasive transitional cell carcinoma of the bladder, and pathology shows metastatic disease in one of the pelvic nodes. The most appropriate management of this patient is
a.   Adjuvant cisplatin-based chemotherapy
b.   Adjuvant radiation therapy
c.   Surveillance
d.   Adjuvant cisplatin-based chemotherapy or surveillance
e.   Adjuvant chemoradiation

110.4   Which of the following statements about chemotherapy for metastatic urothelial carcinoma is *incorrect*?
a.   Cisplatin and carboplatin have equivalent efficacy.
b.   M-VAC (methotrexate, vinblastine, doxorubicin [Adriamycin], cisplatin) represents an appropriate first-line regimen.
c.   The GC (gemcitabine, cisplatin) doublet represents an appropriate first-line regimen.
d.   CMV (cisplatin, methotrexate, vinblastine) represents an appropriate first-line regimen.
e.   The PC (paclitaxel, carboplatin) doublet has never been studied in a completed phase III trial.
f.   There are no phase III trials of second-line chemotherapy.

110.5   Appropriate therapy for bladder cancer invading into the muscularis propria includes all of the following *except*
a.   Radical cystectomy
b.   Cystoprostatectomy
c.   Aggressive transurethral resection of the tumor followed by combined therapy using chemoradiation
d.   Intravesical BCG
e.   Partial cystectomy

111.1   Which of the following factors has *not* been associated with an increased risk of developing prostate cancer?
a.   Being of African American race
b.   Having a father with prostate cancer
c.   Having benign prostatic hypertrophy (BPH)
d.   Being of older age
e.   Eating a high-fat diet

111.2   In determining risk of recurrence after treatment of a patient with newly diagnosed prostate cancer, all of the following are useful *except*
a.   Biopsy Gleason score
b.   Serum prostate-specific antigen (PSA)
c.   Clinical stage
d.   Percentage of biopsy cores involved
e.   Percentage of free-to-total PSA in serum (% free PSA)

111.3   Which of the following is a *rarely* seen complication of external beam radiotherapy?
a.   Erectile dysfunction
b.   Urinary incontinence
c.   Mild rectal irritation
d.   Acute cystitis
e.   Mild fatigue during treatment

111.4   All of the following are acceptable methods of hormonal therapy for a patient with newly diagnosed metastatic prostate cancer *except*
a.   Leuprolide alone
b.   Leuprolide plus flutamide
c.   Flutamide alone
d.   Diethylstilbestrol (DES)
e.   Bilateral orchiectomy

111.5   Chemotherapy is best considered for use in which of the following clinical states?
a.   Newly diagnosed patient being considered for radical prostatectomy
b.   Adjuvant use in a patient at high risk of recurrence after radical prostatectomy
c.   Asymptomatic patient with a rising PSA test and negative bone scan after radiation therapy
d.   Metastatic disease currently responding to hormonal therapy
e.   Symptomatic disease no longer responding to hormonal therapy

112.1   **Options for treatment of biopsy-proven superficial squamous carcinomas of the penis include**
a.   Local surgical excision
b.   Topical chemotherapy
c.   Laser surgery
d.   Mohs' micrographic surgery
e.   All of the above

112.2   **The most important prognostic factor in the management of squamous carcinoma of the penis is**
a.   Involvement of the corpora cavernosa
b.   Tumor grade
c.   Lymphatic crossover at the base of the penile shaft
d.   Tumor involvement of the inguinal nodes
e.   Obstructive voiding symptoms

112.3   **With respect to female urethral carcinoma,**
a.   Squamous carcinoma is the most common histologic type
b.   Tumor grade markedly influences prognosis and metastatic spread
c.   Urethral tumors are more common in non-Caucasian women
d.   Undifferentiated carcinoma is the second most common histopathology
e.   Transitional cell carcinoma and adenocarcinoma are extremely rare in the female urethra

112.4   **Which of the following is *not* a characteristic of the majority of male urethral cancers?**
a.   They arise in the bulbar urethra.
b.   They are squamous cell carcinomas.
c.   They commonly produce obstructive symptoms.
d.   They may be associated with urethral stricture disease.
e.   Metastases from distant sites are common.

113.1   **A 25-year-old patient presents with a painless mass in his right testis. An orchiectomy reveals a yolk sac tumor and a teratoma. Staging work-up reveals an ipsilateral 7 cm right-sided retroperitoneal mass. Results of a chest computed tomography (CT) scan are normal. Physical examination reveals a fullness in the abdomen but is otherwise completely normal. Serum human chorionic gonadotropin (hCG) is normal; α-fetoprotein preorchiectomy is 800 ng/mL and postorchiectomy is 1,000 ng/mL. He is treated with three courses of BEP (bleomycin, etoposide, cisplatin). The abdominal mass reduces in size to 5 cm, and the α-fetoprotein returns to normal. A postchemotherapy retroperitoneal lymph node dissection reveals a mature teratoma.**

    Follow-up remains normal until 7 years later. A routine annual evaluation revealed a serum α-fetoprotein of 500 ng/mL; a repeat count is 550 ng/mL. His history and physical examination are completely normal. An abdominal and pelvic CT scan reveals a 5 cm right pelvic mass but is otherwise normal. Results of a chest CT scan are normal. What is the optimal therapy for this patient?
a.   Salvage chemotherapy with platinum and ifosfamide–based salvage chemotherapy
b.   Salvage chemotherapy with high-dose chemotherapy and peripheral stem cell rescue
c.   Four courses of cisplatin and etoposide
d.   Surgical resection of the residual pelvic mass

113.2   **A 27-year-old patient presented with a left testicular mass. Orchiectomy revealed pure embryonal cell carcinoma. His pre-orchiectomy hCG was 120 mIU/mL, and α-fetoprotein was 90 ng/mL. One week later his hCG was normal and his α-fetoprotein was 130 ng/mL. Results of a chest CT scan were normal. An abdominal and pelvic CT scan revealed a 3 × 3 cm left para-aortic node. Your recommendation for this patient would be to undergo**
a.   Repeat serum markers in 1 week and make a decision at that time
b.   Nerve-sparing retroperitoneal lymph node dissection
c.   Three courses of chemotherapy with BEP
d.   Four courses of chemotherapy with cisplatin and etoposide

113.3   **Using the International Staging System for nonseminomatous germ cell tumors, which of the following does *not* constitute advanced disease (poor risk)?**
a.   Histology of pure choriocarcinoma
b.   Serum α-fetoprotein > 10,000 ng/mL
c.   Presence of cutaneous metastases
d.   Primary mediastinal yolk sac tumor with an 8 cm anterior mediastinal mass as the only evidence of disease

FEMALE REPRODUCTIVE ORGANS

114.1 **Treatment of basal cell carcinoma of the vulva is**
  a. Radical vulvectomy with inguinal femoral lymphadenectomy
  b. Radical vulvectomy alone
  c. Simple vulvectomy
  d. Wide local excision
  e. Laser vaporization of lesion

114.2 **Treatment of a large verrucous vulvar carcinoma is**
  a. Preoperative radiation with radical vulvectomy
  b. Radical vulvectomy with nodal sampling
  c. Radical vulvectomy alone
  d. Radical vulvectomy and postoperative radiation
  e. Simple vulvectomy

114.3 **The most frequent nonsquamous cell malignancy of the vulva is**
  a. Sarcoma
  b. Paget's disease
  c. Melanoma
  d. Verrucous carcinoma
  e. Bartholin's gland carcinoma

114.4 **Lymphatic drainage of the lower one-third of the vagina is directly to the**
  a. Pelvic lymph nodes
  b. Aortic lymph nodes
  c. Inguinal lymph nodes
  d. Obturator lymphoses
  e. Sentinel lymph nodes

114.5 **The cambian zone is associated with which vaginal malignancy?**
  a. Squamous cell
  b. Embryonal rhabdomyosarcoma
  c. Endodermal sinus tumor
  d. Melanoma
  e. Clear cell adenocarcinoma

115.1 **Which of the following statements concerning carcinoma of the cervix is correct?**
  a. Carcinoma of the cervix is the most common cancer among women worldwide.
  b. The incidence and mortality rates in developing countries in Latin America are similar to incidence and mortality rates reported in Spain, Canada, and China.
  c. In the United States, the incidence rates for cervical cancer have declined in the past 45 years because of the introduction of screening with the Pap smear and the treatment of precancerous conditions.
  d. The American Cancer Society as well as the American College of Obstetricians and Gynecologists have reliable data on the prevalence and incidence of precancerous cervical lesions occurring annually in the United States.
  e. In the United States, the incidence rates for invasive cervical cancer show no significant racial-ethnic differences.

115.2 **Which of the following risk factors has the most significant epidemiologic research evidence supporting an etiologic role in cervical neoplasia?**
  a. Herpes simplex virus type 2
  b. Multiple sexual partners
  c. Human papillomavirus (HPV)
  d. Cigarette smoking
  e. Early age of first sexual intercourse

115.3 **Which of the following statements concerning adenocarcinoma of the cervix is correct?**
  a. Adenocarcinomas represent approximately 5% of all invasive cervical carcinomas today.
  b. Well-differentiated villoglandular adenocarcinomas follow an aggressive clinical course and are best treated with concomitant chemotherapy and external beam and intracavitary radiation therapy.

c.   Adenoid basal carcinomas consist of small uniform cells resembling basal cell carcinomas and have a clinical course similar to small cell neuroendocrine carcinomas.

d.   Papillary serous adenocarcinomas occur in the endometrium and ovary. A histologically identical lesion arising in the cervix has not been encountered.

e.   Adenocarcinomas with an endometrioid pattern represent the second most common type of primary endocervical adenocarcinoma.

115.4   Which of the following statements concerning small cell carcinoma of the cervix is correct?

a.   It is frequently associated with hypercalcemia.

b.   It is more common in women older than 60 years.

c.   It is resistant to external beam and intracavitary radiation therapy.

d.   It is a very aggressive cancer and systemic spread is frequently present at the time of initial diagnosis.

e.   It is more sensitive to chemotherapy than oat cell carcinoma of the lung.

115.5   Which of the following statements concerning the human papillomavirus is correct?

a.   The viral infection can be eliminated by any of three outpatient therapies to the cervix: cryotherapy, laser vaporization, or loop electrosurgical excision procedure (LEEP).

b.   HPV deoxyribonucleic acid (DNA) of the intermediate-risk and high-risk types are found with the same frequency in patients with either high-grade squamous intraepithelial lesions or adenocarcinoma in situ.

c.   During infection, HPV integrates its high-risk DNA into the host genome of cervical cancer cells and such integration leads to an increased expression of E6 and E7, which are virus-encoded proteins that can disrupt the cell regulatory process.

d.   Following the initial infection with HPV and expression of E6 and E7 proteins, the damage is continuous and such increased expression is not necessary for maintaining the infected cell in the transformed state.

e.   The development of effective vaccines for prevention of precancerous lesions of the cervix focus on virus-encoded proteins found in the long control region of the HPV genome.

115.6   Which of the following statements concerning the spread of carcinoma of the cervix is correct?

a.   Skip metastases to aortic lymph nodes, bypassing the pelvic nodes, is more common in patients with stage IB1 cancers than in patients with IB2 cancers.

b.   The degree of cellular differentiation and the depth of stromal invasion of the cervix are more important prognostic factors than the presence of multiple positive low pelvic lymph nodes.

c.   Magnetic resonance imaging (MRI) is the preferred method of defining lymph node metastases according to Fédération Internationale de Gynécologie et d'Obstétrique (FIGO) guidelines.

d.   The FIGO staging guidelines are based on the findings of surgical documentation of the extent of the disease.

e.   The finding of carcinoma in a pelvic lymph node by fine-needle aspiration (FNA) does not change the clinical stage of a carcinoma according to FIGO guidelines.

115.7   Which of the following statements concerning external beam radiation therapy in the treatment of patients who have invasive carcinomas of the cervix is correct?

a.   Linear accelerators provide a wide range of high-energy electrons that are superior to high-energy photons in the treatment of carcinoma of the cervix.

b.   External beam radiation therapy with 4 mV photons is threefold more effective than gamma rays emitted from a cobalt 60 unit in the treatment of an obese patient with an anterior-posterior pelvic diameter measuring 30 cm.

c.   High-energy linear accelerators emit a photon beam that has a greater skin-sparing effect than gamma rays emitted by a cobalt 60 unit.

d.   The four-field technique may be used only with 15 to 25 mV machines emitting photons, and the four-field technique cannot be used with cobalt 60 or 4 to 6 mV photon units.

e.   The use of the four-field technique is contraindicated when concurrent chemotherapy is being administered.

115.8   Which of the following statements concerning normal tissue's sensitivity to ionizing radiation is correct?

a.   Ionizing radiation damages the small arteries and induces an occlusive effect.

b.   The mucosa of the stomach and duodenum are resistant to ionizing radiation because there are no stem cells in the mucosa.

c.   The vascular occlusive effects of collagen diseases or arteriosclerosis are not accelerated by ionizing radiation.

d.   The acute diarrhea that occurs in patients receiving whole pelvis external beam radiation is due to a hypermotility syndrome that has no relationship to stem cell function or height of the villi lining the distal small bowel.

e.   The endarteritis induced by ionizing radiation is a reversible process.

115.9   A 32-year-old otherwise healthy patient (gravida 4, para 4) with a tubal ligation had an abnormal Pap smear and a small biopsy of the exocervix that revealed a squamous cell carcinoma invading 2 mm into the cervical stroma. No vascular space involvement was identified. There was no visible lesion on the cervix. Which of the following statements is correct?

a.   The logical treatment would be to proceed directly to a modified radical hysterectomy and pelvic lymph node lymphadenectomy.

b.   Treatment options based on the available information would include external beam radiation plus brachytherapy.

c.   Conization of the cervix with endocervical curettage would be an unnecessary step in the management of this patient.

      d.   The FIGO stage of this invasive carcinoma would be a stage IB1.
      e.   None of the above are correct.

115.10   **Which of the following statements is correct in reference to the use of chemotherapy for patients with squamous cell carcinoma of the cervix?**
      a.   Combination chemotherapy involving three agents is superior to single-agent chemotherapy in patients who have distant metastases because the disease-free survival and overall survival is increased threefold by the use of the three-drug combination.
      b.   Combination *cis*-platinum plus fluorouracil intravenous chemotherapy is the treatment of choice following node-positive radical hysterectomy and pelvic lymphadenectomy.
      c.   Single-agent carboplatinum induces a complete clinical response rate of 30% in patients with metastatic squamous carcinoma versus single-agent *cis*-platinum's complete response rate of 10 to 12%.
      d.   Neoadjuvant chemotherapy is recommended for patients with 5 cm cervical carcinomas when a radical hysterectomy and pelvic lymphadenectomy are part of the treatment plan.
      e.   None of the above are correct.

116.1   A 55-year-old female with a grade 3 adenocarcinoma diagnosed by office biopsy undergoes an exploratory laparotomy, peritoneal washings, hysterectomy, bilateral salpingo-oophorectomy, and a pelvic and aortic lymphadenectomy. Intraoperatively, there is no gross evidence of extrauterine disease. The final pathology reveals a grade 3 endometrioid adenocarcinoma with 70% myometrial invasion. The tumor is 3 cm in diameter and occupies the lower uterine segment; it invades the stroma of the cervix. The lymph nodes show no evidence of tumor; however, the peritoneal washings reveal malignant cells. The International Federation of Gynecology and Obstetrics (FIGO) surgical stage of this patient is
      a.   IC
      b.   IIB
      c.   IIIA
      d.   IB
      e.   IIIB

116.2   **Which of the following is *not* a risk factor associated with endometrial cancer?**
      a.   Nulliparity
      b.   Obesity
      c.   Hypertension
      d.   Granulosa-theca cell tumor of the ovary
      e.   Oral contraceptive use

116.3   **Incidence of progression to carcinoma in patients with complex atypical hyperplasia is**
      a.   1%
      b.   3%
      c.   8%
      d.   29%
      e.   49%

116.4   **Which is the most common histologic subtype in endometrial carcinoma?**
      a.   Endometrioid adenocarcinoma
      b.   Adenosquamous carcinoma
      c.   Uterine papillary serous carcinoma (UPSC)
      d.   Endometrial papillary adenocarcinoma
      e.   Clear cell carcinoma

116.5   **Which of the following statements is *not* true regarding treatment of stage I adenocarcinoma of the endometrium?**
      a.   Exploratory surgery (laparotomy or laparoscopy), peritoneal washings, and hysterectomy/bilateral salpingo-oophorectomy should be performed in stage I grade 1 tumors.
      b.   Exploratory surgery (laparotomy or laparoscopy), peritoneal washings, hysterectomy/bilateral salpingo-oophorectomy, and selective pelvic and aortic lymphadenectomy should be performed for stage I grade 3 tumors.
      c.   Lymphadenectomy should be performed for the following high-risk factors regardless of stage: > 50% myometrial invasion, clear cell or papillary serous histology, adnexal masses, lymph-vascular space invasion, cervical invasion.
      d.   The hysterectomy should be intrafascial.

117.1   A 46-year-old female undergoes an exploratory laparotomy for a 5 cm complex left adnexal mass diagnosed by ultrasonography. Intraoperatively the patient is found to have a normal-appearing left adnexa; however, the left fallopian tube is enlarged and densely adherent to the pelvic side wall. Frozen section assessment of the left fallopian tube reveals a poorly differentiated adenocarcinoma. The patient undergoes a total abdominal hysterectomy, bilateral salpingo-oophorectomy, pelvic and aortic lymphadenectomy, omentectomy, and abdominal peritoneal biopsies. Results of peritoneal washings are negative. The final pathology reveals a poorly differentiated papillary serous adenocarcinoma of the left fallopian tube extending to the submucosa. The omentum, lymph nodes, and pelvic and aortic lymph nodes are free of tumor. What is the International Federation of Gynecology and Obstetrics (FIGO) surgical stage of this patient?

a. IA
b. IIA
c. IIB
d. IIIA
e. IIIB

117.2 **Which of the following statements is *not* a diagnostic criterion for carcinoma of the fallopian tube?**

a. Grossly, the main tumor is in the tubes and arises from the endosalpinx.
b. In the presence of microscopic ovarian metastases, the tumor arising from the endosalpinx must be > 1 cm.
c. Histologically, the pattern reproduces the epithelium of the tubal mucosa (papillary pattern).
d. A transition from benign to malignant tubal epithelium is demonstrated.
e. The ovaries and endometrium are normal or have a much smaller tumor volume than that of the tube.

117.3 **The most consistent prognostic factor in the literature associated with survival from fallopian tube carcinoma is**

a. Stage
b. Amount of residual disease after cytoreduction
c. Histologic grade
d. Extent of tubal invasion
e. Presence of ascites

117.4 **The most active chemotherapy regimens in the treatment of fallopian tube carcinoma are**

a. Cisplatin-based regimens
b. Cyclophosphamide-based regimens
c. Hormonal-based regimens
d. Melphalan-based regimens

117.5 **The incidence of nodal metastases in apparent stage I fallopian tube carcinoma is**

a. 5%
b. 15%
c. 33%
d. 50%
e. 66%

118.1 **A 54-year-old woman is diagnosed with stage III epithelial ovarian cancer. After her initial surgery, a sample of tissue is evaluated that reveals overexpression of the *HER2/neu* oncogene. The finding is most directly associated with which of the following?**

a. Response to chemotherapy
b. Overall prognosis
c. Tumor grade
d. Stage of disease

118.2 **Following initial surgery, a 50-year-old woman with stage III epithelial ovarian cancer underwent Southern blot analysis of ovarian tissue, which disclosed a mutated *P53* tumor suppressor gene. This finding has been found to correlate positively with**

a. Patient age
b. Stage of disease
c. Exposure to asbestos
d. Family history of ovarian cancer
e. Histologic type of ovarian cancer

118.3 **A 37-year-old woman with a CA 125 measurement of 89 IU is diagnosed with a unilateral solid adnexal mass. The patient wishes to preserve her fertility. At exploratory laparotomy, a mixed cystic solid ovarian tumor is removed. There is no evidence that there is any other disease in the upper abdomen and retroperitoneal spaces, and the contralateral ovary appears entirely normal. Examination of a frozen section reveals a borderline serous tumor, apparently confined to the removed ovary. Of the following, which is the most appropriate therapy for this patient?**

a. Unilateral salpingo-oophorectomy
b. Bilateral salpingo-oophorectomies
c. Bilateral salpingo-oophorectomies and total abdominal hysterectomy
d. Bilateral salpingo-oophorectomies, total abdominal hysterectomy, pelvic and para-aortic lymphadenectomy, and omentectomy

118.4   A 38-year-old woman presents with amenorrhea, breast atrophy, acne, hirsutism, clitorimegaly, a deepening voice, and a receding hairline. On pelvic examination, a 9 cm firm mobile right adnexal mass is palpated. Of the following, which is the most likely diagnosis?
   a.   Immature teratoma
   b.   Endodermal sinus tumor
   c.   Sertoli-Leydig cell tumor
   d.   Granulosa-theca cell tumor
   e.   Mucinous cystadenocarcinoma

118.5   A 9-year-old premenarchal girl presents with an apparently rapid enlarging abdominopelvic mass. Results of a computed tomography scan suggest a large solid ovarian tumor. α-Fetoprotein serum concentration is 38 ng/dL, and human chorionic gonadotropin is 1,500 IU/mL. Of the following lesions, which is the most likely diagnosis?
   a.   Embryonal carcinoma
   b.   Immature teratoma
   c.   Choriocarcinoma
   d.   Dysgerminoma

118.6   A 55-year-old woman presents with a 12 cm adnexal mass. An exploratory laparotomy is performed, and an intact unilateral cystic ovarian tumor is found. There is no evidence of ascites and no palpable evidence of disease outside of the ovary. During removal, the mass is ruptured. Results of a frozen section are consistent with a well-differentiated (stage I) serous adenocarcinoma of the ovary without capsular penetration or surface excrescenses. A comprehensive staging laparotomy, including a pelvic and para-aortic lymphadenectomy, is performed; all biopsies are normal. Of the following, what is the best management of this patient?
   a.   No further treatment
   b.   Postoperative radiation
   c.   Intraoperative radiocolloid
   d.   Postoperative chemotherapy

118.7   A 65-year-old woman presents with postmenopausal bleeding. Pelvic examination shows a normal-size uterus with an 8 cm left adnexal mass. Endometrial biopsy results are consistent with a well-differentiated adenocarcinoma of the endometrium. Which of the following malignancies is most likely to be a synchronous ovarian tumor?
   a.   Brenner tumor
   b.   Immature teratoma
   c.   Serous cystadenocarcinoma
   d.   Mucinous cystadenocarcinoma
   e.   Endometrioid cystadenocarcinoma

119.1   The most common site of metastasis with gestational trophoblastic tumors is the
   a.   Ovary
   b.   Vagina
   c.   Lung
   d.   Liver
   e.   Brain

119.2   Patients with persistent gestational trophoblastic tumors with small vaginal metastases and low human chorionic gonadotropin (hCG) levels (low-risk stage II) are generally treated with
   a.   Radiation therapy
   b.   Surgical resection
   c.   Single-agent chemotherapy
   d.   Combination chemotherapy
   e.   Surgical resection and adjuvant chemotherapy

119.3   Patients with persistent gestational trophoblastic tumors with large lung metastases and high hCG levels are generally treated with
   a.   Single-agent chemotherapy
   b.   Surgical resection and chemotherapy
   c.   Surgical resection alone
   d.   Combination chemotherapy
   e.   Radiation therapy

119.4   Patients who have nonmetastatic gestational trophoblastic tumors and desire to retain fertility are generally treated with
   a.   Local uterine resection
   b.   Local uterine resection and adjuvant single-agent chemotherapy

    c.   Intracavitary radiation
    d.   Single-agent chemotherapy
    e.   Combination chemotherapy

120.1   **Sarcomas of the uterus comprise what percent of uterine tumors?**
    a.   1 to 2%
    b.   3 to 5%
    c.   6 to 8%
    d.   10 to 15%

120.2   **The classification of uterine sarcomas by the Gynecologic Oncology Group (GOG) includes**
    a.   Stromal sarcomas and leiomyosarcoma
    b.   Rhabdomyosarcoma and carcinosarcoma
    c.   Chondrosarcoma, osteosarcoma, and carcinosarcoma
    d.   Leiomyosarcoma, endometrial stromal sarcoma, and carcinosarcoma

120.3   **The most active single agent for treatment of carcinosarcoma is**
    a.   Ifosfamide
    b.   Cisplatin
    c.   Doxorubicin
    d.   Etoposide

120.4   **The most active single agent for leiomyosarcoma is**
    a.   Ifosfamide
    b.   Cisplatin
    c.   Doxorubicin
    d.   Etoposide

120.5   **The primary treatment for sarcomas of the uterus is**
    a.   Radiation therapy
    b.   Chemotherapy
    c.   Radiation followed by surgery
    d.   Surgery

THE BREAST

121.1   **Which of the following statements most accurately describes the behavior of breast cancer in the United States?**
    a.   Breast cancer has the highest mortality of any tumor in US women.
    b.   The risk of developing breast cancer for women of any age is 1 in 8.
    c.   The percentage of women who die from their breast cancer has increased by 5% during the past 10 years.
    d.   Thirty percent of women who have breast cancer ultimately die from their disease.
    e.   The percentage of patients who are initially seen with invasive ductal carcinoma has increased because of the influence of mammography.

121.2   **Which of the following statements concerning ductal carcinoma in situ (DCIS) is *not* correct?**
    a.   The frequency of this diagnosis has been increasing with wider use of mammography for screening purposes.
    b.   Of the many subtypes, the comedocarcinoma DCIS has the worst prognosis and least favorable histologic pattern.
    c.   HER2/neu protein overexpression, a poor prognostic indicator, has not been observed in the papillary and cribriform subtypes of DCIS.
    d.   A high labeling index has been observed in the case of comedocarcinoma DCIS.
    e.   Evaluation of estrogen receptor (ER) and progesterone receptor (PR) status is an important prognostic indicator for DCIS.

121.3   **A well-educated 45-year-old woman has been diagnosed with breast cancer and is being evaluated for surgical treatment. She is aware of the importance of lymph node status as a prognostic indicator. Which of the following statements is correct?**
    a.   Even after excising the first six lymph nodes, the more lymph nodes that are removed, the easier it becomes to assess prognosis.
    b.   Nodal metastasis is no longer believed to be the most significant prognostic factor in determining risk of relapse after 5 and 10 years because of the description of factors such as *P53* tumor suppressor gene content, *BRCA1/BRCA2* mutations, and HER2/neu protein overexpression.
    c.   The presence of sinus histiocytosis in the lymph nodes is always a poor prognostic indicator.
    d.   The relapse rate at 5 years but not at 10 years is significantly greater for patients with ≥ four nodes with metastases as compared with patients who have one to three nodes.
    e.   The National Surgical Adjuvant Breast Project (NSABP)-04 trial demonstrated that after mastectomy, histologic grade and tumor size are helpful in further determining prognosis at 5 and 10 years in patients who have ≥ four nodes with metastases.

121.4 A 57-year-old American woman began menstruating at age 12, went into menopause at age 52, and had her first child at age 34. She currently uses estrogen replacement therapy. She has one glass of wine with dinner every night and has a 50 pack-year history of smoking. Which of the following statements regarding her risk of developing breast cancer is true?

a. The administration of even low doses of estrogen increases the risk of developing breast cancer at least fourfold in postmenopausal women. This effect is less prominent in premenopausal women.
b. Alcoholic beverages may have a protective effect regarding breast cancer, provided the drinking is not excessive.
c. Cigarette smoking, especially with a greater than 40 pack/year exposure, has been demonstrated to increase the likelihood of breast cancer.
d. Menarche at age 12 confers twice the risk of breast cancer as does menarche at age 13.
e. Women who have children in their thirties may still have less risk of developing breast cancer than women who remain nulliparous. This is believed to be related to the fact that nulliparous women will have more ovulatory cycles.

121.5 Studies of the biology of breast cancer have led to the discovery of various growth factors and hormones, as well as several oncogenes, which might play a role in the behavior of the malignant cells that define this disease. Which of the following statements regarding the preceding is *not* true?

a. In experimental systems, ER-negative cells are more sensitive to the effects of the inhibitory factor tumor growth factor β (TGF-β) than are ER-positive cells.
b. Autostimulation of breast cancer cells by autocrine and paracrine modulation of estrogen-induced growth factors may favor tumor growth.
c. Antiestrogens have a cytocidal effect because of their ability to arrest cells in the S phase.
d. Families who have mutations in the tumor suppresser gene *P53* are prone to breast cancer as well as other tumors.
e. Transgenic mice that express the oncogenes *myc, ras*, and *HER2/neu* in a tissue-specific pattern have an increased incidence of both benign and malignant breast pathology.

121.6 Which of the following histologic subtypes of invasive breast cancer is associated with the worst prognosis?

a. Infiltrating ductal carcinoma
b. Medullary carcinoma
c. Tubular carcinoma
d. Colloid carcinoma
e. Papillary carcinoma

121.7 A 67-year-old woman who has invasive ductal carcinoma of the right breast is found to have 2 of 10 lymph nodes that contain cancer at the time of her axillary lymph node dissection. The metastatic work-up is negative. Which of the following statements concerning this patient's therapeutic course is accurate?

a. The benefit of tamoxifen therapy beyond 6 months is unclear.
b. If tamoxifen is used as the only therapy, the patient's chances for long-term survival will not be increased.
c. Toxicities (cumulative) limit the long-term use of tamoxifen.
d. Tamoxifen will increase the risk of atherosclerotic heart disease by raising the circulating levels of cholesterol.
e. Use of tamoxifen is associated with a slight increase in the risk of uterine cancer.

121.8 A 65-year-old woman is seen with a large fungating chest wall mass and metastatic bone lesions. She is diagnosed with stage IV breast cancer. As her oncologist, you know that in this situation one of the following statements is *not* correct. Which one?

a. The fact that her tumor was ER-positive on review of the pathologic specimen and that her Cancer and Leukemia Group B (CALGB) performance score was 0 (highest) predicts that she will have a good response to a combination chemotherapy regimen that includes doxorubicin.
b. Although complete remission rates are approximately 10 to 20%, patients who receive combination chemotherapy have a median survival of 2 years.
c. The cyclophosphamide, Adriamycin (doxorubicin), 5-fluorouracil (CAF) combination may actually be slightly more effective than cyclophosphamide, methotrexate, and 5-fluorouracil (CMF); however, the toxicity is greater.
d. If the initial therapy does not yield a response, the total response rate to salvage regimens, even when these consist of combinations of drugs, is approximately 20 to 30%.
e. In metastatic disease, a strategy of stopping chemotherapy after six to eight cycles is no better than continuing chemotherapy constantly until the disease progresses.

121.9 A 63-year-old woman was diagnosed with stage IV breast cancer 2 years ago and was found to have an ER- and PR-positive tumor. Tamoxifen therapy was started and caused a partial response associated with a minimal tumor burden and no progression. The patient returns to your office for routine follow-up and asks you whether it is time to start her on chemotherapy in addition to her tamoxifen. How would you answer this question?

a. The majority of studies addressing this question show no advantage of combination endocrine/chemotherapy treatment.
b. You recommend chemotherapy because the patient has had only a partial response. The addition of chemotherapy to her treatment will thus enhance her chances of a more prolonged survival.

c. Hormonal agents are contraindicated in patients receiving chemotherapy because these agents induce a quiescent chemoresistant state in the cancer cells.

d. You recommend the administration of estrogen to prime the cancerous cells. This can result in an increase in the S-phase fraction, during which the cells are more chemosensitive, and therefore a greater cell kill ensues when cytotoxic drugs are administered.

e. Postmenopausal women may paradoxically have a recrudescence of their tumors when chemotherapy is added to a successful hormonal chemotherapy.

121.10 **On performing a routine breast examination, it is possible to encounter a number of findings that must be interpreted with caution. Which of the following interpretations of different physical signs is true?**

a. The presence of a bloody discharge almost always means that there is an underlying breast cancer, and therefore this finding warrants further investigation.

b. Regarding palpation of axillary lymph nodes, clinical judgment is inaccurate, with 75% false-negative findings and 50% false-positive findings.

c. The presence of pain is most common in the diagnosis of breast cancer. Therefore, a pathologic specimen needs to be obtained from the painful tissue to exclude the presence of neoplastic cells.

d. On palpation, fibrocystic disease seems to blend into the surrounding tissue, whereas cancerous lumps usually have well-defined borders and are fairly fixed into the rest of the glandular structure.

e. Cyclic breast pain is uncommon in premenstrual women. This symptom usually is due to perimenopausal hormonal surges and is commonly associated with an underlying carcinoma that flares with the endocrine stimulus.

121.11 **Many studies have been carried out analyzing the indications for mammography as a screening tool for breast cancer. These studies have been plagued by different weaknesses and criticisms, and their meaning is still debated today. Other trials are still ongoing in the attempt to clarify this complex issue. Which of the following statements is correct?**

a. Studies that report survival rates or average survival time are likely to be particularly accurate because they avoid biases that commonly occur when studying breast cancer incidence and mortality in response to mammography screening.

b. Lead-time bias refers to the fact that the date of death of a woman from breast cancer will be delayed with the influence of mammography, therefore causing a bias in the interpretation of the results.

c. Length-time bias refers to bias incurred due to the discovery of more slow-growing tumors in the screened group, whereas patients who have more rapidly growing tumors will be diagnosed at other times. Thus, the screened group will seem to be doing better because of the less biologically malignant nature of their disease.

d. Counting the number of deaths from breast cancer in both group studies (screening and not screened) is prone to lead-time and length-time bias and should be avoided.

e. Length-time bias refers to bias incurred due to the fact that screened women are diagnosed with larger or more progressed tumors that have been growing longer. This makes the issue of improved survival from screening efforts difficult to interpret.

121.12 **Which of the following statements regarding the proper use of screening procedures for early detection of breast cancers is *not* correct?**

a. Women over the age of 50 and under the age of 74 years should have yearly mammographic examinations because this has been shown to reduce their risk of dying from breast cancer by 70%.

b. Although it has not been conclusively demonstrated that women between the ages of 40 and 49 years should undergo yearly mammography, this issue should be decided between a patient and her physician in view of the particulars of her case.

c. The role of self-breast examination (SBE) is not entirely clear because there are no data to show that this practice definitely prolongs survival, even though it has been shown to lead to earlier detection. In spite of this, SBE is recommended routinely.

d. The interpretation of data regarding the efficacy of mammography screening in women 40 to 49 years old requires a longer follow-up (at least 8 years) to begin to detect different survival times between screened and nonscreened groups.

e. Women who have a positive history of a first-degree relative with breast cancer should have their first mammography between 30 and 35 years of age.

121.13 **A 48-year-old woman had a stage II (lymph-node positive) breast cancer treated by lumpectomy and radiotherapy, followed by adjuvant chemotherapy with CAF. The cancer was strongly ER- and PR-positive. Following the chemotherapy, she started receiving tamoxifen therapy. During the chemotherapy, her menstrual periods ceased, and she developed severe hot flashes before the onset of tamoxifen therapy. The hot flashes became debilitating. Which of the following would you recommend?**

a. Replacement estrogen therapy

b. A barbiturate

c. A progestational agent

d. Reassurance

e. Synthroid

121.14 **A 64-year-old man is found to have multiple bilateral pulmonary nodules as revealed by chest radiography 4 years after a right radical mastectomy for breast cancer. Results of a bone scan are normal, and a search for other primary sources of cancer is not productive. This patient's second marriage occurred 6 months ago. The preferred method of management would be**

a. Stilbestrol, nonenteric coated, 5 mg tid

b. Medroxyprogesterone

c. CAF chemotherapy
d. Bilateral orchiectomy
e. Luteinizing hormone–releasing hormone analogues

121.15 Carcinoma of the breast in men
a. Generally has a better prognosis than similar stage disease in women
b. Is typically treated in a similar fashion as in women
c. Can be predicted by the presence of *BRCA1* and *BRCA2* gene mutations
d. Is clinically evident by unilateral gynecomastia in most men
e. Accounts for 5% of malignancies in men

121.16 Which of the following is a true statement regarding cystosarcoma phyllodes?
a. They are a variant of lobular carcinoma in situ.
b. Most lesions are malignant and tend to spread rapidly to the regional lymph nodes.
c. They have a high grade of multifocality and are often bilateral.
d. Wide local excision or simple mastectomy is usually sufficient for therapy.
e. Preoperative chemotherapy is typically indicated for large primary lesions, followed by salvage mastectomy.

121.17 Which of the following statements regarding ductal carcinoma in situ (DCIS) and lobular carcinoma in situ (LCIS) of the breast is true?
a. They are derived from similar cell types of the breast.
b. They have an equal risk of subsequent invasive malignancy.
c. They have an equal incidence of bilateral occurrence.
d. DCIS is typically associated with subsequent development of invasive disease. Patients with LCIS typically have occult invasion at the time of presentation.
e. The risk of synchronous invasive cancer is higher in patients with DCIS, and patients with LCIS may have bilateral disease.

121.18 A 46-year-old woman is seen with a 2.5 cm right upper outer quadrant breast mass and is noted on a mammogram to have diffuse microcalcifications throughout the same breast. Needle-directed biopsy demonstrates DCIS. The management of this lesion should be
a. Segmental resection, with evaluation of the surgical margins in order to determine if segmental resection alone is proper therapy
b. Lumpectomy followed by postoperative external beam radiotherapy to the remaining breast
c. Segmental resection with follow-up mammography in order to determine the change in the calcification overtime
d. Total mastectomy
e. Lumpectomy and axillary lymph node dissection

121.19 The management of DCIS of the breast is controversial. Several new molecular markers have been developed in order to determine which patients have a worse prognosis. These include all *but*
a. HER2/neu protein overexpression
b. Flow cytometry in order to determine S-phase fraction of the tumor
c. Sialyl-Tn expression
d. Chromosome I aneusomy
e. *P53* tumor suppressor gene overexpression of the primary tumor

121.20 A 52-year-old woman is seen with an ill-defined right breast mass and dimpling of the skin. Biopsy of the skin demonstrates lymphatic invasion with adenocarcinoma. Results of a metastatic work-up with chest radiography, computed tomography (CT) scan of the abdomen, and bone scan were normal. The therapy at this point should be
a. Modified radical mastectomy with postoperative cyclophosphamide, methotrexate, and 5-fluorouracil (5-FU)(CMF)
b. Preoperative external beam radiotherapy and lumpectomy followed by postoperative CMF
c. Combination chemotherapy with cyclophosphamide, doxorubicin, and 5-FU (CAF) followed by modified radical mastectomy if the patient responds to initial therapy, followed by postoperative radiotherapy
d. Four cycles of preoperative chemotherapy and, if there is a response, bone marrow transplantation with high-dose chemotherapy
e. High-dose chemotherapy with stem-cell transplantation, followed by salvage mastectomy

121.21 A patient with a history of breast cancer who was treated with lumpectomy and axillary node dissection, followed by postoperative radiotherapy 5 years earlier, develops a recurrence in the ipsilateral breast. At this point, the patient should be treated with
a. Lumpectomy with additional postoperative radiotherapy
b. Systemic chemotherapy
c. Total mastectomy
d. Tamoxifen alone
e. Additional radiotherapy isolated to the recurrence

THE SKIN

122.1   **A 45-year-old man is evaluated with a 8 mm black nevus on the abdominal wall. Excisional biopsy demonstrated a Clark III 1.5 mm thick nodular melanoma. What should be the next step in management?**
a.   The patient should receive adjuvant interferon-α over a 1-year course.
b.   The margins of wide excision vary according to the primary site, and in this case 4 cm margins are appropriate.
c.   The primary should be excised with 2 cm margins, and the patient should be considered for lymphatic mapping and sentinel lymphadenectomy.
d.   No further therapy is necessary.

122.2   **A 50-year-old active man has a history of a Clark level V 4 mm thick melanoma of the right arm. Four years after treatment of the primary disease, this patient is found to have two asymptomatic pulmonary metastases in the right upper lobe. Both tumors are 2 cm in size. The next step in management should be to**
a.   Complete the staging evaluation, and if otherwise negative, proceed with pulmonary resection
b.   Obtain whole body positron emission tomography (PET) scan and treat with outpatient 5-FU–based chemotherapy regimen
c.   Treat with single-agent dacarbazine (DTIC)
d.   Consider the patient for hospice home care as stage IV melanoma is not curable
e.   Complete the patient's staging work-up, and if otherwise negative, treat with interferon-α 5 million units subcutaneously administered weekly for 48 weeks

122.3   **A 64-year-old man presents after excisional biopsy of a Clark level V 6 mm thick melanoma of the right temporal scalp. The next step in management should be**
a.   External beam radiation of 5,000 cGy to the scalp and right neck
b.   Mohs' surgical resection of the scalp primary
c.   Wide surgical resection employing 2 cm margins with skin graft repair
d.   Staging evaluation with computed tomography (CT) scans of the neck, chest, abdomen, and pelvis followed by DTIC-based chemotherapy
e.   Wide surgical resection followed by prophylactic radiation to the right neck

122.4   **A 30-year-old woman presents after biopsy of a Clark level II 0.55 mm thick melanoma of the back. She has had numerous dysplastic nevi removed from her torso in the past. The next step in management should be**
a.   Wide excision of the melanoma with 1 cm margins and continued close follow-up as she likely has the familial atypical mole-melanoma syndrome
b.   Genetic analysis to examine this patient for chromosome alterations on the short arm of 1
c.   Screening of other family members for dysplastic nevi, melanoma, and pancreatic cancer
d.   Observation
e.   Treatment with a melanoma differentiation antigen peptide vaccine

122.5   **A 45-year-old man has a history of a Clark level IV 4.25 mm thick melanoma of the left heel. Three years after wide excision of the primary melanoma, this patient develops approximately 50 dermal metastases on the calf and distal thigh. Staging evaluation demonstrates no other sites of metastases. The next step in management should be**
a.   Left superficial groin dissection and hyperthermic isolated limb perfusion with melphalan
b.   Excision and hyperthermia of the skin lesions
c.   High-dose bolus interleukin-2 administered as 600,000 IU/kg every 8 hours for 5 consecutive days
d.   DTIC-based chemotherapy
e.   Intralesional injection of the skin lesion with bacille Calmette-Guérin

123.1   **Which molecular signaling pathway has been found to be perturbed in hereditary and sporadic basal cell carcinomas?**
a.   Wint
b.   Sonic hedgehog
c.   *ras*
d.   Stat-Jak
e.   None of the above—no pathway is determined for sporadic tumors

123.2   **What is the treatment of choice for dermatofibrosarcoma protuberans (DFSP)?**
a.   Wide excision with 3 cm margins
b.   Wide excision with adjuvant radiation
c.   Wide excision with sentinel lymph node examination
d.   Mohs' micrographic surgery with margin control
e.   Intralesional interferon

123.3 A female patient presents with multiple perioral skin-colored papules on her face that have been diagnosed as trichilemmomas. What is the appropriate work-up?
a. Genetic screening for *PTEN* mutation
b. Mammography
c. Gastrointestinal endoscopy
d. Laser ablation of lesions by a cosmetic surgeon
e. Mohs' micrographic surgery of lesions

123.4 A patient is referred to you with a single yellowish 5 mm papule on the left cheek of several months' duration. Results of a shave biopsy reveal sebaceous carcinoma. You should inform the patient that
a. A single lesion of this type is not concerning
b. A wide excision is necessary to prevent metastasis
c. Mohs' surgery is required to prevent recurrence
d. Surgery and radiation are required
e. A systematic work-up for internal malignancy is warranted

123.5 A cutaneous squamous cell carcinoma (SCC) on which of the following locations has the highest rate of mestasis?
a. Lip
b. Eyelid
c. Ear
d. Penis
e. Scalp

BONE AND SOFT TISSUE

124.1 Most classic high-grade osteosarcomas are at which stage on presentation?
a. IA/IB
b. IIA
c. IIB
d. III

124.2 Giant cell tumor of the bone would be the diagnosis for which of the following patients?
a. 10-year-old male with a diaphyseal radiolucent lesion
b. 50-year-old female with a lesion in the iliac wing
c. 25-year-old female with a radiolucent lesion in her distal femur
d. 35-year-old male with a lesion in the middle phalange
e. 14-year-old male with a lesion in the humeral head

124.3 Aspirin relieves pain most dramatically in which type of tumor?
a. Osteoid osteoma
b. Osteoblastoma
c. Osteosarcoma
d. Ewing's sarcoma
e. Lymphoma

124.4 Adjuvant chemotherapy for a typical chondrosarcoma includes which of the following?
a. Methotrexate
b. Ifosfamide
c. Doxorubicin
d. Dactinomycin
e. None of the above

124.5 Which tumor is in the Ewing's family of tumors?
a. Langerhans cell histiocytosis
b. Primitive neuroectodermal tumor
c. Lymphoma
d. Myeloma
e. Clear cell sarcoma

125.1 All of the following have been associated with the development of human soft tissue sarcoma *except*
 a. Mutation of the *P53* gene
 b. Rous sarcoma virus infection
 c. Polyvinyl chloride exposure
 d. Radiation exposure
 e. Immunosuppression

125.2 A 46-year-old man is seen with abdominal fullness and a palpable 6 cm lower abdominal mass. Work-up demonstrates a low-density mass in the retroperitoneum, and biopsy suggests a low-grade liposarcoma. The most appropriate therapy is
 a. Preoperative chemotherapy followed by resection and postoperative external beam radiotherapy
 b. Preoperative chemotherapy followed by resection
 c. Complete surgical resection, if possible
 d. Preoperative chemotherapy based on chemosensitivity of the primary lesion; then complete surgical resection followed by postoperative radiotherapy
 e. Partial resection for palliation of symptoms followed by postoperative external beam radiotherapy

125.3 A patient with a retroperitoneal sarcoma has been followed up with routine computed tomography (CT) scans of the abdomen after having complete surgical resection 2 years previously. The CT scan reveals a mass in the retroperitoneum adjacent to the left kidney. The patient is asymptomatic, and treatment should be
 a. Surgical resection in order to reduce the tumor burden and hopefully to prevent further recurrences
 b. Preoperative external beam radiotherapy combined with intraoperative radiotherapy and resection
 c. High-dose external beam radiotherapy alone in order to preserve the kidney
 d. Observation and resection only if the patient is symptomatic from disease
 e. High-dose methotrexate

125.4 A 35-year-old man is seen with a large (8 × 10 cm) mass on the proximal thigh. Which of the following is true regarding biopsy of this lesion?
 a. Because the patient has not noticed a change in the lesion in 6 months, a follow-up visit should be scheduled in 6 months to determine if a biopsy is indicated for this stable lesion.
 b. An experienced pathologist can diagnose malignant sarcomas by fine-needle biopsy.
 c. Excisional biopsy of this large lesion is indicated because it is probably malignant, and an incisional biopsy would only disseminate disease.
 d. A transverse biopsy excision is preferred over incisional biopsies of extremity soft tissue sarcoma.
 e. Frozen-section analysis is not justified if at least a 1 cm specimen is sent for permanent section review.

125.5 Which statement best reflects our understanding of soft tissue sarcomas?
 a. The AJCC classification of soft tissue sarcomas reflects the universal organization of sarcomas based on anatomic site of the primary.
 b. The AJCC staging system for soft tissue sarcomas is based on TNM status, with tumor size the only important prognostic factor.
 c. There is no universally accepted classification system for soft tissue sarcomas.
 d. The AJCC clinicopathologic staging system for soft tissue sarcoma depends primarily on tumor size and lymph node status.
 e. Histogenetic classification of sarcomas has been accepted because sarcomas have one cell type and are easily distinguishable.

125.6 Which of the following statements regarding the treatment of extremity soft tissue sarcomas is *not* correct?
 a. Internal hemipelvectomy can be performed for attempted limb salvage even if sarcoma is invading the ilium.
 b. Brachytherapy is most effective for low-grade tumors because it improves local control by 65% when compared with surgery alone.
 c. Adjuvant chemotherapy is well established for osteosarcoma and Ewing's sarcoma.
 d. Advances in multimodality therapy and improved operative techniques have allowed limb salvage for more than 90% of extremity soft tissue sarcomas.
 e. The role of preoperative radiotherapy limb salvage is more pronounced for those with large tumors.

125.7 Which of the following statements concerning soft tissue tumors is *not* correct?
 a. Liposarcoma is one of the most common soft tissue tumors.
 b. Desmoid tumors are treated with local excision and brachytherapy.
 c. The potential for metastasis of malignant fibrous histiocytoma (MFH) is directly related to the size and grade of the primary tumor.
 d. Alveolar rhabdomyosarcoma carries an extremely poor prognosis.
 e. Patients who have classic Kaposi's sarcoma have a higher incidence of secondary malignancies such as lymphoma.

HEMATOPOIETIC SYSTEM

127.1 **Which is the *least* important prognostic factor in patients with acute myelogenous leukemia (AML)?**
   a.   Immunophenotype
   b.   Cytogenetics
   c.   Age
   d.   White count at presentation
   e.   Lactate dehydrogenase (LDH) level at presentation

127.2 **Which of the following is the *least* important risk factor for the development of AML?**
   a.   Having undergone therapeutic radiation
   b.   Having undergone alkylating agent chemotherapy
   c.   Etoposide use
   d.   History of rheumatoid arthritis
   e.   Benzene exposure

127.3 **Which of the following agents is used to limit renal damage from tumor lysis syndrome in the treatment of patients with acute leukemia?**
   a.   Omeprazole
   b.   Ranitidine
   c.   Allopurinol
   d.   Ciprofloxacin
   e.   Furosemide

127.4 **Which of the following chemotherapeutic regimens is most effective in the postremission management of patients with AML?**
   a.   High-dose cytarabine
   b.   Idarubicin plus continuous infusion cytarabine
   c.   Daunorubicin, etoposide, and cytarabine
   d.   Etoposide plus cytarabine
   e.   High-dose etoposide and busulfan

127.5 **Over two-thirds of patients with acute promyelocytic leukemia (APL) can expect to enjoy prolonged disease-free survival based on therapy with which of the following strategies?**
   a.   Standard induction chemotherapy followed by allogeneic transplantation
   b.   Standard induction chemotherapy followed by autologous transplantation
   c.   Induction therapy with retinoic acid alone followed by consolidation chemotherapy
   d.   Concomitant retinoic acid and chemotherapy during induction, chemotherapy consolidation, and maintenance with retinoic acid
   e.   Concomitant retinoic acid plus chemotherapy during induction and consolidation chemotherapy

128.1 **A 56-year-old white man is found by his hematologist to have a white blood cell count of 56,000/µL and a differential count entirely consistent with chronic myelogenous leukemia (CML). The spleen is enlarged 3 cm below the left costal marginal. Two tests for the Philadelphia chromosome are negative. What is your next step?**
   a.   Change cytogeneticists
   b.   Determine Bcr-Abl
   c.   Tell the patient he does not have CML
   d.   Tell the patient he has a variant of CML

128.2 **A 25-year-old woman with a matched male sibling donor asks your opinion with respect to the treatment of CML in this era of imatinib therapy. Although there is a great variation in opinion, the majority of experienced hematologists would suggest**
   a.   A bone marrow and allogeneic transplantation be performed
   b.   A 6-month trial of imatinib followed by transplantation if necessary
   c.   Treatment with imatinib plus interferon plus cytarabine
   d.   Treatment with interferon alone

129.1 **At least 70% of children who have acute lymphoblastic leukemia are likely to be cured; however, only approximately one-third of adults who are seen with the same disease will have such a favorable outcome. Which of the following is the most important reason for this discrepancy?**
   a.   Adults are more likely to have lymphoblasts harboring a t(9;22) abnormality.
   b.   Adults who have acute lymphocytic leukemia (ALL) are more likely to have lymphoblasts that harbor a t(8;14) abnormality.
   c.   Adults are more likely to have central nervous system disease.

d. Adults have higher white blood cell counts than do children.

e. It is more difficult to administer full-dose chemotherapy to adults.

129.2 **In general, for a given cancer, the younger the patient the better the prognosis. Which of the following statements regarding this issue is _not_ correct?**

a. There are two age peaks for the incidence of ALL: childhood and age over 50 years.

b. Current protocols for ALL produce cure rates of 60 to 70% in children and 15 to 40% in adults.

c. The greater curability of younger patients is due primarily to their better tolerance of chemotherapy.

d. Cytogenetic, immunophenotyping, and molecular biology studies indicate that ALL is heterogeneous.

e. Hyperdiploidy occurs more commonly in pediatric ALL than in adult ALL.

130.1 **Which of the following combinations represents the characteristic immunophenotypic features of chronic lymphocytic leukemia (CLL)?**

a. CD19+, CD20+, CD5–, CD23–, CD103+, CD25+, sIg (bright)

b. CD19+, CD20+, CD5+, CD23–, sIg (bright)

c. CD19+, CD20+, CD5+, CD23–, sIg (bright)

d. CD19+, CD20+, CD5+, CD23+, sIg (dim)

130.2 **Which of the following combinations of features is associated with poor prognosis in CLL?**

a. del 13q, CD38+, trisomy 12, absence of IgVh gene mutations

b. del 13q, CD38–, del 11q, presence of IgVh gene mutations

c. del 17p, CD38+, del 11q, absence of IgVh gene mutations

d. del 17p, CD38+, trisomy 12, absence of IgVh gene mutations

130.3 **Which of the following is the correct statement regarding an immune disorder in CLL?**

a. The incidence of hypogammaglobulinemia increases with disease progression.

b. Autoimmune hemolytic anemia (AIHA) is common in CLL and mostly associated with cold antibodies.

c. Fludarabine is the treatment of choice for autoimmune hemolytic anemia in CLL.

d. Prophylactic γ-globulin therapy has been shown in a randomized clinical trial in CLL patients to reduce the incidence of infections and increase the survival time.

130.4 **Which of the following is _not_ a valid indication for starting systemic treatment for CLL?**

a. Disease-related symptoms such as weight loss, night sweats, and fever

b. Marked hypogammaglobulinemia

c. Anemia and/or thrombocytopenia

d. Lymphocyte doubling time of < 6 months with hyperlymphocytosis

130.5 **Which of the following statements is correct with regard to treatment of CLL?**

a. CLL is a curable disease with the presently available chemotherapy agents.

b. Fludarabine, as initial therapy, has proven to be superior to chlorambucil in achieving objective responses but has not resulted in significant improvement in overall survival in CLL.

c. Monoclonal antibodies such as rituximab or alemtuzumab, either used as single agents or in combination with fludarabine, have significantly increased the overall survival time in CLL.

131.1 **Hairy cell leukemia (HCL) is best characterized by which one of the following combinations of clinical manifestations?**

a. Splenomegaly and adenopathy

b. Pancytopenia and splenomegaly

c. Hepatomegaly and adenopathy

d. Pancytopenia and hepatomegaly

e. Pancytopenia and adenopathy

131.2 **Complications of the clinical course of HCL include all _except_ which one of the following?**

a. Atypical mycobacterial infections

b. Lytic bone lesions

c. Vasculitic skin lesions

d. Hematuria

e. Splenic rupture

131.3 **The immunophenotype for hairy cells is best characterized as**

a. CD5–, CD11c+, CD25+

b. CD5–, CD11c–, CD25–

    c.   CD5–, CD19+, CD103–

    d.   CD5–, CD19+, CD25–

    e.   CD11c+, CD19+, CD25–

131.4   The best treatment for a middle-aged man who has a palpable spleen, pancytopenia, and an absolute neutrophil count of 500/mm^2 is

    a.   Splenectomy

    b.   Interferon

    c.   Cladribine

    d.   Fludarabine

    e.   Cytarabine

131.5   Administration of interferon therapy is indicated in patients who have bone marrow that is

    a.   Hypercellular

    b.   Hypocellular

    c.   Unobtainable

    d.   Packed with hairy cells

    e.   Packed with metastatic carcinoma

132.1   Which of the following represents a newly generated mediator of mast cell inflammation?

    a.   Neutral proteases

    b.   Chondroitin sulfate

    c.   Biogenic amines

    d.   Peroxidase

    e.   Prostaglandin D$_2$

132.2   A 35-year-old female patient is known to have multiple discrete hyperpigmented nodular papule lesions that, at biopsy, are proven to be owing to infiltration with mature mast cells. The patient feels well, and her complete blood count and radiographic evaluation reveal no other sites of disease. Which of the following physical findings is most likely to be associated with this condition?

    a.   Flushing

    b.   Pruritus after showering

    c.   Urticaria wheals after mechanical trauma

    d.   Pleural rub

    e.   Systolic murmur augmented with deep inspiration

132.3   An activating mutation in which of the following genes is responsible for independent growth of mast cells in systemic mastocytosis?

    a.   c-*abl*

    b.   Platelet-derived growth factor receptor β

    c.   c-*kit*

    d.   *FLT3*

    e.   *ras*

133.1   Splenectomy may be performed as part of the staging for Hodgkin's disease. Patients at highest risk of postsplenectomy sepsis are

    a.   Those who have splenectomy as a result of trauma, idiopathic thrombocytopenic purpura (ITP), or hereditary spherocytosis

    b.   Those who have splenectomy for metastatic nonhematopoietic disease

    c.   Those with Hodgkin's disease and other diseases of the reticuloendothelial system

    d.   Those who have coexisting bowel problems

    e.   Those receiving chronic antibiotic prophylactic therapy

133.2   Which of the following statements concerning the epidemiology of Hodgkin's disease is *not* correct?

    a.   Non-Hodgkin's lymphoma is increasing in incidence and is now more common than Hodgkin's disease.

    b.   Hodgkin's disease in patients over 40 years is more likely to be lymphocyte predominant or of mixed cellularity.

    c.   Patients with Hodgkin's disease who are less than 16 years old are likely to be males with lymphocyte-predominant histology.

    d.   Like non-Hodgkin's lymphoma, Hodgkin's disease occurs in increasing incidence in immunosuppressed patients, including patients undergoing transplantation.

    e.   In developing countries, Hodgkin's disease tends to occur frequently in young patients.

133.3   Which of the following statements regarding Hodgkin's disease is *not* correct?

    a.   Lymphocyte-predominant Hodgkin's disease is seen more often in males either under 15 years of age or over 40 years, is often localized to a single node, and is indolent in nature.

    b.   Patients with mixed cellularity more often have constitutional symptoms and stages III and IV disease compared with patients who have the lymphocyte-predominant or nodular-sclerosing types.

c.   Nodular sclerosis represents 70% of Hodgkin's disease cases in economically developed countries but is less common in developing countries.

d.   Granulomatous lesions in a lymph node increase the risk that Hodgkin's disease will be found elsewhere.

e.   Granulomatous lesions in an involved node are an adverse prognostic factor for patients with Hodgkin's disease.

133.4   **Which of the following statements concerning Hodgkin's disease is *not* correct?**

a.   Part or all of the Epstein-Barr virus (EBV) genome is found in the Reed-Sternberg (RS) cells of up to 50% of patients who have Hodgkin's disease.

b.   There is a direct correlation between the abundance of lymphocytes in the lymph nodes of patients with Hodgkin's disease and a slow rate of progression of the disease.

c.   The RS cells of lymphocyte-predominant Hodgkin's disease are CD15 positive, whereas the RS cells of the mixed cellularity and nodular sclerosis types are CD15 negative.

d.   Although the lymphoid infiltrate in a Hodgkin's lymph node may be polymorphous, cytogenetic and molecular studies indicate clonality of the RS cells.

e.   Patients with the lymphocytic-depleted subtype have a relatively poor prognosis.

133.5   **Which of the following statements regarding the RS cell is *not* correct?**

a.   Both B- and T-cell antigens have been demonstrated on the RS cell.

b.   The RS cell may express immunoglobulin and/or T-cell receptor gene rearrangements.

c.   Hodgkin's disease is characterized by the t(14;18) translocation that results in amplification of *bcl-2* oncogene products.

d.   The CD15 antigen can rarely be demonstrated on RS cells.

e.   RS cells frequently express activation antigens such as interleukin-2 (IL-2) receptors.

133.6   **Which of the following statements regarding the immune response in Hodgkin's disease is *not* correct?**

a.   The immune defect is present at the time of diagnosis and presumably precedes the onset of the disease.

b.   Cellular immunologic deficits persist even in patients who achieve long-term remissions with radiotherapy and/or chemotherapy.

c.   Herpes zoster appears most commonly within the first year after treatment.

d.   Systemic infection with encapsulated organisms such as pneumococci and *Haemophilus influenzae* appear predominantly in splenectomized patients.

e.   Pneumococcal vaccine should be given following splenectomy.

133.7   **Which of the following statements regarding Hodgkin's disease is *not* correct?**

a.   It tends to involve central rather than peripheral lymph nodes.

b.   The disease spreads by contiguity to adjacent lymph nodes.

c.   Hematogenous spread may account for stage IV disease.

d.   Relapse at pretreatment sites of tumor after complete remission is more likely in patients who have Hodgkin's disease compared with those who have non-Hodgkin's lymphoma.

e.   The liver is generally involved in the presence of splenic involvement.

133.8   **Which of the following statements is *not* correct regarding nitrogen mustard, vincristine (Oncovine), procarbazine, prednisone (MOPP) or doxorubicin (Adriamycin), bleomycin, vinblastine, dacarbazine (ABVD) therapy for Hodgkin's disease?**

a.   Patients who relapse after combination chemotherapy with MOPP or ABVD have a much lower response to retreatment with the original combination treatment compared with the alternative combination.

b.   ABVD is superior to MOPP in that infertility and secondary tumors are less frequent.

c.   In comparative studies, downward dose modification with MOPP occurs more commonly than with ABVD.

d.   Hybrid regimens derived from MOPP and ABVD, as well as alternating MOPP-ABVD therapy, have proved superior to MOPP or ABVD with regard to disease-free and overall survival.

e.   In comparative studies, ABVD is equivalent to MOPP in terms of disease-free survival.

134.1   **A 70-year-old man presents with a 4-week history of a rapidly growing right-sided neck mass causing tracheal compression. An excisional biopsy shows diffuse large B-cell lymphoma. Staging shows a localized mass in the right lower neck and a normal complete blood count (CBC) and lactate dehydrogenase (LDH) level but no evidence of disease elsewhere, including a negative bone marrow biopsy. He has a history of a myocardial infarction 9 years prior but has preserved left ventricular function. The optimal treatment option is**

a.   Local radiation

b.   CHOP (cyclophosphamide, doxorubicin [hydroxydaunomycin], vincristine [Oncovin], prednisone) for three cycles followed by involved field radiotherapy

c.   CHOP for eight cycles

d.   CHOP for eight cycles followed by involved field radiotherapy

e.   CVP (cyclophosphamide, vincristine, prednisone)

134.2 A 40-year-old man presents with a 2-week history of abdominal discomfort and bloating. He is found by his physician to have a right-sided abdominal mass, confirmed by results from a computed tomography (CT) scan. He undergoes a core needle biopsy, the results of which are consistent with Burkitt's lymphoma. His staging CT shows no other disease; his CBC shows mild anemia with a hematocrit (Hct) of 34. His LDH level is 4,000 (laboratory upper limit is 250), and a bone marrow aspirate and biopsy shows about a 15% involvement with classic vacuolated cells. The optimal treatment option is

   a. CHOP for eight cycles
   b. CHOP plus rituximab for eight cycles
   c. CHOP for eight cycles with high-dose methotrexate
   d. CODox-M alternating with IVAC (two cycles of each)
   e. CHOP for eight cycles followed by autologous stem cell transplantation

134.3 A 65-year-old woman presents with pruritus, diffuse lymphadenopathy, hepatosplenomegaly, skin lesions, and B symptoms. A CBC shows an Hct of 33 and eosinophilia. What is the most likely histologic subtype of lymphoma?

   a. Hodgkin's disease
   b. Follicular lymphoma
   c. Diffuse large B-cell lymphoma
   d. Peripheral T-cell lymphoma
   e. Adult T-cell leukemia/lymphoma

134.4 A 63-year-old man presents with slight left-sided flank pain and peripheral lymphadenopathy. A biopsy of a cervical node reveals follicular small cleaved cell lymphoma. He has multiple 2 to 3 cm peripheral nodes, and a CT scan shows left retroperitoneal lymphadenopathy with a mass measuring about 8 × 10 cm. His LDH is normal; a CBC shows a white blood cell count of 12,000 with 20% fissured lymphs, an Hct of 32, and a platelet count of 120,000. His bone marrow biopsy shows about a 30% involvement of the intratrabecular space. Treatment options include

   a. CHOP
   b. CHOP with rituximab
   c. Rituximab as a single agent
   d. CVP
   e. Close observation

135.1 The most common immunophenotype for mycosis fungoides (MF) is

   a. CD4–, CD20+, CD30–
   b. CD4–, CD20+, CD30+
   c. CD4+, CD8–, CD7–
   d. CD4+, CD8–, CD7+

135.2 The most common site of presentation for early-stage MF is the

   a. Face and scalp
   b. Upper extremities
   c. Chest
   d. Bathing trunk area
   e. Lower extremities

135.3 A characteristic microscopic change noted in biopsies of MF is

   a. A prominent grenz zone
   b. A prominent infiltrate of eosinophils in the dermis
   c. Epidermotropism
   d. Epidermal ulceration and abscess formation
   e. Reed-Sternberg-like cells as a component of the dermal infiltrate

135.4 For patients with MF who have generalized cutaneous tumors, the most effective single therapy is

   a. Topical nitrogen mustard
   b. Psoralen plus ultraviolet A (PUVA)
   c. Total skin electron beam therapy
   d. Doxorubicin-based combination chemotherapy
   e. Systemic bexarotene

135.5 A common complication of total skin electron beam therapy for MF is

   a. Neutropenia
   b. Mild to moderate nausea and vomiting
   c. Diarrhea

    d.   A transient decrease in pulmonary function

    e.   Onychoptosis

136.1   **A 57-year-old construction worker is seen by his primary care physician for lower back pain. On physical examination he appears well, without localizing symptoms. Laboratory studies reveal a hemoglobin level of 15 g/dL with normal differential and platelet counts. Plain films of the lumbosacral spine are all normal. His chemistries, including renal function and calcium tests, are all normal. A serum protein electrophoresis (SPEP) reveals 2 g/L of a monoclonal immunoglobulin (Ig) G. Which of the following is the most likely diagnosis?**

    a.   Multiple myeloma

    b.   Waldenström's macroglobulinemia

    c.   Monoclonal gammopathy of uncertain significance (MGUS)

    d.   Non-Hodgkin's lymphoma

136.2   **Several prognostic variables have been identified in multiple myeloma. The single most predictive prognostic factor in the presence of normal renal function is**

    a.   Durie and Salmon staging

    b. β_2-Microglobulin

    c.   Plasma cell labeling index

    d.   Chromosome 13 deletion

    e.   Plasmablastic morphology

136.3   **The single most active agent in the treatment of myeloma is**

    a.   Vincristine

    b.   Thalidomide

    c.   Dexamethasone

    d.   Melphalan

    e.   Doxorubicin

136.4   **Renal failure in myeloma is caused by**

    a.   Myeloma kidney

    b.   Dehydration

    c.   Hypercalcemia

    d.   Hyperuricemia

    e.   Infection

    f.   All of the above

136.5   **Bisphosphonate therapy in myeloma**

    a.   Improves overall survival

    b.   Improves disease-free survival

    c.   Decreases morbidity by reducing skeletal events

    d.   Results in all of the above

137.1   **Which one of the following is essential for the diagnosis of polycythemia vera (PV) in routine clinical practice?**

    a.   The exclusion of conditions known to cause secondary or relative polycythemia

    b.   The demonstration of increased granulocyte expression of the polycythemia rubra vera 1 (*PRV1*) gene

    c.   The demonstration of spontaneous erythroid colony formation in vitro

    d.   The demonstration of decreased megakaryocyte expression of the thrombopoietin receptor (c-*mpl*) by bone marrow immunohistochemistry

137.2   **Which one of the following statements is *false* regarding treatment in essential thrombocythemia?**

    a.   Cytoreductive treatment may be necessary in the context of a previous thrombosis history.

    b.   Aspirin therapy has been shown to prevent deep venous thrombosis.

    c.   Observation alone is a reasonable management option for a pregnant women without a history of thrombohemorrhagic complications.

    d.   Treatment with anagrelide has not been shown to be either safer or more efficacious than treatment with hydroxyurea.

137.3   **In which one of the following disorders does substantial bone marrow fibrosis *not* occur?**

    a.   Myelofibrosis with myeloid metaplasia (MMM)

    b.   Chronic myeloid leukemia (CML)

    c.   Myelodysplastic syndrome (MDS)

    d.   ET

NEOPLASMS IN AIDS

138.1   Treatment for acquired immunodeficiency syndrome (AIDS)-related Kaposi's sarcoma (KS) should always include
   a.   Cytotoxic chemotherapy
   b.   Antiherpesvirus agents
   c.   Antiretroviral therapy
   d.   Radiation therapy

138.2   KS is an inexorably progressive malignant process inevitably requiring chemotherapy to prevent major organ damage. True or false?

138.3   KS herpesvirus (KSHV) infection is highly prevalent in North America, and transmission is associated with casual contact. True or false?

138.4   AIDS related non-Hodgkin's lymphoma has unique features including
   a.   A high incidence of extranodal involvement
   b.   A rare association with indolent or low-grade histology
   c.   The frequent presence of Epstein-Barr virus genome in the tumor
   d.   The need to consider prophylaxis for opportunistic infection during chemotherapy
   e.   All of the above

UNKNOWN PRIMARY SITE

139.1   A 65-year-old women develops a right lower quadrant abdominal pain and increasing abdominal girth. She has been previously healthy and has had no previous abdominal surgery. Physical examination reveals ascites; a computed tomography (CT) of the abdomen/pelvis shows ascites, several 2 to 3 cm peritoneal-based masses, and enlarged retroperitoneal lymph nodes. Results of a chest radiography are normal. Laboratory evaluation reveals a normal chemistry profile, a cancer antigen 125 level of 400, and a carcinoembryonic antigen level of 10. A thoracentesis is performed and yields exudative fluid with cytology positive for poorly differentiated adenocarcinoma. Optimal management should now include
   a.   Upper gastrointestinal endoscopy with endoscopic retrograde cholangiopancreatography
   b.   Laparoscopy with biopsy
   c.   Laparotomy with maximal surgical cytoreduction
   d.   Chemotherapy with paclitaxel and carboplatin
   e.   Chemotherapy with 5-fluorouracil, leucovorin, and irinotecan

139.2   A 55-year-old male with a long history of cigarette smoking develops a painless right neck mass. Physical examination reveals an isolated firm movable 2 cm lymph node in the right jugulodigastric area. Further evaluations including complete blood counts, chemistry profile, and chest radiography are normal. A CT scan of the neck shows the palpable lymph node as well as three other lymph nodes in the upper neck, all ranging from 1 to 2 cm. A complete ear, nose, and throat (ENT) examination including endoscopy is unrevealing. The next procedure performed should be
   a.   Excisional biopsy of the palpable right cervical node
   b.   Needle aspiration of the palpable right cervical node
   c.   Right radical neck dissection
   d.   Bone marrow aspiration and biopsy
   e.   Fiberoptic bronchoscopy

139.3   A 55-year-old previously healthy woman develops an asymptomatic 3 cm left axillary mass. Physical examination including breast examination is normal, except for several movable firm left axillary nodes, ranging from 1 to 3 cm in size. Mammography and magnetic resonance imaging (MRI) of the left breast are unrevealing of any suspicious abnormalities. Needle biopsy of an enlarged left axillary lymph node shows poorly differentiated adenocarcinoma, with negative results for estrogen/progesterone receptor and HER/2. Complete staging examination including bone scan and CT scans of the chest, abdomen, and pelvis are normal. A left axillary node dissection is performed, which reveals 4 of 15 lymph nodes involved by metastatic poorly differentiated adenocarcinoma. Management should now include
   a.   Observation without further treatment
   b.   Radiation therapy to the left axilla
   c.   Chemotherapy with paclitaxel, carboplatin, and etoposide
   d.   A left mastectomy
   e.   Chemotherapy with docetaxel, doxorubicin, and cyclophosphamide followed by radiation therapy to the left breast

139.4 A 64-year-old male presents with fatigue, low back pain, anorexia, and a recent 9 kg weight loss. Physical examination reveals a firm 3 cm left supraclavicular lymph node, as well as two pathologic lymph nodes in the left inguinal area, each measuring 2.5 cm. CT scan of the chest is normal. CT scan of the abdomen shows bulky retroperitoneal adenopathy, with a conglomerate mass measuring 6 × 6 cm, and two small abnormalities in the liver suggestive of metastases. Excisional biopsy of the left supraclavicular lymph node reveals "anaplastic neoplasm, favor carcinoma." Results of immunoperoxidase staining are positive for cytokeratin, negative for leukocyte-common antigen, negative for HMB-45, positive for chromogranin, positive for synaptophysin, and negative for vimentin. The most likely diagnosis is

a. Small cell lung cancer
b. Poorly differentiated sarcoma
c. Anaplastic lymphoma
d. Poorly differentiated neuroendocrine carcinoma
e. Metastatic carcinoid tumor

139.5 **Optimal management of the patient in question 4 now includes**
a. Fiberoptic bronchoscopy
b. Treatment with octreotide
c. Treatment with 5-fluorouracil and streptozocin
d. Treatment with a platinum- and etoposide-based chemotherapy
e. Palliative radiation therapy to the symptomatic retroperitoneal lymph nodes

ANSWERS

CENTRAL NERVOUS SYSTEM

83.1 **Answer: (a)** Anaplastic astrocytomas are less cellular and contain fewer mitoses than GBM and do not exhibit necrosis. Oligodendrogliomas are characterized by uniform round cells with "chicken wire" vasculature, frequent calcifications, and artifactual perinuclear halos around the oligodendroglioma cells ("fried egg" appearance). Medulloblastomas are composed of a predominant population of round to oval undifferentiated small blue cells and occasionally contain Homer Wright rosettes. Ependymomas consist of uniform polygonal cells in a collagenous background with well-defined cytoplasmic borders; they form rosettes.

83.2 **Answer: (e)** Standard treatment for GBM involves conformal fractionated radiation treatments to a standard dose of 60 Gy. A phase III study demonstrated no survival benefit to hyperfractionated irradiation to 72 Gy compared with standard single-fraction irradiation. There is also no benefit with whole brain irradiation to a focal glioblastoma lesion compared with conformal radiotherapy.

83.3 **Answer: (c)** Although there are molecular aberrations associated specifically with some primary brain tumors (eg, loss of chromosome 10 in GBM), they do not predict response to chemotherapy. The allelic loss of chromosomes 1p and 19q is the molecular signature of oligodendrogliomas. Patients with oligodendrogliomas that contain these molecular aberrations respond to the chemotherapy regimen PCV (procarbazine, lomustine [CCNU], and vincristine) and have better outcomes than is seen in those without these aberrations.

83.4 **Answer: (c)** The most consistent molecular aberration in meningioma is deletion of the *NF2* gene, which is located on chromosome 22q; it is thus a prominent brain tumor type along with schwannoma that is associated with *NF2*. Benign (grade I) meningiomas occur more commonly in females, although anaplastic (grade III) meningiomas occur more frequently in males. Recurrence rates decrease with more extensive resection, not only of the tumor but also of its dural attachment to bone. Meningiomas on MRI do enhance homogeneously and often have the dural tail sign, but are extra-axial in location. This allows them to be distinguished from gliomas, which are almost always located intra-axially.

84.1 **Answer: (a)** Although the other primaries have a greater propensity to bleed, they are much less common than lung cancer.

84.2 **Answer: (c)** Radiosurgery can be used for brain metastases from any primary, but the lesions must be 3 cm or less in diameter. Radiosurgery should be avoided in patients whose metastases have marked edema because it can exacerbate edema and worsen the patient's neurologic symptoms. No more than three lesions should be treated with the radiosurgical technique.

84.3 **Answer: (c)** Evidence of controlled trials indicates that prophylactic anticonvulsants do not prevent the development of seizures in patients with brain tumors and, thus, are not indicated. If the patient subsequently develops seizures, an anticonvulsant drug should be given. Dexamethasone almost never causes a rash other than acne.

84.4 **Answer: (a)** Randomized trials indicate that surgery is superior to whole brain radiation in promoting survival, and that radiation following surgery is superior to surgery without radiation in preventing central nervous system recurrence.

THE EYE

85.1 **Answer: (b)** See Table 85-1.

85.2 **Answer: (b)** Although the 5-year mortality rate of American patients with retinoblastoma is 5% or less, in some parts of the developing world, 5-year mortality rates remain a dismal 50%.

85.3 **Answer: (d)** The absence of drusen has been demonstrated to be a risk factor for progression of a choroidal nevus into a melanoma. Drusen, the byproducts of retinal pigment epithelial cell metabolism, are typically considered the mark of a benign lesion. See Table 85-8.

ENDOCRINE GLANDS

86.1 **Answer: (d)** Microadenomas causing Cushing's disease can be difficult to detect on MRI. If clinical suspicion is strong and laboratory evaluation is consistent with the disease, then surgical planning requires cavernous sinus sampling to help lateralize the location of the tumor.

86.2 **Answer: (b)** The patient exhibits signs and symptoms of elevated serum GH. Although this condition is most likely to result from a GH-secreting pituitary adenoma, an ectopic source of GH can be ruled out by obtaining an MRI of the sella. In addition to the obvious cosmetic deformities caused by elevated GH, this condition also leads to orthopedic problems as well as an increased mortality rate in comparison to age-matched controls. The patient should therefore be advised to undergo further evaluation and treatment.

86.3 **Answer: (c)** In general, by the time a patient with acromegaly comes to medical attention, the tumor is large enough to be detected by MRI. Therefore, a search for an ectopic source of GH secretion is indicated in this patient. Very rarely, a GH-secreting microadenoma can elude detection on MRI. In this setting, with an ectopic source of GH ruled out, cavernous sinus sampling can be undertaken to attempt to establish a pituitary microadenoma as the source of the elevated GH. If a gradient of GH is found in the cavernous sinus sampling, this test will also provide useful information to the surgeon about which side the tumor is on.

86.4 **Answer: (b)** Sudden visual loss in the context of a known macroadenoma constitutes pituitary apoplexy, which is a surgical emergency. The fact that restitution of normal PRL levels is unlikely to result from surgery is irrelevant. The patient must undergo immediate surgery to decompress his optic chiasm in the hope of reversing the visual loss. Hydrocortisone should be administered for the sudden hypopituitarism that results from an acute hemorrhage into a macroadenoma.

86.5 **Answer: (d)** Bitemporal hemianopsia results from continued pressure on the optic chiasm. Surgical debulking of the tumor will decompress the chiasm, although it will not cure a tumor that has already invaded the cavernous sinuses. Adjuvant radiotherapy, therefore, should follow surgical debulking of the tumor.

87.1 **Answer: (c)** The most cost-effective diagnostic test to perform on a patient with a solitary thyroid nodule is a fine-needle aspiration. False-positive and false-negative results occur in fewer than 5% of cases. Levels of serum thyroglobulin are generally normal in patients with thyroid carcinoma who have an intact thyroid gland present, and they can be elevated in patients with common benign conditions, such as thyroiditis. Ultrasonography and radioiodine scanning lack definitive findings that are diagnostic of malignancy and can only occasionally rule out the presence of a malignancy. Ultrasonography-guided fine-needle aspiration is best reserved for re-aspiration attempts if an initial nonguided aspiration yields inadequate or nondiagnostic material.

87.2 **Answer: (c)** Based on the information available, this 35-year-old patient has at least a T2N1Mx extent of disease, and further operative and postoperative staging data may indicate a greater extent of disease. Given her palpable nodal metastases, an ipsilateral modified radical neck dissection would reduce her likelihood of cervical recurrence. To administer adjuvant radioiodine therapy, which likely would also reduce her recurrence risk, a total thyroidectomy would also be required. Given her young age, adjuvant external beam radiotherapy would be unlikely to affect her risk of either recurrence or mortality. A radical neck dissection would be disfiguring without evidence of improved disease control.

87.3 **Answer: (b)** Given the likely extent of disease, with extensive pulmonary and bony metastases from follicular thyroid carcinoma, systemic therapy with radioactive iodine is indicated. Despite the lack of palpable disease, the primary site is within the thyroid gland, and a total thyroidectomy would be required prior to administration of radioiodine. For the locations of metastases, a high initial empiric activity of radioiodine would commonly be used, at least 150 to 200 mCi. In the setting of high-risk metastatic disease, thyroid hormone suppression therapy may improve disease control. Bone pain from metastatic lesions often responds to focal radiotherapy, and this therapy should be considered as well. Cytotoxic chemotherapy is not administered at initial presentation given the lack of a curative regimen and the efficacy of less toxic treatments in disease control.

87.4 **Answer: (d)** A mutation of the *P53* tumor suppressor gene can be identified in the majority of cases of anaplastic thyroid cancer. In the sequence of somatic mutations, generally the acquisition of a *P53* mutation in a differentiated thyroid carcinoma leads to dedifferentiation and development of the anaplastic phenotype. *RET* proto-oncogene mutation is associated with medullary and papillary carcinomas, not anaplastic. Ionizing radiation increases the risk of developing papillary carcinoma. Radioactive iodine therapy for Graves' disease is not associated with the development of thyroid malignancies. TSH suppression therapy improves disease-free survival for patients with differentiated thyroid carcinoma but does not appear to affect the risk of developing anaplastic transformation.

87.5 **Answer: (a)** The patient appears to have a familial form of medullary thyroid carcinoma, most likely of the MEN-IIa variety. Given the multifocal nature of this disease, initial surgical therapy should include complete thyroid resection with removal of the central neck lymph nodes as well. Lateral node compartments may be spared at initial surgery if they do not appear to be involved, but further resection eventually may be necessary. Given the risk of hyperparathyroidism and pheochromocytoma in MEN-IIa, screening studies for these two diagnoses should be performed before any further surgical intervention is planned. After thyroidectomy, thyroid hormone replacement therapy will be required; TSH-suppressive treatment is not indicated for medullary carcinoma. Chemotherapy is reserved for patients with progressive and/or symptomatic disease and generally is not indicated at the time of initial presentation.

88.1 **Answer: (d)** Cases of adrenal cancer have been described in families with a hereditary cancer syndrome who exhibit mutations in tumor suppressor genes. One such condition is the Li-Fraumeni syndrome, characterized by sarcoma, breast cancer, brain tumors, lung cancer, laryngeal carcinoma, leukemia, and adrenal cortical carcinoma (although adrenal cancer occurs infrequently in this syndrome). The deleterious genotype in these cases has been expressed through several generations and found in both children and adults. This syndrome appears to be related to mutations in the *P53* tumor suppressor gene. Deletions have been noted in chromosomal region 2q22–q34, a locus that corresponds to the inhibin α-subunit and in region 17p TP53, a tumor suppressor gene locus. This deletion may explain the changes in the *P53* tumor suppressor gene and its 53 kD protein. Some of these changes were point mutations in exons 5 through 8 and resulted in a single amino acid change, leading to synthesis of a protein with an altered half-life. A germline mutation of the *P53* gene was found in a patient with an incidentally found adrenal cortical carcinoma. This mutation resulted in a premature stop codon. However, mutations at the P53 loci are not found only in malignant adrenal tumors; they have also been found in benign adrenal adenomas and pheochromocytomas. Another study showed alteration in the *P53* gene product in about 50% of cases of adrenal cortical carcinoma but was unable to show that the *P53* status had any effect on long-term survival. Other genetic markers examined in adrenal cortical carcinoma have included the H19, the *IGF-II*, and the $P57^{kip2}$ genes. These genes have been mapped to chromosome 11p15.5 and appear to be important for fetal growth and development. The levels of expression of the H19 and *IGF-II* genes are very high in human fetal adrenal glands, but they subsequently decrease by 50% in adults. The gene product for $P57^{kip2}$, a member of the P21CIP1 cyclin-dependent kinase family, appears to regulate cell proliferation, exit from the cell cycle, and maintenance of differentiated cells. This gene product is usually found to be high in most normal human tissues. H19 and $P57^{kip2}$ gene expression is adrenocorticotropic hormone dependent, and regulation of the $P57^{kip2}$ gene appears to be related to the cyclic adenosine monophosphate–dependent protein kinase pathway. A markedly reduced expression of the H19 gene has been found in both non-functioning and functioning adrenal cortical carcinomas, especially in tumors that produce cortisol and aldosterone, and loss of activity of the $P57^{kip2}$ gene product has been detected in virilizing adenomas and adrenal cortical carcinomas, suggesting that this gene product plays a role in the normal maintenance of adrenal cortical differentiation and function. In contrast, *IGF-II* gene expression has been shown to be high in adrenal cortical carcinomas. Finally, the c-*myc* gene has been evaluated for a possible role in adrenal tumorigenesis. c-*myc* gene expression is relatively high in neoplasms, and it is often linked to poor prognosis; however, in contrast to other neoplasms, adrenal cortical carcinomas have a low expression of c-*myc,* approximately 10% of that found in normal adrenal tissue.

88.2   **Answer: (b)**   Silent adrenal cortical carcinomas do not present with recognizable symptoms of excessive hormone production and are detected when they attain large size and cause local symptoms. Some of these tumors, however, may be detected incidentally in the course of investigation of unrelated abdominal complaints. A hormonal profile should also be obtained on patients with apparently silent adrenal tumors. Some of these tumors produce biosynthetic steroid pathway intermediates such as progesterone and 11-deoxycortisol. It is important to determine the level of these steroids prior to surgical resection of the tumor because these hormones can be used as biochemical markers in the postoperative follow-up.

88.3   **Answer: (c)**   The mitotic rate is an important criterion not only for distinguishing malignant from benign tumors but also for predicting the clinical virulence of adrenal cortical carcinomas. Patients with carcinomas with a high mitotic rate (> 20 mitoses per 10 high-power fields [HPF]) have a shorter disease-free survival period compared with those with low mitotic rates (< 20 mitoses per 10 HPF).

88.4   **Answer: (b)**   The metabolic changes associated with excessive hormonal production can cause significant morbidity and shortened life expectancy in patients with residual disease that does not respond to antitumor therapy. Inhibitors of adrenal function have been used to suppress steroid hormone production and improve the clinical manifestations of the disease. The most commonly used inhibitors are ketoconazole and aminoglutethimide.

88.5   **Answer: (e)**   Surgical resection, even if incomplete, should be considered the initial step in therapy. If there is local extension into other structures, tumor debulking should be carried out to the maximum degree possible. It is frequently necessary to remove the adjoining kidney en bloc with the tumor because of invasion of the upper pole. In cases of liver metastases, a partial lobectomy or segmentectomy, with resection of the involved portion of the liver, has led to long-term remission. Adherence or invasion of the wall of the inferior vena cava may require resection of that portion of the wall and a patch. These aggressive efforts to excise all grossly visible tumor are justified because chemotherapy appears to be most effective when the tumor burden is minimal. Resection of metastases is also recommended when their number is limited and they are surgically accessible (eg, in lung or liver). Resection of these lesions should be considered especially in patients who have had long disease-free intervals after resection of the primary tumor and have favorable tumor biology.

     Chemotherapy has resulted in only temporary improvement. Chemotherapeutic agents used in the treatment of metastatic adrenal carcinoma include doxorubicin, cisplatin, etoposide, paclitaxel, 5-fluorouracil, vincristine, and cyclophosphamide.

     Mitotane has been used in the treatment of patients with metastatic adrenal cortical carcinoma, as monotherapy or in combination with other chemotherapeutic drugs, but there is no complete consensus regarding its efficacy. In a series of reports, mitotane has been associated with partial or complete response in 33% of patients with adrenal cancer.

HEAD AND NECK

90.1   **Answer: (d)**   The strength and consistency of the association between smoking and SCCHN has been demonstrated in numerous case-control and cohort studies with significant relative risks or odds ratios in the 3- to 12-fold range (also stated as 200–1200% increased risk). Furthermore, a dose-response effect is consistently shown in these studies between the duration and dose of smoking with increasing risk of SCCHN, and between the time since quitting and the decreasing risk of SCCHN.

90.2   **Answer: (c)**   Slaughter's classic 1953 report on oral cancer proposed that UADT carcinogenesis is a process of "field cancerization"—the repeated exposure of a region's entire tissue area to carcinogenic insult (eg, tobacco and alcohol), which increases the tissue's risk of developing multiple independent premalignant and malignant foci. This concept (also called *field carcinogenesis* or *condemned-mucosa syndrome*) may explain the clinical occurrence of multiple primary and second primary tumors in SCCHN. Epidemiologic studies have consistently shown that this rate of second primary is 4 to 7% per year, which is supported by more recent studies of *P53* mutations.

90.3   **Answer: (c)**   Although surgical excision alone has been the mainstay of treatment of oral cavity lesions, combined surgery and adjuvant radiation therapy to include the primary site and regional nodes is commonly used for most advanced cancers (stages III and IV) and is being used increasingly for small stage II cancers that exhibit pathologic indicators of lymph node metastasis or perineural invasion. Although select tumors can be managed with radiation alone, to achieve control rates comparable to those with surgery and postoperative radiotherapy, doses as high as 80 to 85 Gy with interstitial implants are needed; this would result in an unacceptably high risk of loss of function and osteo-radionecrosis of the mandible.

90.4   **Answer: (d)**   To date there has been no consistent overall improvement in locoregional control or survival using sequential chemotherapy. However, there have been several large randomized studies that have shown a reduction in the incidence of distant metastases, even though the basic intent of those studies was different. Although various studies have perhaps shown a trend toward decreased distant metastases, this benefit has not been reflected in improved survival, perhaps because of the development of, for example, second primaries or comorbidities.

90.5   **Answer: (d)**   Although the VACSP study shows that induction chemotherapy plus radiotherapy is as effective as the previous standard treatment of surgery and postoperative radiotherapy, the question of what role chemotherapy actually plays has been raised. Answers (a) and (b) are clearly wrong as, not only did chemotherapy with radiotherapy not improve survival, it actually had a higher local failure rate. Most of those patients who failed were salvaged effectively with laryngectomy, and there was no detriment to survival owing to the delay of the laryngectomy. The morbidity associated with this approach was felt to be justified by the increased laryngeal preservation rate. One major criticism of the VA study has been the fact that it did not consider the function of the larynges; therefore, answer (c) is wrong.

91.1   **Answer: (c)**   The ameloblastoma is a locally aggressive lesion that requires a resection margin of approximately 1 cm. When large, it tends to penetrate the bone and invade the soft tissues, thereby mandating the removal of an additional soft tissue margin. Odontomas, ossifying fibromas, and adenomatoid odontogenic tumors are usually slow-growing lesions that are easily removed by enucleation or enucleation and curettage. They tend not to recur.

91.2   **Answer: (d)**   The odontogenic fibroma is usually associated with the root of a tooth at its apex and is unilocular or multilocular if large. It is predominantly radiolucent but may contain some radiopaque flecks. The ameloblastoma and the clear cell odontogenic tumor are both aggressive destructive radiolucent lesions. The calcifying epithelial odontogenic tumor (Pindborg tumor) most commonly presents with a mixed pattern of radiodensity and may be nearly opaque.

91.3   **Answer: (a)**   The malignant ameloblastoma is deemed to be malignant by virtue of its development of metastasis. The histology of the metastatic lesion is the same as that of the primary lesion, and both are benign histologically. Both the malignant ameloblastoma and the ameloblastic carcinoma tend to metastasize to the lungs. The ameloblastic carcinoma has the histologic presentation of an epithelial malignancy. There is no specific immunofluorescent pattern for these lesions, and neither one is known to have a predilection for causing hypercalcemia.

91.4   **Answer: (b)**   The various dysplasias are actually reactive bone lesions, although in the past some were considered to be neoplastic. The only true tumor in this group is the cemento-ossifying fibroma, also called *ossifying fibroma* or *cementifying fibroma,* and *cementoblastoma.* There is also the entity of central odontogenic granular cell tumor, of which only 21 examples have been reported. This latter lesion behaves like an ameloblastic fibroma.

91.5   **Answer: (a)**   The order of frequency of metastatic lesions to the jaw in men is lung, prostate, kidney, bone, and adrenal gland. In women it is breast, adrenal gland, colorectal then genitourinary sites, and thyroid.

THE THORAX

92.1   **Answer: (e)**   Each of the methods can assist in the evaluation of a new nodule. All patients with pulmonary nodules should have any and all old films reviewed. Repeat imaging is an appropriate method, especially when old films are unavailable and the risk of malignancy is low (nonsmoker). PET scanning is quickly becoming the standard initial method of diagnosis where available. Wedge resection is the most aggressive method but is also very cost effective when the risk of malignancy is high.

92.2   **Answer: (c)**   The tumors in (a) and (b) are both T4N0 tumors. Resection by an experienced thoracic surgeon can lead to 5-year survival approaching 40% in these stage IIIB tumors. Option (d) is a T3N1 tumor, which could be approached surgically. Option (c) is also a T4N0 tumor, but the presence of a malignant pleural effusion makes aggressive local therapy with surgery a poor choice for treatment.

92.3   **Answer: (c)**   Recent CT screening trials have not included a control group; therefore, no information regarding the impact on disease-specific mortality reduction can be obtained. In the Mayo lung project, which evaluated the benefit of plain chest radiography, there was a significant improvement in lung cancer survival; however, at the end of the study and at long-term follow-up, there has been no impact on disease-specific mortality. This discrepancy is explained by a number of biases inherent in screening studies that affect a disease-specific survival end point, but not a disease-specific mortality end point. CT screening is highly sensitive but not specific.

92.4   **Answer: (b)**   Radiation can cure NSCLC. Historically, treatment techniques that do not explicitly account for tissue inhomogeneity and tumor motion have limited our ability to detect a radiation dose response beyond about 70 Gy.

93.1   **Answer: (d)**   This patient has a pleural effusion of unknown etiology. An infectious cause as well as tuberculosis is unlikely in the absence of fever. Lung cancer is a possibility in view of the smoking history, but the lack of a parenchymal lesion on chest CT scan and the normal bronchoscopy make this possibility unlikely. However, a peripheral adenocarcinoma cannot entirely be ruled out. The most important information here is the history of shipyard work in the distant past, indicating occupational asbestos exposure. Malignant mesothelioma is a strong possibility, rather than benign asbestos effusion, which usually occurs sooner after asbestos exposure. Pleural fluid cytology and needle-pleural biopsy often have negative results in malignant pleural mesothelioma, which is currently an important cause of "idiopathic" pleural effusion. The best approach is therefore to perform a thoracoscopy; this allows the diagnosis of malignant mesothelioma in > 80% of cases, and rules out benign asbestos effusion as well as other carcinomas. It would be inappropriate to use a sclerosing agent or give a course of corticosteroids without an established diagnosis. Repeating the chest radiography in 3 months is also inappropriate because the effusion can recur quickly in patients with malignant mesothelioma. Thoracoscopy is less aggressive than thoracotomy. Even if surgery might be contemplated in this case, it is still preferable to obtain a firm diagnosis first.

93.2 **Answer: (e)** So-called benign pleural mesotheliomas are fibrous tumors of the visceral or parietal pleura and are usually not related to asbestos exposure. The most common associated signs are clubbing and/or osteoarthropathy, but pleural effusion is exceptional. Surgical excision is curative.

93.3 **Answer: (c)** Cigarette smoking acts synergistically with asbestos exposure to produce lung cancer. According to Selikoff, compared with death rates for lung cancer in individuals who neither smoked nor worked with asbestos, rates were 5 times greater for men who worked with asbestos but did not smoke, 11 times greater for those who smoked but did not work with asbestos, and 53 to 90 times greater for those exposed to both cigarettes and asbestos. Smoking has not been shown to increase the risk of malignant mesothelioma, however.

94.1 **Answer: (d)**

94.2 **Answer: (e)**

94.3 **Answer: (d)**

94.4 **Answer: (c)**

95.1 **Answer: (b)**

95.2 **Answer: (c)**

95.3 **Answer: (d)**

96.1 **Answer: (b)** Hematologic neoplasia has been uniquely associated with mediastinal nonseminomatous germ cell tumors. The i(12p) chromosomal abnormality typical of germ cell tumors is shared by hematologic neoplasia, indicating a common origin.

96.2 **Answer: (b)** Complete surgical resection is sometimes appropriate for small asymptomatic anterior mediastinal masses. Although surgical resection is potentially curative in mediastinal seminoma, the outcome of therapy is improved by the addition of postoperative mediastinal irradiation. The exquisite radiosensitivity of seminoma allows a relatively low dose (30 Gy) of radiation therapy to be administered. This treatment approach is curative in more than 90% of patients with small surgically resectable mediastinal seminomas. Initial surgical resection of larger tumors is not indicated because the chance of cure is low, and more effective treatments with combination chemotherapy are delayed.

96.3 **Answer: (d)** This patient has a typical presentation of primary mediastinal seminoma, with a large symptomatic anterior mediastinal mass and normal hCG/AFP levels. A core needle biopsy usually provides sufficient material for pathologic examination; with a mass of this size, documentation of metastatic disease does not change the treatment approach. Initial combination chemotherapy produces better results than does radiation therapy, and it would act at least as fast as radiation therapy in relieving this patient's superior vena cava syndrome.

96.4 **Answer: (a)** This patient with a mediastinal nonseminomatous germ cell tumor has had complete normalization of serum tumor markers and is left with a residual mediastinal mass after completion of four courses of standard chemotherapy. In this setting, the majority of patients do not have residual active tumor but have either only a necrotic tumor remaining or benign teratoma. Therefore, further chemotherapy at this point is not indicated. This patient should undergo a resection of the mediastinal mass, with subsequent treatment based on the surgical findings.

97.1 **Answer: (a)** A clinically detectable solitary lung nodule carries a 0.4 to 9% probability of malignancy in patients without a history of malignancy and a 25% probability in patients with known malignancy.

97.2 **Answer: (c)** Prior reception of induction chemotherapy does not exclude a patient from being a candidate for surgical resection. If a patient receives induction chemotherapy, the surgery should be delayed at least 4 weeks to allow the bone marrow to recover. Criteria that should be evaluated prior to surgical resection include excluding extrathoracic disease, controlling the primary disease, making sure the lesion is resectable, determining the disease-free interval and TDT, and the number of metastases. The number of metastases is not a contraindication to surgical resection in and of itself; it should be evaluated with other criteria as well.

97.3 **Answer: (a)** TDT should be calculated using chest radiography only because CT scans may transect a metastasis a few millimeters differently in sequential examinations and give inconsistent size measurements. TDT should be determined on the most aggressive lesion, that is, the fastest-growing lesion. TDT has not been found to be related to the tumor histology as shown by many studies. TDT has been studied as a criteria for pulmonary metastasectomy, particularly with melanoma. A TDT of at least 40 to 60 days has been recommended as optimal.

97.4   **Answer: (d)**   There are studies confirming improved survival in selected patients with all the cancer types listed except pancreatic carcinoma.

97.5   **Answer: (b)**   If resection of the primary lesion is not feasible, there is usually no need to resect the pulmonary metastasis because of limited survival benefit to the patient. Patients with bilateral metastases should undergo resection of the *least* involved side first. In this way, the true extent of any residual disease on the less involved side is known at the time of thoracotomy on the worse side, when one may be faced with a major pulmonary resection such as bilobectomy or pneumonectomy. The patient will also have more adequate pulmonary function for the second procedure than if the bilobectomy or pneumonectomy is done first. VATS has been studied as a way to resect pulmonary metastases, but several studies have reported high recurrence rates and high missed lesion rates. Reports of extended resections of pulmonary metastases have shown favorable 5-year survival rates in selected patients.

GASTROINTESTINAL TRACT

98.1   **Answer: (a)**   The most common histology worldwide is squamous cell carinoma. In North America and Western Europe, adenocarcinoma has become the most common histology, partly because of changing risk factors including dietary changes and increased gastroesophageal reflux.

98.2   **Answer: (d)**   The most common presentation of esophageal cancer is dysphagia, which is often associated with an advanced stage because of involvement of the entire esophagus or the presence of a large polypoid obstructing mass. The next most common symptoms are pain (25%) and gastroesophageal reflux (40%).

98.3   **Answer: (d)**   EUS is the most accurate means of determining tumor depth. EUS depicts the normal esophagus as five alternating hyperechoic and hypoechoic layers reperesenting the mucosa/lamina propria, muscularis mucosae, submucosa, muscularis propria, and adventitia. EUS is operator dependent and must be performed by an experienced endoscopist to be accurate.

98.4   **Answer: (a)**   Although surgery alone can result in cures in all of the stages listed, the earliest stage disease has the best chance (stage I) of success because of a low likelihood of micrometastic disease. Multimodality treatment schemes with chemotherapy, radiation therapy, and surgery have been evaluated in more advanced stages (II–IVA) because of the high chance of locoregional and distant recurrence with surgery alone.

98.5   **Answer: (a)**   The optimal treatment for this group of patients is controversial. Surgery alone is associated with a high rate of locoregional and distant failure, and multiple strategies combining radiation therapy, chemotherapy, and surgery have been evaluated. Preoperative and postoperative radiation therapy have not shown clear survival benefits compared with surgery alone, perhaps because both modalities focus primarily on locoregional disease and fail to address micrometastic disease.

99.1   **Answer: (b)**   Lesions up to 3 cm in diameter have been successfully managed in large series. Signet ring histology is a marker of aggressive histology with submucosal spread common. Ulceration usually is associated with at least invasion to the submucosa. T2 lesions, because of involvement of the muscle layers and chances of nodal disease, are not candidates for EMR.

99.2   **Answer: (c)**   Survival of gastric cancer patients in the United States after gastrectomy remains suboptimal. Recent analyses by the American College of Surgeons and American Cancer Society showed the staged-stratified 5-year survival to be as follows: IA 78%, IB 58%, II 34%, IIIA 20%, IIIB 8%, and IV 7%. Postoperative chemoradiotherapy as carried out in the INT0116 trial has improved progression-free survival and overall survival and is recommended.

99.3   **Answer: (b)**   This is a typical case of diffuse gastric cancer. Peritoneal carcinomatosis is the most common site of distant metastasis. Ovarian metastases (Krukenberg's tumors) and periumbilical nodules are common. Gastric cancers of this type frequently spread submucosally within the stomach and may only be found on deep biopsies. Early satiety is owing to decreased gastric wall compliance. Tumor markers are nonspecific in this setting. CA 125 may become elevated with peritoneal carcinomatosis. CEA can be elevated in a number of cancers.

100.1   **Answer: (d)**   Ablation with alcohol or radiofrequency in a cirrhotic liver is effective and preserves normal liver function. In patients with advanced cirrhosis, with small "incidental" hepatomas, transplantation can be successful. Chemoembolization or embolization alone is offered to patients with hepatoma, although its utility is unproven. Patients with cirrhosis do not tolerate a major hepatic lobectomy, although a small-wedge resection may be feasible.

100.2   **Answer: (c)**   Incidence and mortality rates are steadily increasing for both cancers in the United States and much of the developed world. In HCC, this is thought to reflect the impact of chronic hepatitis B and C virus infections. The cause of the increase in cholangiocarcinoma remains unknown.

100.3   **Answer: (a)**   Alcoholic cirrhosis, particularly in the presence of chronic hepatitis C virus infection, is a very strong risk factor for development of HCC. Oral contraceptives have been associated with the development of hepatic adenomas, and there is no evidence that they protect against HCC. Tobacco use is higher among men in most populations, but the evidence for its association with development of HCC is weak.

101.1 **Answer: (b) and (c)**

101.2 **Answer: (b)**

101.3 **Answer: (c)**

101.4 **Answer: (d)**

101.5 **Answer: (c) and (d)**

103a.1 **Answer: (d)** Hypertension is not a presenting symptom of pancreatic cancer. A primary tumor in the pancreatic head often obstructs the pancreatic duct and can therefore result in pancreatic exocrine insufficiency and subsequent frequent loose bowel movements. The resulting malabsorption combined with the anorexia and cachexia that characterize pancreatic cancer often result in weight loss. The hyperglycemia associated with pancreatic cancer is both an early manifestation of the disease and possibly a predisposing factor. This is discussed at length in the text. The pain associated with pancreatic cancer is owing to tumor involvement of the mesenteric and celiac plexus. This is an autonomic pain of foregut origin, and is therefore poorly localized to the mid- and upper abdomen and back. Cancer of the exocrine pancreas occurs most commonly in the pancreatic head and, depending on the exact location of the tumor, may cause biliary obstruction owing to compression or invasion of the intrapancreatic portion of the bile duct.

103a.2 **Answer: (c)** Current epidemiologic studies suggest that 25% of pancreatic cancer can be attributed to cigarette smoking. An additional 15% of pancreatic cancers may be attributable to obesity and inactivity. High insulin concentrations in the microenvironment of the pancreatic duct cell (secondary to the intake of frequent large meals) may contribute to malignant transformation. It is possible that as many as 40% of pancreatic cancer cases are preventable through avoidance of tobacco use and obesity by living an active healthy lifestyle.

103a.3 **Answer: (b)** Although all of these tests are commonly used in patients with pancreatic cancer, CT can often accurately delineate the location of a tumor within the pancreas, and, most importantly, it can determine whether the patient has localized potentially resectable disease, locally advanced disease, or metastatic pancreatic cancer. At selected institutions MRI may be preferred over CT. Transabdominal ultrasonography is a reasonable first test to demonstrate the presence of intra- and extrahepatic biliary dilatation in patients with obstructive jaundice. Invasive upper endoscopy to include ERCP or EUS should not be performed until CT imaging has been completed. Procedure-related pancreatitis can make it impossible to accurately stage a patient with possible pancreatic cancer and can obscure the diagnosis in the absence of high-quality CT performed prior to ERCP and/or EUS.

103a.4 **Answer: (b)** The most common technique for management of the jaundiced patient is endobiliary decompression via ERCP. As noted above, it is important that the patient be accurately staged with high-quality CT imaging prior to undergoing ERCP or any other form of endoscopic or operative intervention. For patients with locally advanced and metastatic pancreatic cancer, biliary decompression is routinely performed with ERCP-placed endobiliary stents. For patients with localized potentially resectable disease, the placement of preoperative biliary stents remains somewhat controversial. Clearly, in those patients who may experience a delay in surgery (eg, because of the delivery of protocol-based neoadjuvant therapy); in those with profound symptoms of pruritus, fatigue, and anorexia; or in those with a poor performance status; endobiliary decompression is necessary. Nasobiliary decompression is rarely performed, and placement of a percutaneous transhepatic catheter remains a reasonable alternative in those patients who, for technical reasons, cannot be successfully stented endoscopically.

103a.5 **Answer: (c)** In the current (6th) edition of the *AJCC Cancer Staging Manual*, stage III is reserved for patients with locally advanced nonmetastatic disease (as assessed radiographically or at operation), and stage IV is reserved for those patients with extrapancreatic metastatic disease (M1). A patient who has undergone a compete resection but is found to have a positive regional lymph node (or lymph nodes) is accurately staged at stage IIB.

103b.1 **Answer: (b)** Given the location of these tumors, the majority of patients with periampullary neoplasms develop biliary obstruction and present with hyperbilirubinemia. Because these patients develop biliary obstruction, patients are often diagnosed early in the course of their disease with small tumors, which may contribute to their improved survival when compared with patients with pancreatic cancer.

103b.2 **Answer: (a)** Although the presence of regional lymph node metastases in a patient with ampullary carcinoma is associated with a less favorable outcome after surgery compared with patients who have no nodal involvement, it is not as powerful a prognostic factor as is seen with pancreatic adenocarcinoma. The presence of lymph node metastases is not a contraindication to potentially curative surgery. These patients should be considered for adjuvant therapies with chemotherapy and/or chemoradiation.

103b.3 **Answer: (c)** Preoperative staging of periampullary neoplasms should start with computed tomography, and if there is no evidence of distant metastatic disease, one should perform upper endoscopy with EUS. The overall accuracy of EUS in staging depth of invasion (T stage) ranges from 74 to 82%. The overall accuracy for detection of lymph node metastases (N stage) is in a similar range. If a tumor is not visible and the bile duct is obstructed, endoscopic retrograde cholangiopancreatography (ERCP) should be performed. At the time of diagnostic ERCP, we routinely place endoscopic stents to prevent cholangitis in these patients. Endoscopic stents are also placed in patients with biliary obstruction in whom surgery is delayed because of the planned delivery of neoadjuvant therapy.

103b.4   **Answer: (b)**   Local excision of periampullary neoplasms is rarely performed because of the difficulty in excluding invasive adenocarcinoma preoperatively by EUS or endoscopic biopsy, the inability to accurately define depth of invasion, and the frequent development of local recurrence, even with benign lesions. For these reasons, we rarely consider local excision of a periampullary neoplasm. Small benign tumors without evidence of high-grade dysplasia on endoscopic biopsy or intraoperative frozen section analysis may be considered for local resection with close endoscopic surveillance postoperatively. However, unless contraindicated by medical comorbidities or performance status, the gold standard for resection of nonmalignant and particularly malignant periampullary neoplasms is pancreaticoduodenectomy.

103b.5   **Answer: (a)**   Although duodenal polyps develop in 50 to 90% of patients with FAP, only about 5% of patients with duodenal polyps eventually develop periampullary carcinoma. The adenoma-carcinoma sequence for periampullary lesions is well established, although progression of duodenal polyps to invasive cancer is uncommon in the lifetime of FAP patients. Current regimens for upper gastrointestinal tract surveillance in FAP patients vary with respect to the age at which to begin endoscopies and the recommended interval for examinations. Most authors advocate the first endoscopic evaluation with random biopsies at the age of 20 to 25 years. The frequency of endoscopic surveillance is determined by the severity of the duodenal adenomatosis. Most investigators advocate endoscopy every 3 years for Spigelman stages I and II, every 2 years for stage III, and every 6 to 12 months for stage IV disease. Surgical options for duodenal polyps involve local excision and pancreaticoduodenectomy (the pylorus-preserving Whipple procedure or the pancreas-sparing technique of duodenal resection). Because of the multifocal nature of the duodenal polyps in patients with FAP, local excision (polypectomy, ampullectomy) usually results in early recurrence. For patients with severe duodenal adenomatosis (Spigelman stage III or IV) or a family history of duodenal carcinoma, a more radical surgical approach to include complete resection of the duodenum is indicated.

104.1   **Answer: (e)**   Leiomyoma is the most symptomatic benign tumor of the small bowel, accounting for approximately 20% of all benign small bowel tumors.

104.2   **Answer: (d)**   Regional enteritis, nontropical sprue, celiac disease, and Crohn's disease have all been shown to be associated with an increased risk of adenocarcinoma of the small bowel.

104.3   **Answer: (e)**   In a large series reported by Moertel of surgically confirmed carcinoids, 3% were in the duodenum, 5% in the jejunum, 32% in the proximal ileum, and 60% in the distal ileum.

104.4   **Answer: (c)**   GI stromal tumors express the mutated c-*kit* tyrosine kinase. Several mutations have been identified. Targeting of this mutated tyrosine kinase by specific tyrosine kinase inhibitors is currently being evaluated.

104.5   **Answer: (d)**   Imatinib mesylate (Gleevec) was first prescribed for patients with *bcr-abl* positive leukemias. This drug has also been shown to inhibit the c-*kit* tyrosine kinase. Promising results have been seen in patients, with more than 50% of patients demonstrating objective responses; this contrasts the < 10% response rates with traditional chemotherapy.

105.1   **Answer: (b)**   Carcinoid tumors are the most common appendiceal tumor, comprising 32 to 77% of appendiceal neoplasms.

105.2   **Answer: (b)**   Current recommendations for carcinoid tumors are that tumors < 2 cm require only appendectomy. Those > 2 cm require hemicolectomy. Some authors advocate hemicolectomy for patients with primary tumors between 1.5 and 2 cm in diameter. The rationale for hemicolectomy in appendiceal carcinoids is to remove metastatic nodal disease.

105.3   **Answer: (c)**   A recent report of 385 patients with peritoneal surface spread of appendiceal malignancy demonstrated that complete cytoreduction in conjunction with intraperitoneal chemotherapy was associated with an 86% 5-year survival if the tumor demonstrated adenomucinosis. If there was hybrid pathology, there was approximately a 50% 5-year survival. Incomplete cytoreduction had a survival of 20% at 5 years and 0% at 10 years.

105.4   **Answer: (c)**   The extent of tumor invasion is the most important factor when determining treatment of appendiceal adenocarcinoma because these tumors behave in a fashion similar to that of colonic adenocarcinoma, a tumor felt to be best treated with the same aggressive surgical approach. For any lesion with invasion beyond the mucosa, right hemicolectomy with resection of draining lymph nodes is advocated. In the presence of such invasion, the 5-year survival after right hemicolectomy is 60% compared with 20% after appendectomy alone.

106.1   **Answer: (c)**   All of the above except gender are risk factors for colorectal cancer. Colorectal cancer incidence increases after age 50 years and after each subsequent decade. However, this does not mean that colorectal cancer is not common in individuals < 50 years of age. In the Surveillance, Epidemiology, and End Results statistics for the period 1995 to 1999, colorectal cancer incidence for individuals ages 40 to 49 was 48/100,000. Any person who presents with symptoms and signs of colorectal cancer should be evaluated irrespective of his or her age. Prior history of adenomas as well as family history of adenomas and colorectal cancer are risk factors for colorectal cancer; colorectal cancer incidence is increased two- to threefold in individuals who have an affected first-degree relative. The earlier the colorectal cancer is diagnosed, the higher the risk. Affected second-degree relatives also influence the individual risk of colorectal cancer but not as much as first-degree relatives. A personal history of adenomas also influences the risk of colorectal cancer: Peutz-Jeghers syndrome, an autosomal dominant syndrome, predisposes not only to colorectal cancer but also to gastric, pancreatic, breast, and uterine carcinomas, as well as ovarian sex cord tumors, Sertoli cell tumors, and adenoma malignum of the cervix.

106.2   **Answer: (e)**   Although TP53, MSI, and 18q deletion have been used to correlate prognosis in colorectal cancer, none of these markers is currently used routinely in the clinical setting. TP53 mutations correlate with response to preoperative radiation and neoadjuvant chemoradiation for rectal adenocarcinoma. Tumors with mutated *P53* appear to be more resistant to treatment than tumors with wild-type *P53*. It has been reported that stage II colorectal tumors with 18q deletion behave more like stage III tumors. This difference has also been reported in stage II tumors. However, despite a majority of studies confirming these results, there are several studies in which the difference in survival was not noted. MSI is present in 80 to 85% of hereditary nonpolyposis colorectal cancer tumors, whereas it is present in approximately 10 to 15% of sporadic colorectal cancer. In two population-based studies, patients whose tumors had MSI had a better survival rate than patients whose tumors did not have MSI, independently of other prognostic factors.

106.3 **Answer: (e)**   Patients with unresectable metastatic disease are commonly asymptomatic or have minimal symptoms with regard to the primary tumor. In such a situation the management of the primary tumor should be individualized. Surgery may not necessarily be the best treatment option. Performing less than an en bloc resection for tumors adhered to adjacent organs or structures compromises cure rates and increases recurrences. Resection of the primary colorectal tumor is not contraindicated in the presence of a hepatic metastasis(es), especially if the latter is (are) resectable. The presence of a synchronous hepatic metastasis has been reported to be an adverse factor after hepatic resection, but it is not a contraindication for hepatic resection; therefore, if the patient has a potentially resectable hepatic metastases, the primary tumor should be resected and the hepatic metastases should be dealt with at the time of the primary surgery or later. Obstruction and perforation of the primary colorectal tumor have been shown to be adverse prognostic factors.

106.4 **Answer: (c)**   In the Dutch Mesorectal Trial, at a median of 24.9 months, patients who received preoperative radiation therapy had a local recurrence rate of 2.4% compared with those who did not receive preoperative radiation. In the United States, two cooperative group trials evaluating preoperative chemoradiation versus postoperative chemoradiation for resectable rectal cancer closed because of lack of accrual. Although the German CAO/ARO/Arbeitsgemeinschaft Internistische Onkologie randomized trial has been completed, results have not been published; this latter trial may indeed determine which approach is better. In randomized controlled studies, both preoperative and postoperative radiation therapy have been shown to decrease local recurrence. Radial margins of excision as well as expertise of the surgeon have been reported to influence the outcome after rectal cancer surgery.

106.5 **Answer: (d)**   Adjuvant therapy for colon cancer has been demonstrated to be effective in stage III colon cancer patients. In these patients, adjuvant chemotherapy has been shown to decrease recurrence rate by about 30 to 40% and to increase survival rate by approximately 30%. Six months of 5-fluorouracil/leucovorin has been proven to be as effective as 12 months of 5-fluorouracil/levamisole (Table 106-4). The role of chemotherapy in stage II colon cancer is controversial. At the present time, it is not recommended to administer adjuvant chemotherapy to stage II colon cancer patients outside of a clinical trial or a high-risk colon cancer (T4). There is no role for adjuvant chemotherapy in stage I colon cancer.

107.1 **Answer: (b)**   There is strong evidence for HPV being a causative agent, including the relationship of this virus to genital warts and the common history of genital warts in these patients with anal cancer. There is a high prevalence of deoxyribonucleic acid (DNA) in these tumors from HPV type 16. Although HIV has been suggested as a causative agent in homosexual men, a large study of 435 HIV-associated tumors in Italy demonstrated that, among intravenous drug abusers, anal tumors were extremely rare.

107.2 **Answer: (a)**   Almost every large trial has had at least one patient who has died of thrombocytopenia or who has experienced life-threatening thrombocytopenia. For this reason, many trials have been attempting to replace mitomycin-C with cisplatin.

107.3 **Answer: (c)**   Published results in many studies with at least 40 patients reported overall survival rates of 75 to 80%, with a few studies as high as 85%.

107.4 **Answer: (a)**   A superficial and deep groin dissection has a high morbidity and has not been effective in the treatment of inguinal lymph nodes. Multimodality chemoradiotherapy has been the most effective treatment for positive groin nodes.

107.5 **Answer: (c)**   Tumor thickness is the major determinant of prognosis for melanomas of the anal canal, just as it is for melanomas in other locations.

GENITOURINARY TRACT

108.1 **Answer: (b)**

108.2 **Answer: (c)**

108.3 **Answer: (c)**

108.4 **Answer: (b)**

108.5 **Answer: (c)**

109.1 **Answer: (c)**

109.2 **Answer: (b)**

109.3   **Answer: (c)**

109.4   **Answer: (c)**

109.5   **Answer: (a)**

110.1   **Answer: (c)**   Black race is associated with a lower incidence of bladder cancer among both males and females. In contrast, male gender is associated with a threefold higher risk of bladder cancer. Cigarette smoking is associated with an increased risk of bladder cancer and is thought to be responsible for about 50% of cases in the United States. Heavy smokers have a risk of bladder cancer three to five times higher than that in nonsmokers. Infection with *S. haematobium*, a parasite that takes up residence in the pelvic veins and the venous plexus surrounding the bladder, is associated with a higher risk of bladder cancer, particularly squamous cell carcinoma. The eggs of the parasite penetrate into the bladder wall and provoke inflammation and granulomata, and this is thought to be responsible for the higher incidence of bladder cancer seen in endemic areas. The incidence of bladder cancer is three times higher in those who have been infected with *S. haematobium* than in those who have not. Occupational studies have shown that exposure to aromatic amines is associated with an increased risk of bladder cancer. Aromatic amines are found in cigarette smoke and in materials used by those who work with dye, leather, rubber, and paint.

110.2   **Answer: (e)**   Intravesical 5-fluorouracil has not been shown to affect recurrence or progression rates in patients with urothelial carcinomas. In contrast, intravesical BCG, mitomycin-C, doxorubicin, and thiotepa following transurethral resection (TUR) have all been shown to reduce recurrence rates compared with TUR alone. However, only BCG appears to lower the risk of progression from nonmuscle-invasive to muscle-invasive disease, and BCG has been shown to be more effective than thiotepa, doxorubicin, and epirubicin at reducing recurrence rates. Intravesical chemotherapy, as opposed to intravesical BCG, has never been shown to reduce the risk of progression.

110.3   **Answer: (d)**   Five-year disease-free survival is about 60 to 70% for all patients following radical cystectomy, and only 20 to 35% for patients with lymph node metastases. As a result, several randomized controlled trials have studied adjuvant chemotherapy. The three trials that used cisplatin-based chemotherapy showed a significant improvement in relapse-free survival but no statistically significant difference in overall survival. All three trials were severely underpowered and showed a statistically nonsignificant trend toward improvement in overall survival. The small size of the trials and other major flaws in how they were carried out make it impossible to reach a conclusion as to whether adjuvant chemotherapy offers a survival benefit in patients with locally advanced bladder cancer. Therefore, a large international study is comparing immediate adjuvant chemotherapy to surveillance in patients with a high risk of relapse following cystectomy; if this trial reaches its accrual goals, it will be adequately powered to establish or rule out a clinically meaningful overall survival benefit. Although many experts in bladder cancer recommend against adjuvant chemotherapy, until it is proven that there is an overall survival benefit, practicing oncologists frequently use adjuvant chemotherapy based on the demonstration of improved relapse-free survival and the nonsignificant trend toward an improvement in overall survival. About 75% of relapses following cystectomy are distant rather than local recurrences, so there is no clear rationale for adjuvant radiation therapy, nor are there any randomized trials showing a survival benefit with such therapy.

110.4   **Answer: (a)**   The only chemotherapy regimens that have been shown to increase survival include cisplatin. These regimens include M-VAC and CMV. GC was compared with M-VAC in a large phase III trial, and no difference in survival was seen. The trial was not adequately powered to rule out a small advantage to M-VAC, but GC has, nonetheless, become a widely accepted first-line regimen as a result of that trial, partly because it is better tolerated than M-VAC. Thus, M-VAC, CMV, and GC have all been tested in phase III trials and are all considered standard first-line regimens.

PC has never been tested in a completed phase III trial, and it is unknown how its efficacy compares with that of M-VAC, CMV, or GC. Thus, it is unknown whether PC results in any improvement in survival, and PC is not considered a standard first-line regimen. Carboplatin has never been shown to be equivalent to cisplatin, and the available data indicate that carboplatin is probably inferior to cisplatin. Two small comparative trials have randomized patients to either a cisplatin-based regimen or a carboplatin-based regimen. Both trials reported a significantly higher response rate in the cisplatin arm, and one trial reported a longer disease-specific survival in the cisplatin arm. Neither trial was adequately powered to address overall survival, but all available clinical data indicate that carboplatin is less active than cisplatin in urothelial carcinomas. Optimal second-line chemotherapy remains poorly defined, and there are no published phase III trials in this setting.

110.5   **Answer: (d)**   Intravesical therapy using BCG is appropriate for carcinoma in situ for tumors invading the lamina propria but not the muscularis propria (ie, T1 tumors), and for high-grade or recurrent low-grade noninvasive cancers (Ta). Intravesical therapy is not appropriate for muscle-invasive disease. For muscle-invasive cancers in which there is no evidence of metastases, the standard options are (1) radical cystectomy (which in men is also referred to as a *cystoprostatectomy* because the prostate is removed in a radical cystectomy; both operations include bilateral pelvic lymph node dissections), and (2) bladder-sparing approaches, which include chemoradiation and, in carefully selected cases, partial cystectomy. Chemoradiation is preceded by a very aggressive transurethral resection of the tumor; after about 40 Gy of radiation has been delivered, cystoscopy is repeated and biopsies of the tumor site are taken. If any residual tumor is detected at that point, bladder sparing is aborted and the patient undergoes radical cystectomy.

111.1   **Answer: (c)**   BPH, like prostate cancer, occurs in older men and can cause similar symptoms including urinary outflow obstruction. However, no convincing studies have demonstrated any causal relationship between BPH and a higher risk of developing prostate cancer. African Americans have among the highest risk of prostate cancer in the world, and a family history of a first-degree relative with prostate cancer increases an individual's risk by two- to threefold. Age is a strong risk factor for prostate cancer, with up to 70% of men over age 80 years having histologic evidence of prostate cancer in autopsy series. High-fat diets have been implicated in multiple epidemiologic studies and may account for some of the geographic differences in prostate cancer risk around the world.

111.2 **Answer: (e)** In most studies that have evaluated this question, prognosis for localized prostate cancer after treatment is based on clinical stage, serum PSA at diagnosis, and biopsy Gleason score. Recent studies have also shown that the percentage of biopsy cores that have cancer present, as well as the maximum amount of cancer on each core, provides additional prognostic information in some patients. However, % free PSA has not been demonstrated to provide any additional prognostic value for recurrence, above that provided by the total PSA itself; it is a useful test for helping determine whether cancer is present in the first place, in men with a PSA between 4 and 10 ng/mL. A lower % free PSA in these patients predicts for a higher likelihood that cancer will be found on biopsy.

111.3 **Answer: (b)** Urinary incontinence is an uncommon complication of external beam radiotherapy. It occurs more often after radical prostatectomy, usually in the form of mild stress incontinence. Erectile dysfunction is common after both procedures, although much controversy exists over the optimal technique to preserve erectile function. Urinary symptoms including cystitis, hematuria, and urethral strictures are seen during or after radiation therapy, but often resolve over time. Similarly, mild fatigue is often noted by patients during radiation but seldom persists.

111.4 **Answer: (c)** Androgen-deprivation therapy is the standard treatment for patients with metastatic prostate cancer. Traditionally surgical castration with bilateral orchiectomy or chemical castration with estrogens such as DES were considered equivalent options. Luteinizing hormone–releasing hormone (LH-RH) agonists such as leuprolide were shown in randomized trials to be an acceptable alternative to DES. Combined androgen blockade with LH-RH agonists plus an antiandrogen such as flutamide have not been convincingly shown to have a significant advantage over LH-RH agonists alone, but it remains an option to use both drugs simultaneously. Flutamide alone, however, is not an acceptable alternative because a randomized trial comparing flutamide to LH-RH agonists showed an inferior survival rate with flutamide alone.

111.5 **Answer: (e)** The use of cytotoxic chemotherapy has been extensively evaluated in hormone-refractory prostate cancer, and palliative benefits have been demonstrated in randomized trials. Although many ongoing clinical trials are studying the potential value of chemotherapy in earlier disease states (eg, neoadjuvant, adjuvant, rising PSA, newly metastatic disease), no proven role exists yet for chemotherapy in these patients.

112.1 **Answer: (e)** Treatment of penile cancer is based on the extent of the primary tumor and its tumor grade, established by biopsy of the lesion. Antibiotic therapy is begun prior to biopsy and continued through surgical therapy and for 4 to 6 weeks afterward. Once the tissue diagnosis is confirmed, small superficial tumors may be successfully treated with local surgical excision, topical chemotherapy, laser surgery, Mohs' micrographic surgery, or superficial radiation therapy.

112.2 **Answer: (d)** The national Surveillance, Epidemiology, and End Results database (1973–1987; 1,101 patients) shows a relative survival rate of 95% for patients with carcinoma in situ and 70% for all stages. Relative survival for localized tumor was 80%, with survival rates of 52% for regional (nodal) disease and 18% for distant disease. Horenblas and colleagues reported a 93% 5-year survival when nodes were negative versus 50% in patients with clinically positive nodes. Srinivas and colleagues reported a crude 5-year survival rate of 28% in patients with proven inguinal metastases. Patients with minimal nodal disease (N1, N2) had 5-year survivals of 50 to 80%, whereas those with N3/N4 disease had a much graver outcome, with survivals of 4 to 12%. Patients with negative groins had a 74% 5-year survival. The outcome of patients with pelvic metastases has been very poor.

112.3 **Answer: (a)** The histopathology of female urethral cancer depends on the tissue of origin. Squamous carcinoma is the most common comprising about 50% of all tumors. Transitional cell carcinoma and adenocarcinoma are the next most common and occur with roughly equal frequency. Unlike in penile cancers, tumor grade does not appear to influence either propensity for metastasis or prognosis. Female urethral cancers occur more often in Caucasian women than in Blacks. Mixed tumors, undifferentiated carcinomas, melanoma, cloacagenic anal carcinoma, and clear cell adenocarcinoma have also been reported.

112.4 **Answer: (e)** Fifty to 75% of male urethral cancers arise in the bulbar urethra. The remainder occur predominantly in the fossa navicularis. Some 90% of male tumors demonstrate squamous cell carcinoma histology. Often there is an association with stricture of the urethra. Infrequently, transitional cell carcinoma or undifferentiated tumor may predominate at the bladder neck or within the prostatic urethra. Poorly differentiated transitional cell cancers may show some squamous characteristics. Rarely adenocarcinoma may arise in the glands of Littre or the prostatic utricle. Metastases from distant tumor sites to the penis also occur infrequently.

Obstructive symptoms are common in more proximal lesions, whereas urethral bleeding and palpation of a mass herald more distal lesions. In general, the more proximal a tumor, the later its development and the higher its stage at diagnosis.

113.1 **Answer: (d)** These patients are rarely, if ever, curable with any form of salvage chemotherapy. The only indication for chemotherapy would be to reduce the size of the mass to facilitate surgery. This patient should undergo pelvic resection and begin routine follow-up as these types of patients are at risk of early and late relapse. The surgery would be expected to reveal both a yolk sac tumor and a teratoma.

113.2 **Answer: (c)** This patient has a rising α-fetoprotein and pure embryonal cell carcinoma. There would be a very high expectation that chemotherapy alone would cure this disease. A previous randomized study by the Eastern Cooperative Oncology Group demonstrated an inferiority of three courses of cisplatin and etoposide (VP-16) versus three courses of cisplatin, etoposide, and bleomycin. Another attractive and reasonable alternative would be to treat him with four courses of etoposide and cisplatin.

113.3 **Answer: (a)** Histology is not an independent prognostic variable. *Any* nonpulmonary visceral metastasis, α-fetoprotein > 10,000 ng/mL, or primary mediastinal nonseminomatous germ cell tumor constitutes poor-risk disease.

FEMALE REPRODUCTIVE ORGANS

114.1   **Answer: (d)**   Basal cell carcinoma of the vulva is locally invasive nonmetastatic carcinoma. The treatment consists of a wide local excision.

114.2   **Answer: (e)**   Verrucous vulvar carcinoma grows slowly and invades locally, rarely spreading to regional nodes. Radiation therapy or radical surgery with node sampling is not indicated. Treatment is a simple vulvectomy or wide local excision.

114.3   **Answer: (c)**   Melanoma of the vulva is the most frequent nonsquamous cell malignancy. There are approximately 400 cases per year with an overall survival of 33%.

114.4   **Answer: (c)**   The upper vagina drains to the pelvic nodes. The lower one-third of the vagina drains directly to the inguinal lymph nodes.

114.5   **Answer: (b)**   The cambian zone is a subepithelial zone caused by the infiltration of an embryonal rhabdomyosarcoma of the vagina.

115.1   **Answer: (c)**   The incidence and mortality rates for cancer of the cervix in the United States have decreased by 70% over the past 45 years. Such declines have not occurred in developing countries that do not have screening programs, facilities, and personnel to treat precancerous lesions.

115.2   **Answer: (c)**   HPV is currently thought to be a significant factor in promoting unregulated cell proliferation by neutralizing the tumor repressor functions of *P53* and the retinoblastoma gene.

115.3   **Answer: (e)**   Adenocarcinomas comprise 20% of cervical carcinomas diagnosed today. The endometrioid adenocarcinoma is the second most common primary adenocarcinoma of the cervix.

115.4   **Answer: (d)**   Small cell carcinoma of the cervix resembles oat cell carcinoma of the lung and is a very aggressive cancer. System spread is frequently common at the time of diagnosis, accounting for the poor survival rate.

115.5   **Answer: (c)**   E6 and E7 are HPV-related virus-encoded proteins that inactivate the *P53* tumor suppressor gene and the retinoblastoma tumor suppressor gene.

115.6   **Answer: (e)**   A positive FNA is useful in planning therapy but is not allowed when the FIGO clinical staging guidelines are used.

115.7   **Answer: (c)**   The skin-sparing effect of high-energy linear accelerators is superior to cobalt or to 6 mV photons.

115.8   **Answer: (a)**   The vascular occlusive effect is essential in the tumor eradication properties of ionizing radiation and is not reversible.

115.9   **Answer: (e)**   A single biopsy is insufficient evaluation in this patient. Conization plus endocervical curettage is recommended. If the lesion invaded no more than 3 mm in the final specimen and had clear margins and no vascular space involvement, the patient would be adequately treated with an abdominal or vaginal hysterectomy.

115.10   **Answer: (e)**   Neoadjuvant chemotherapy has not been of proven benefit in randomized studies, and the complete response rates and overall survival are similar for either single-agent or combination chemotherapy. Chemotherapy with radiation has proven advantages in certain clinical situations.

116.1   **Answer: (c)**   Historically, endometrial cancer staging was a clinical exercise based on physical examination, noninvasive radiographic testing, and measurement of the depth of the uterine cavity. However, inaccuracies in this system lead to the possibility of undertreating a significant proportion of stage I cancers. The Gynecologic Oncology Group (GOG) inaugurated a pilot study to perform staging laparotomy in the course of initial surgical treatment of patients with clinical stage I endometrial carcinoma. This study noted that 16 of 140 patients evaluated had cancer in their lymph nodes despite the fact that preoperative clinical evaluation indicated an earlier stage of disease. In a subsequent expansion of this pilot study, it was noted that 9.6% of 843 patients with clinical stage I disease had lymph node metastasis. In addition, extensive surgical staging detected extrauterine disease in 23.2% of patients with apparent preoperative clinical stage I disease. These observations strengthened the impetus for more precise staging, and in 1988 the FIGO introduced the requirement for surgical staging of patients with endometrial carcinoma. The latest modifications of the surgical staging system were promulgated in 1994 to 1995 and are presented in Tables 116-4 and 116-5 of the text. This system requires the performance of total abdominal hysterectomy, bilateral salpingo-oophorectomy, and washings for cytologic examination for all patients and complete staging for those with high-risk features as noted in Figure 116-2.

116.2   **Answer: (e)**   A previous list of conditions thought to increase the risk of endometrial cancer included body size, obesity, hypertension, diabetes, nulliparity, a history of colon and/or breast carcinoma, syndromes of ovulation failure, syndromes of increased endogenous estrogen exposure, and exposure to exogenous estrogen.
        Recently, the list was refined and focused, based on an improved understanding of the underlying pathophysiology. Nulliparity as compared with multiparity of five or more births, menopause after age 53 years, and 23 kg of excess weight are all important risk factors that can increase a woman's probability of endometrial cancer by five to 10 times compared with patients without these risk factors. Multivariate

analysis controlled for age and obesity has verified the association between endometrial cancer and diabetes but not hypertension. The obesity observed in the typical phenotype associated with the endometrial cancer patient is related to a higher level of circulating estrogen than in cohorts of thinner patients. This results from peripheral aromatization in the fat of estrogen precursors. Investigators have observed an increased risk of endometrial carcinoma in diabetic patients with normal body mass indices with an increasing body mass index (BMI).

There are pathologic variants in women that are associated with an increased risk of endometrial cancer, and these features have in common the production of increased levels of estrogen or the requirements for exogenous estrogen supplementation. It is known that patients with granulosa-theca cell tumors of the ovary have clinical manifestations of increased estrogen exposure. Gusberg and Kardon reviewed the endometrial histology of 115 patients with these ovarian tumors and found that 21% developed endometrial carcinoma and 43% had benign changes that were thought to be precancerous, such as adenomatous hyperplasia. Others have not found the same incidence of adenocarcinoma but have identified a high incidence of atypical hyperplasia.

The Centers for Disease Control and Prevention reported that oral contraceptive use for at least 12 months diminished the risk of endometrial cancer by 50% compared with that for women who had never used oral contraception. Nulliparous women seemed to benefit most, and the protection lasted for a decade following the discontinuation of oral contraceptive use.

116.3 Answer: (d) Patients with atypical hyperplasia are more likely to develop carcinoma than are those with benign lesions of the endometrium, although the potential is difficult to quantify. Cytologic atypia is the only morphologic feature distinguishing endometrial lesions with invasive potential from benign ones. The classic study of Kurman, outlined in Table 116-2 of the text, followed 170 patients with all grades of endometrial hyperplasia without hysterectomy being performed for at least 1 year and with no irradiation therapy administered. Only 1.5% of patients with nonatypical hyperplasia progressed to carcinoma compared with 8% with simple atypical hyperplasia and 29% with complex atypical hyperplasia.

116.4 Answer: (a) Endometrioid adenocarcinoma is the most common of the endometrial cancer histologies. It is characterized by the disappearance of stroma between abnormal glands that have infoldings of their linings into the lumens, disordered nuclear chromatin distribution, nuclear enlargement, and a variable degree of mitosis, necrosis, and hemorrhage. This classic variety accounts for 60 to 65% of adenocarcinomas.

Adenosquamous cancer has malignant elements from both its squamous component and its adenomatous component. It usually accounts for 7% or less of adenocarcinomas of the endometrium. Although data are still maturing, it is suggested that when this convention is followed, adenosquamous cancer does not behave differently from endometrioid adenocarcinomas of the same stage and grade.

Described by Hendrikson in 1982, UPSC comprises 5 to 10% of stage I endometrial carcinomas and is characterized by an expansive papillary architecture with a fibrovascular matrix, marked cytologic atypia, bizarre nuclei, and widespread nuclear pleomorphism. The lesion is highly virulent, is usually found with deep myometrial penetration at the time of diagnosis, is often extrauterine in location in patients with clinical early-stage disease, and is almost always incurable when the disease has left the uterus.

Endometrial papillary adenocarcinomas must be distinguished from UPSCs because of their different behavior. They are characterized histologically as being usually well-differentiated papillary features composed of very slender papillations, orderly neoplastic epithelial cells, few mitoses, and less cellular disorder than UPSCs. The endometrial carcinomas with papillary features behave identically to the endometrioid adenocarcinomas.

Clear cell cancers have been described in detail by Kurman and Scully. Histologically, although there are a variety of patterns, a presentation of polygonal or flattened cells with clear cytoplasm accounts for more than half of the cells. This group constitutes approximately 6% of endometrial carcinomas and occurs more frequently in older women. The 5-year overall survival is approximately 40%, but this may be because of the increased age of the patients and the fact that clear cell carcinomas are generally found in patients with higher stages of cancer. Clear cells often appear in histologic mixtures when tumors are assigned to a different category based on the prevalent cell type, and their presence usually confers a diminished prognosis.

116.5 Answer: (d) The adoption of a surgical staging system has created controversy regarding what constitutes an adequate staging procedure, which patients should be surgically staged, and whether extensive staging or lymphadenectomy has therapeutic value. Selective pelvic and para-aortic lymphadenectomy refers to removal or biopsy of some but not all lymph nodes within the external iliac, internal iliac, obturator, hypogastric, and common iliac groups as well as the para-aortic groups. Adverse risk factors necessitating lymph node dissection include grade 2 or grade 3 lesions with > 50% myoinvasion; clear cell, papillary serous, and squamous and undifferentiated cell types; adnexal metastasis; lymph-vascular space invasion and/or cervical invasion; > 50% of uterine cavity involvement; and suspicious nodes.

The therapeutic benefit of node dissection has been described by several investigators. Most recently Trimble and colleagues reported on the impact of pelvic node sampling in 10,066 women from the National Cancer Institute Surveillance, Epidemiology, and End Results program with stage I and II endometrioid adenocarcinomas. They found an improved 5-year relative survival only in patients with stage I grade 3 tumors. However, data on adjuvant postsurgical treatment was not available in this population.

Regardless of stage, extrafascial not intrafascial hysterectomy is employed in the treatment of endometrial carcinoma.

117.1 Answer: (c) Until 1991 there was no universally accepted staging system for patients with tubal carcinoma. In 1967 Erez and colleagues proposed a clinical staging system based on prognostic observations. This was modified in 1970 by Dodson and colleagues to conform with the FIGO surgical staging system for ovarian cancer. The subsequent year Schiller and Silverberg modified the Dodson system to emphasize the importance of disease confined to the tubal lumen and the prognostic importance of invasion through the tubal wall to spread beyond the serosa. These staging systems were prevalent in most of the reports during the past 20 years, and in 1991 FIGO officially promulgated a staging system for tubal carcinoma (see Table 117-2 of text). The new staging system takes into account observation of the hollow viscus, the importance of ascites, and the impact of lymphatic spread.

Because fallopian tube cancer is rarely diagnosed preoperatively, the surgeon is usually confronted with the diagnosis intraoperatively. The new FIGO staging system requires a surgical exercise similar to that mandated for ovarian carcinoma. This includes cytologic analysis of either ascitic fluid or pelvic and abdominal washings, abdominal hysterectomy and bilateral salpingo-oophorectomy, omentectomy, and selective (or therapeutic) pelvic and para-aortic lymphadenectomy with selective peritoneal biopsies.

117.2   Answer: (b)   Although more than 90% of fallopian cancers are papillary adenocarcinomas, the synchronous presentation of the same histology in multiple pelvic sites recommends the establishment of diagnostic criteria that will identify primary fallopian tube cancer. The criteria established by Hu and colleagues and later modified slightly by Sedlis have been widely accepted (see Table 117-1 of text).

117.3   Answer: (a)   In view of the inherent difficulties of studying such a rare disease, the role of prognostic factors assumes a great importance. Stage is the most consistent prognostic factor associated with survival. Although initial tumor burden does not have predictive significance regarding survival, residual disease after cytoreduction is a strong prognostic factor of survival. Other clinical prognostic factors include the presence of ascites. Recently Rosen and colleagues reported on prognostic factors in 143 women with primary fallopian tube carcinoma. FIGO stage, histologic grade, and presence of residual tumor had an independent prognostic impact in multivariate analysis. Several histologic factors are prognostic of survival, most notably the extent of tubal invasion. The observation that extent of tubal invasion was associated with a poorer prognosis was first reported by Schiller and Silverberg. Peters and colleagues, analyzing stage I disease, observed a statistically significant increase in the risk of death with invasion of > 50% of the tubal muscle.

117.4   Answer: (a)   Because of similarities in the appearance of papillary carcinomas of the tube and ovary, in the past it was logical to apply to patients with tubal carcinoma the cytotoxic agents known to be active against ovarian carcinoma. Cyclophosphamide, melphalan, and thiotepa were among the frequently used single agents in the early cytotoxic treatment of tubal carcinoma. Response rates to single alkylating agents were generally < 20% in small series of patients with disparate stages and prognostic features. With the introduction of cisplatin-containing regimens, complete clinical responses were noted for patients with advanced disease and were confirmed by second-look surgery. Peters and colleagues demonstrated that multiagent chemotherapy with cisplatin achieved an 81% objective response rate, whereas multiagent therapy without cisplatin achieved a 29% response rate and single-agent therapy (other than cisplatin) achieved a 9% response rate. In the cisplatin group, there were 12 complete surgical responses in 20 patients.

117.5   Answer: (c)   Studies from the literature indicate that the pattern of spread of fallopian tube carcinoma is similar to ovarian carcinoma with both intraperitoneal and lymphatic spread commonly encountered. However, because older staging systems did not mandate lymphadenectomy, there are few data concerning the incidence of lymph node metastases at the time of presentation. Tamimi and Figge reviewed 15 patients treated over a 12-year period in their institution. Lymph node sampling was not routine at the time of initial surgery, yet 4 of their patients had positive para-aortic nodes at the time of presentation, and overall 8 of their patients had lymph node involvement either at the time of presentation or at the time of recurrence shortly after treatment. Semrad and colleagues studied patterns of recurrent disease and noted a 71% incidence of extraperitoneal metastases, suggesting a strong probability of unrecognized lymphatic invasion at the time of initial therapy. More recently, di Re and colleagues, studying the lymphatic spread of fallopian tube carcinoma in 17 patients undergoing surgical staging, observed an increase in nodal metastases rates with stage of disease and grade. Of note, the percentage of patients with positive nodes was 33%, 66%, and 80% for stages I, II, and III to IV disease, respectively. Overall, patients with negative nodes had a median survival of 76 months, compared with only 33 months if nodal metastases were found.

118.1   Answer: (b)   Studies have shown that the overexpression of *HER2/neu* is associated with a poorer prognosis (shorter median and overall survivals) than for those patients whose tumors do not overexpress the oncogene. This finding appears to be independent of the stage and grade of the tumor. In addition, although many of these patients initially respond to chemotherapy, they tend to relapse faster than do patients whose tumors do not overexpress *HER2/neu*.

118.2   Answer: (b)   *P53* is the most commonly mutated tumor suppressor gene in solid tumors and in ovarian cancer. Low-stage tumors have a lower rate of mutation than do high-stage tumors. The other factors listed do not correlate well with the presence of mutations of *P53*.

118.3   Answer: (a)   The prognosis of women with low-stage borderline serous tumors is excellent, with 10-year survivals being close to 100%. Therefore, conservative management (preservation of the uterus and the contralateral ovary and uterine tube) is appropriate in these patients.

118.4   Answer: (c)   Of these germ cell and stromal lesions of the ovary, the one associated with virilization is the Sertoli-Leydig cell tumor, which is known for its secretion of androgenic steroids.

118.5   Answer: (a)   Of these germ cell ovarian tumors, the one that typically produces α-fetoprotein is the embryonal carcinoma. Endodermal sinus tumors also secrete this protein, and in both instances α-fetoprotein can be a useful marker to determine the clinical course of the disease. Occasionally, mixed germ cell tumors, such as those with elements of dysgerminoma, can also secrete this protein.

118.6   Answer: (a)   The studies show that for well-differentiated stage I ovarian carcinomas, there is no benefit to giving adjuvant chemotherapy as the survival is excellent, 90 to 95% at 5 years, and no improvement is shown with platinum-based chemotherapy. Iatrogenic intraoperative rupture does not appear to worsen the prognosis in these patients.

118.7   Answer: (e)   The coexistence of endometrioid carcinoma of the ovary and endometrioid endometrial cancer is well known; thus, they represent synchronous carcinomas. In these patients with two low-stage carcinomas, the prognosis is excellent and is considerably better than in those patients with carcinoma arising from one of the sites and metastasis to the other.

119.1   **Answer: (c)**   In patients with persistent gestational trophoblastic tumors, the most common sites of metastasis include the lung (70%), vagina (30%), liver (10%), and brain (10%).

119.2   **Answer: (c)**   Patients with persistent gestational trophoblastic tumors and small vaginal metastases are generally treated with primary single-agent chemotherapy, which induces remission in 80 to 90%.

119.3   **Answer: (d)**   Patients with persistent gestational trophoblastic tumors with large lung lesions and high hCG levels (high-risk stage III) are commonly resistant to single-agent chemotherapy. Combination chemotherapy is employed as the primary treatment; almost all patients can anticipate remission.

119.4   **Answer: (d)**   Single-agent chemotherapy induces complete sustained remission in about 90% of patients with nonmetastatic gestational trophoblastic tumors.

120.1   **Answer: (b)**   Even though the female pelvis is richly endowed with blood vessels, connective tissue, and müllerian elements, sarcomas of the vulva, vagina, cervix, uterus, and ovaries account for < 1.5% of the cancers of these organs. The most common site for sarcoma in the female pelvis is the uterus, but only 3 to 5% of uterine cancers are sarcomas.

120.2   **Answer: (d)**   Because of the infrequent occurrence of sarcomas, classification of these cancers was a taxonomic dilemma until Ober, in 1959, proposed a classification that became the basis from which modern modifications have derived. A detailed classification adapted from Kempson and Bari and a functional classification developed by the GOG are presented in Table 120-1.

120.3   **Answer: (a)**   For patients with carcinosarcoma, there are two clearly active agents: ifosfamide and cisplatin (see Table 120-2 of text). Ifosfamide is the most active single agent in the treatment of advanced or recurrent carcinosarcoma of the uterus. Sutton and colleagues conducted a phase II study of ifosfamide (1.5 g/m^2/d for 5 d q4wk) and mesna in 30 patients with advanced or recurrent carcinosarcoma who had no prior chemotherapy. In 28 patients available for response, 5 patients had complete responses (17.9%) and 4 patients had partial responses (14.3%), for a total response rate of 32.1%. However, the response duration ranged from 1.4 to 8.6 months, with a median response duration of only 3.8 months.

120.4   **Answer: (c)**   Of the single agents that have been tested in patients with leiomyosarcoma (see Table 120-2 of text), doxorubicin is the most active. In the two GOG phase III trials comparing doxorubicin-based chemotherapy in combination with dacarbazine (DTIC) or cyclophosphamide in advanced uterine sarcomas, response rates of 25% and 13%, respectively, were observed in patients with leiomyosarcoma treated with doxorubicin alone. Patients with leiomyosarcoma also had a significantly longer survival time than did the other histologic cell types studied (12.1 versus 6.0 mo).

120.5   **Answer: (d)**   The initial therapy for sarcomas of the gynecologic tract is surgical except in cases of embryonal rhabdomyosarcoma (see Figure 120-2 of text). Patients with uterine sarcoma require total abdominal hysterectomy and careful staging. The ovaries may be retained in premenopausal patients with leiomyosarcoma because it appears to improve the patient's prognosis. However, a bilateral salpingo-oophorectomy should be performed in all other patients, including those with low-grade endometrial stromal sarcoma because these tumors may be hormone dependent or responsive, and they have a propensity for extension into the parametria, broad ligament, and adnexal structures. For carcinosarcoma, a high percentage of patients with clinical stage I or II disease are upstaged at the time of laparotomy; thus, it appears reasonable to surgically stage these patients. There is a paucity of data regarding the role of lymph node sampling in patients with leiomyosarcoma and endometrial stromal sarcoma, but it appears that almost all patients with these sarcomas who have lymph node metastases also have evidence of intraperitoneal disease spread.

THE BREAST

121.1   **Answer: (d)**   Lung cancer has surpassed breast cancer as the number one cause of cancer death in US women. A woman's lifetime risk of developing breast cancer is 1 in 8; however, as women grow older, the relative risk decreases. An average healthy 50-year-old woman has a 4.4% risk. The death rate from breast cancer has remained stable for the past half century and is now actually declining. The introduction of widespread screening mammography has actually increased the percentage of women who are diagnosed with ductal carcinoma in situ.

121.2   **Answer: (e)**   The frequency of this diagnosis has been increasing with the wider use of screening mammography. Of the different histologic patterns observed in DCIS, the comedocarcinoma variety has the least favorable histology and the worst prognosis. These tumors have a high labeling index and S-phase fraction, as well. Papillary and cribriform varieties are less aggressive, and this seems to correlate with the absence of HER2/neu overexpression of these cells. The evaluation of ER and PR status in DCIS has not yet been clearly established as an important prognostic indicator.

121.3   **Answer: (e)**   Removing more than six lymph nodes at surgery does not enhance the assessment of patients' prognoses. Nodal metastasis remains the most powerful prognostic indicator to date. Sinus histiocytosis is a good prognostic indicator. Patients who have ≥ 4 nodes clearly have a worse prognosis at 5 and 10 years.

121.4 **Answer: (d)** In underdeveloped countries, menarche may be delayed due to poor nutrition, and this may be one of the factors related to the lower incidence of breast cancer in those areas. Menopause after the age of 55 years confers a twofold risk compared with a menopause age of 45. Cigarette smoking is unrelated to breast cancer. Alcohol has a dose-response relationship to breast cancer, with women who drink three glasses of wine having up to a 50% increase in the risk of developing breast cancer. Women who have children in their late thirties have a higher risk of developing breast cancer than those who have had children before the age of 20. Women who give birth in their thirties have a greater risk than women who remain nulliparous. Low-dose estrogen replacement may be associated with a less than twofold increased risk of breast cancer.

121.5 **Answer: (c)** Tamoxifen has been shown to cause a G_1 cell cycle phase block, behaving more like a cytostatic rather than a cytocidal factor. Families who have Li-Fraumeni syndrome have an increased incidence of several tumor types due to mutations in the *P53* gene.

121.6 **Answer: (a)** The pathologist plays an increasingly important role in the management of patients who have carcinoma of the breast. Initial assessment must include determination of whether the tumor is in situ (no invasion through the basement membrane, confined either to a duct or a lobule) or if the tumor is actually invasive. Of the invasive carcinomas, those that grow in a papillary configuration are rare, but it is rare for these benign-behaving tumors to invade the surrounding stroma; therefore, there is a cure rate of 100% if the lesion is completely excised. Medullary carcinomas, constituting 5 to 10% of breast cancers, are circumscribed lesions that attain large dimensions but demonstrate low-grade barely infiltrating properties. Tubular and colloid carcinoma have similarly favorable neutral histories.

121.7 **Answer: (e)** Tamoxifen is a safe and effective drug both for patients with stage II breast cancer who will be given the drug as adjuvant therapy and for patients who have advanced breast cancer. Tamoxifen is a partial estrogen agonist/antagonist. The weak estrogen-like properties account for a slight decrease in the level of cholesterol in postmenopausal women, some changes in the vaginal cytology, and a few excess cases of uterine cancer (generally low stage) that have been reported. Probably because most postmenopausal patients are ER-positive, most will respond to tamoxifen. Those who have ER-positive disease are much more likely to respond to tamoxifen therapy than are those whose tumors do not express the ER (48 vs 15% response rate). Recent studies establish that the aromatase inhibitors anastrozole and letrozole are at least as active as tamoxifen for metastatic breast cancer; they do not predispose to endometrial cancer.

When used for adjuvant therapy, it appears that prolonged tamoxifen administration is better than brief tamoxifen therapy. Tamoxifen actually confers a survival advantage of up to 4 years in postmenopausal women, and therefore is usually given for 5 years after diagnosis of such patients. The estrogen-like effects of tamoxifen lower the circulating cholesterol in women taking this drug; therefore, even prolonged use is not likely to be associated with coronary disease.

121.8 **Answer: (a)** The CALGB has shown that tumors that are high expressors of *HER2* respond better to doxorubicin-containing regimens when the doxorubicin dose is 60 mg/m^2 every 3 weeks times four than at lower doses. A further increase in dose was not beneficial. The statement as given, however, is incorrect. Although performance status, nonvisceral tumor burden, and absence of prior exposure to chemotherapy increase the chance of a response, ER status does not predict response to chemotherapy; therefore, this statement is wrong. Initial response rate of patients who have stage IV disease is approximately 40 to 70%; however, the complete remission rate is only 10 to 20%. In general, more aggressive and continuous chemotherapy confers a better quality of life because the complications from the cancer itself seem to cause more discomfort than the drugs themselves. The most effective drug for the treatment of breast cancer appears to be doxorubicin. However, the CAF combination does not have a clear advantage over the regimen of CMF, even though some studies do show a small difference in favor of CAF. This is especially important considering that CAF is more toxic. Answers d and e are both correct statements.

121.9 **Answer: (a)** At this time, combination treatment cannot be recommended for stage IV disease because there is no solid clinical evidence supporting this modality. The patient has experienced a partial remission and stable disease with tamoxifen therapy for 2 years. This represents successful hormonal therapy. There is no evidence that giving chemotherapy at this time will enhance the patient's survival. There are also no definitive data suggesting that hormonal therapy is contraindicated, although some experimental studies do show an increased resistance of cancer cells to chemotherapy after treatment with tamoxifen. Although some studies suggest a role for estrogen priming to increase the S-phase fraction, this has yet to be confirmed.

121.10 **Answer: (d)** Cancerous breast masses usually have a well-defined margin as opposed to fibrocystic disease, which blends into the surrounding tissue. Adenomas are well defined but are encapsulated and highly mobile when palpated. The most common cause of bloody nipple discharge is a benign papilloma, although the discharge must always be evaluated. Although palpation of axillary lymph nodes is notoriously inaccurate, the true figures from a large NSABP trial are less dismal, with 38% false-negatives and 25% false-positives. Pain is uncommon but not unknown in the presentation of breast cancer and is usually due to benign disease, especially when cyclic pain is encountered during the perimenstrual period in young women.

121.11 **Answer: (c)** Lead-time bias refers to the fact that with screening patients may be diagnosed earlier, even though their date of death will be the same. This would make it seem that these women have a longer survival time, which is false. The correct way to avoid lead and length bias is to count the deaths from breast cancer in both groups and avoid using indicators such as survival rates and average survival.

121.12 **Answer: (a)** There is enough evidence that mammography reduces mortality in the group of women 50 to 74 years of age to recommend its routine yearly use. However, the reduction in mortality is 30%, not 70%. The rest of the statements are all true.

121.13 **Answer: (c)** A patient who has a receptor-positive breast cancer should not receive estrogen replacement therapy because this treatment could stimulate existing cancer cells. Progestogens are employed (in large doses) for treating advanced breast cancer; there is no evidence that smaller doses stimulate breast cancer. Hence, use of progestogen (20–40 mg/d) in the treatment of disabling menopausal symptoms is appropriate and effective.

121.14   Answer: (c)   Bilateral orchiectomy or other antiandrogen hormonal agents would be effective methods of management. However, chemotherapy also can play a significant role in countering this disease. In view of the patient's recent marriage and a possible desire to maintain sexual prowess, chemotherapy is an appropriate initial therapy. If no response occurs or later after reactivation of the cancer occurs, orchiectomy or luteinizing hormone–releasing hormones could be used.

121.15   Answer: (b)   Breast carcinoma in men accounts for 1% of all breast malignancies. However, this disease is rare and often is detected late because most cases of gynecomastia represent benign disease. Stage for stage, men may have a somewhat worse prognosis than women; however, treatment is typically the same for both sexes. Although the presence of *BRCA1* and *BRCA2* malignant gene mutations indicates a high risk of breast malignancies, neither of these tests is useful for screening a population.

121.16   Answer: (d)   Although cystosarcoma phyllodes histologically resemble benign fibroadenomas, these tumors are typically larger than the average fibroadenoma. It is often difficult to differentiate the lesions by histology alone. However, both the large size and rapid growth rate are more indicative of a cystosarcoma phyllodes. They are not multicentric, multifocal, or bilateral. Like most mesenchymal tumors, they tend to metastasize first by blood-borne pathways rather than by the lymphatic system. In the absence of metastases, wide local excision and, if necessary, total mastectomy are appropriate for management of these lesions.

121.17   Answer: (e)   Although DCIS was once a rare entity, it is becoming increasingly common due to early diagnosis of cancer with mammography. The treatment of DCIS continues to be controversial because patients may have occult invasive disease at the time of presentation. This condition is typically not bilateral. Patients who have LCIS have up to a 70% chance of bilateral disease; LCIS should be considered as a marker of subsequent risk of invasive carcinoma rather than as a malignant or premalignant lesion.

121.18   Answer: (d)   The treatment for DCIS remains controversial. Patients with small tumors and low-grade histologies, including papillary, cribriform, and solid subtypes, can typically be managed with lumpectomy alone. Patients with comedo subtypes and larger primary lesions are at higher risk of multifocal disease and likely should have a lumpectomy with postoperative radiotherapy or, as an alternative, total mastectomy. Patients with tumors greater than 4.5 cm, comedo histology, high-grade tumors, and/or those that involve the surgical margins should not be considered for lumpectomy alone or in combination with postoperative radiotherapy. These patients and those who have suspicious microcalcification after segmentectomy should be treated with mastectomy. The presence of microinvasive disease is rare, and, thus, axillary lymph node dissection is typically not warranted in these patients, but it is indicated in the present case.

121.19   Answer: (e)   Although typically the size, grade, architecture (either cribriform, papillary, or comedo), and degree of differentiation of the lesion have been useful in order to determine therapy, none of these factors has been demonstrated to be independently appropriate for determining the therapeutic approach for those who have DCIS. Newer techniques include determining the presence of *HER2/neu* oncogene overexpression, which is higher in comedo than noncomedocarcinomas. DNA flow cytometry has been used for invasive carcinomas but recently has also been used in order to determine the S-phase fraction of noninvasive lesions. Newer techniques to determine the presence of sialyl-Tn expression have shown this marker to be associated with aneuploid and high-nuclear-grade tumors. Although the *P53* tumor suppressor gene has been associated with breast cancer and may indeed correlate with response to chemotherapy, *P53* overexpression has not been associated with DCIS.

121.20   Answer: (c)   Patients who have locally advanced breast carcinoma (inflammatory breast cancer) with involvement of the subdermal lymphatics have up to a 90% chance of having nodal metastases. Although most patients subsequently die of distant metastases, local disease control is imperative. Most regimens have combined preoperative combination chemotherapy, followed by resection of the primary tumor and axillary lymph node dissection, followed by postoperative radiotherapy and possibly additional chemotherapy. The combination approach allows for less aggressive surgical resection and ultimately may improve local disease control.

121.21   Answer: (c)   Patients with ipsilateral breast recurrence who have been treated by lumpectomy alone can be salvaged with total mastectomy. These patients are particularly at high risk of developing metastatic disease and should be considered for adjuvant therapy following surgical resection of the recurrence. Radiotherapy alone is not indicated, except following resection and perhaps if the recurrence is outside the irradiated field. There is no role for the use of tamoxifen alone in this setting, although it may be useful as an adjuvant therapy after mastectomy.

THE SKIN

122.1   Answer: (c)   Four randomized prospective studies have examined the margins of excision of melanoma based on the potential risk of local recurrence. Local recurrence rates vary according to primary site, increase with thickness, and the presence or absence of tumor ulceration. The margins used in these randomized trials were based on primary thickness. Veronesi and the World Health Organization conducted a multicenter trial comparing 1 and 3 cm margins for patients having primaries up to 2 mm thick. Patients with primaries greater than 1 mm thick had a higher risk of local relapse with narrow margins, but there was no difference in survival in either treatment group. Most investigators now recommend 2 cm margins for primaries greater than 1 mm thick. The American Intergroup trial compared 2 to 4 cm margins for primaries of 1 to 4 mm thick. This study demonstrated no difference in local relapse or survival between the narrow and wide margins, and as a result most surgeons have abandoned 4 cm margins for even thick (> 4 mm) lesions. Excisional biopsy is not accepted therapy for the primary disease.

Sentinel lymphadenectomy is a minimally invasive operative technique that is a highly accurate method for staging the regional lymph nodes and should be considered if patients are to be considered for adjuvant therapy trials for lymph node–positive disease.

Interferon-α has been extensively studied as an adjuvant therapy for melanoma primarily in patients with tumor-positive lymph nodes. There are no data to support interferon-α use in patients with disease limited to the primary site.

122.2 **Answer: (a)** The median survival of patients with American Joint Committee on Cancer (AJCC) stage IV melanoma is approximately 4 to 8 months. Yet it is clear that patients with limited number and sites of metastases have a far better survival than individuals with multiple metastases. Patients with pulmonary and soft-tissue metastases have a better survival than those patients with disease in the liver, bone, or brain. The number of metastatic sites has been shown to be of prognostic importance. Staging evaluation is essential before considering options for treatment. Tafra and associates have demonstrated long-term survivors following complete resection of pulmonary metastases with median survival of 25 months as compared with only 11 months for patients with more advanced disease having an incomplete resection. There is no role for low-dose interferon or 5-FU–based chemotherapy for metastatic melanoma. Hospice home care is appropriate for patients with end-stage disease but is not appropriate for this patient.

122.3 **Answer: (c)** Mohs' surgical resection has been used for treatment of melanoma in situ or thin primaries of the head and neck. The efficacy of Mohs' surgery has never been prospectively compared with wider surgical resection and currently is not considered as standard for control of a 6 mm thick melanoma. Although staging evaluations with CT scans of the neck, chest, abdomen, and pelvis are useful for staging patients with thick primaries, DTIC-based chemotherapy is not used for treatment of the primary lesion or occult metastases. External beam radiation has been advocated for control of lymph node basins but appears to have the greatest benefit for patients with multiple (> 3) lymph node metastases or extracapsular disease. It has not been routinely used for control of the primary or for clinically negative lymph nodes.

122.4 **Answer: (a)** A young patient with a history of multiple dysplastic nevi and a thin melanoma has the familial atypical mole-melanoma syndrome. Usually these patients develop thin melanomas of low metastatic potential. Although other family members should be examined for atypical nevi, there is no clear genetic defect associated with this syndrome. Chromosome 1 alterations are associated with melanoma and *P16* gene mutations have been associated with melanoma and pancreatic cancer. Peptide vaccines are being tested for the treatment of advanced melanoma but their efficacy is unknown. At this time there are no data to suggest a peptide vaccine would be useful for control of primary disease.

122.5 **Answer: (a)** Intransit melanoma metastases occur in 1% of all patients and approximately 8% of patients with primaries of the lower extremities. The management of intransit disease should be based on the number of intransit lesions. Patients with only a few metastases are candidates for surgical excision or ablation with intralesional therapy (ie, interferon-α or bacille Calmette-Guérin). Patients with multiple metastases can be considered for hyperthermic isolated limb perfusion. The most commonly employed agent is melphalan, although both cisplatin and DTIC have been used. Biologics such as interleukin-2 are now being investigated for this purpose but have not been shown to be more effective than melphalan alone. Usually a superficial groin dissection is performed along with hyperthermic limb perfusion to control metastases to the regional lymph node basin.

123.1 **Answer: (b)** Sporadic and hereditary basal cell carcinomas have defects in the Sonic hedgehog pathway. The majority of tumors have specific mutations in the *PATCH* gene, which is the receptor for Sonic hedgehog. *PATCH* normally inhibits the activity of the transmembrane protein SMOOTHENED. Experimentally, the drug cyclopamine blocks SMOOTHENED's function and may therefore represent a novel approach to treating basal cell carcinomas in the future.

123.2 **Answer: (d)** DFSP is a local aggressive CD34-positive dermal tumor with a tendency for extensive subclinical extension. Even with wide local excision, these tumors have a high local recurrence rate and have been known to metastasize after multiple failed excisions. Mohs' micrographic surgery is a technique that examines 100% of the margin as it is excised; it can detect small finger-like extensions of tumor at the periphery of the exision that could be missed with traditional frozen section pathologic examination. Recurrence rates following Mohs' surgery are generally < 5%. There is no role for local radiation or adjuvant chemotherapy in the treatment of this low-grade sarcoma.

123.3 **Answer: (b)** Multiple trichilemmomas are the dermatologic hallmark of Cowden disease. Ductal breast carcinoma has been found in up to one-half of females with this syndrome. Although mutations in the tyrosine phosphatase gene *PTEN* have been found in some families, routine genetic screening is not yet feasible. The cosmetically distressing lesions of Cowden disease can be treated with laser ablation using the pulsed carbon dioxide laser. The differential diagnosis of multiple facial papules includes multiple trichoepithelioma and neurofibromatosis, neither of which carries the high internal malignancy rate of Cowden disease.

123.4 **Answer: (e)** Sebaceous carcinoma is a rare malignancy often occurring on the eyelid in older patients. When not located on the eyelid, standard excisional surgery is usually curative. The detection of a single sebaceous carcinoma is suggestive of Muir-Torre syndrome. This syndrome occurs because of mutations in deoxyribonucleic acid mismatch enzymes, and puts patients at risk of internal malignancies including gastrointestinal and genitourinary tumors. Therefore, a systematic screening, including endoscopy and cystoscopy are usually indicated.

123.5 **Answer: (a)** Australia has one of the highest rates of SCC of the lip and a high associated mortality that can reach rates of 10% or more.

BONE AND SOFT TISSUE

124.1 **Answer: (d)**

124.2 **Answer: (c)**

124.3 **Answer: (a)**

124.4 **Answer: (e)**

124.5 **Answer: (b)**

125.1 **Answer: (b)** The development of human soft tissue sarcomas has been associated with various factors: (1) progression from a benign precursor, such as angiosarcoma developing from chronic lymphedema; (2) genetic mutation, such as von Recklinghausen's disease, Li-Fraumeni syndrome, Werner's syndrome, or Gardner's syndrome; (3) Epstein-Barr virus infection in human immnodeficiency virus (HIV)-positive patients; (4) prior radiation exposure; (5) prior exposure to various chemicals; (6) trauma; and (7) immunosuppression in acquired immunodeficiency syndrome in patients who have Kaposi's sarcoma. Rous sarcoma virus is a simian virus that induces soft tissue sarcomas in chickens.

125.2 **Answer: (c)** Retroperitoneal sarcomas constitute approximately 15% of all soft tissue sarcomas. Most patients are first seen with an abdominal mass and nonspecific symptoms. These tumors are typically liposarcomas and, less commonly, leiomyosarcomas or fibrosarcomas. The differential diagnosis includes lymphomas or metastatic testicular carcinomas in men. Once the diagnosis is made, it is important to determine the potential for curative resection. Complete surgical resection is the primary treatment for retroperitoneal sarcomas; complete resection correlates with overall disease-free survival and long-term outcome. Although soft tissue sarcomas of the extremities respond to chemotherapy and radiotherapy, the toxicity of treatment in the abdominal cavity is significant, and there are no data to support using this combination modality during initial treatment.

125.3 **Answer: (d)** Patients who have retroperitoneal sarcomas should be followed up on a routine basis with CT scan of the abdomen. Some patients with locally recurrent disease will be salvaged with re-resection. The benefit of repeat operation in patients with no symptoms is controversial. There is no role for chemotherapy or radiotherapy alone in this setting. Recent studies suggest there may be a benefit to intraoperative radiotherapy and postoperative external beam treatment, but the data are inconclusive.

125.4 **Answer: (b)** Regardless of the apparent stability of a large extremity mass, adequate histologic study of a biopsy specimen is indicated. Generally, frozen-section examination is required to confirm that the specimen is representative of the lesion and adequate for diagnosis. Excisional biopsy is not indicated for this large lesion but could be used for small tumors less than 3 cm in size. Longitudinal biopsy incision is preferred for extremity lesions due to easy incorporation into subsequent definitive surgical incisions. Fine-needle aspiration is useful in the hands of an experienced pathologist for diagnosis of malignant tumors and sarcomas.

125.5 **Answer: (c)** There is no ideal or universally accepted classification system for soft tissue sarcomas. Problems that arise in distinguishing cell origin include changes induced by metaplasia, several different cell types within the same tumor, and the degree of dedifferentiation. These problems can make histogenetic identification extremely difficult. The current AJCC clinicopathologic staging system depends on the tumor size, lymph node status, evidence of distant metastasis, and histopathologic grade (TNMG). The most important prognostic factors for the majority of sarcomas are histopathologic grade and tumor size.

125.6 **Answer: (b)** Brachytherapy is directed radiotherapy after surgery via deposition of radioactive materials through catheters placed at the time of surgery. This modality's use is particularly beneficial for high-grade sarcomas, improving local control from 65 to 90%. However, brachytherapy has no significant impact on low-grade tumors. Adjuvant chemotherapy has an important role in treating bone sarcomas but has not been of conclusive benefit for soft tissue sarcomas. In recent years, the use of limb-sparing surgery has become accepted practice. Even for larger lesions (0.5 cm), preoperative external beam radiotherapy can make a more limited surgical approach feasible.

125.7 **Answer: (b)** Desmoid tumor or musculoaponeurotic fibromatosis is notorious for local recurrence. The principal treatment for this tumor is wide excision. Brachytherapy is generally not indicated because this is a low-grade malignant neoplasm. Like other soft tissue sarcomas, MFH carries a prognosis that is dependent on size and grade of the primary lesion. Although rhabdomyosarcoma is chemoresponsive, complete tumor eradication can rarely be achieved. Even in the typical elderly (non–HIV-infected) patient with classic Kaposi's sarcoma, secondary malignancies do occur with higher than expected frequency.

HEMATOPOIETIC SYSTEM

127.1 **Answer: (a)** By far the two most important prognostic factors in patients with AML are the patient's age and cytogenetics. Cytogenetic abnormalities in AML fall into three categories: good prognostic abnormalities characterized by translocations that reflect mutations in transcription factors t(8;21) inversion 16 or t(15;17); poor prognostic abnormalities (involving abnormalities of chromosome 5 and/or 7 or multiple abnormalities); and intermediate prognosis abnormalities (usually a normal karyotype, or all cytogenetic abnormalities not in the good or poor prognostic categories). Older patients fare poorly. A relatively soft but important prognostic factor includes clinical evidence of a high disease burden at presentation, including a high white count and high serum LDH. Performance status is also a very important factor for outcome.

127.2 **Answer: (d)** Although the vast majority of patients with AML develop their disease spontaneously, particularly if they are over the age of 60 years, certain exposures may predispose to this disease. Deoxyribonucleic acid (DNA) damage is the common thread that links these exposures. Autoimmune diseases such as Sjögren's syndrome or rheumatoid arthritis are not risk factors because stimulation of the immune system appears to be more important in the generation of lymphoid, rather than myeloid, neoplasms. There are two types of therapy-related leukemias. The classic type is alkylating agent induced, which occurs with an incubation period of 3 to 8 years and is associated with chromosomal abnormalities of 5 and 7. A more recognized type is the so-called topoisomerase II inhibitor secondary leukemia often characterized by a shorter incubation period and abnormalities of chromosome 11 at the q23 region.

127.3 **Answer: (c)** The rapid cell turnover occurring at leukemic presentation that is made worse after the use of cytotoxic chemotherapy results in the generation of DNA metabolism byproducts. Purine confabulates are converted to uric acid, which is relatively insoluble in renal tubules. Allopurinol inhibits the enzyme that catalyzes the final step in uric acid metabolism, the conversion of xanthine and hypoxanthine by xanthine oxidase to uric acid. Hydration and alkalization of the urine by administration of intravenous sodium bicarbonate are also adjunctive treatments that can prevent the precipitation of uric acid crystals in renal tubules and the concomitant interstitial nephropathy, which was a former common cause of mortality in patients undergoing antileukemic therapy.

127.4 **Answer: (a)** Randomized studies conducted by the Cancer and Leukemia Group B (CALGB) and the Eastern Cooperative Oncology Group demonstrated the value of high-dose cytarabine in the postremission management of patients with AML. The CALGB study of 8,525 patients compared high-dose cytarabine versus intermediate-dose cytarabine versus low-dose cytarabine in patients who achieved remission. High-dose cytarabine led to significant improvement in disease-free and overall survival in patients under age 60 years. Unfortunately this benefit was not translated to patients over the age of 60 years. An overall long-term survival of 45% in patients in first remission who have been exposed to high-dose cytarabine is comparable to results with allogeneic bone marrow transplantation.

127.5 **Answer: (d)** Reports in the late 1980s documented that retinoic acid could produce remissions via differentiation in patients with advanced acute promyelocytic leukemia. It was thereafter shown that similar results could be obtained in newly diagnosed patients but that, without the addition of chemotherapy, all patients relapsed. Several randomized trials, most notably the French APL 93 trial showed that the best approach was to give retinoic acid and chemotherapy together during induction and to use retinoic acid again during the maintenance phase. The addition of antimetabolite therapy to retinoic acid maintenance seems superior, but this notion is being confirmed by ongoing clinical trials. Arsenic trioxide, a very active agent in advanced APL early in the disease, is being evaluated.

128.1 **Answer: (b)** Five percent of patients with the typical phenotype of CML do not have the Philadelphia chromosome but do have the Bcr-Abl rearrangement. The latter is diagnostic.

128.2 **Answer: (a)** The consensus would indicate that in young individuals, < age 30 years, with a matched unrelated donor, the risk-to-reward ratio is sufficient to justify an immediate transplantation without evaluating response to imatinib therapy. Obviously, this may change as additional information is gathered with respect to the results of imatinib therapy.

129.1 **Answer: (a)** ALL in adults is a different disease biologically than ALL in children. This biologic difference is best exemplified by a 25 to 33% incidence of the Philadelphia chromosome [t(9;22)] in adults yet less than a 5% incidence in children. The cytogenetic abnormality suggests that the leukemia has arisen from primitive hematopoietic elements, is associated with chemotherapy resistance, and presents an essential impossibility of cure without an allogeneic bone marrow transplantation. All balanced translocations are adverse prognostic signs in ALL. The incidence of L-3, or Burkitt's subtype, associated with the t(8;14) cytogenetic abnormality, is also higher in adults than in children. However, even in adults, this finding is relatively unusual, occurring in less than 5% of those who have ALL. Children have a higher likelihood of presenting at some point in their course with central nervous sytem involvement; however, the use of central nervous system prophylaxis, including cranial radiotherapy and/or intrathecal chemotherapy, has diminished the impact of this clinical problem. Although approximately 90% of adults under age 60 years who have ALL will enter remission with newer more intensive regimens, most of these patients are destined to relapse. Unfortunately, allogeneic bone marrow transplantation in adults with ALL in first remission has not been shown to be clearly superior to chemotherapy alone. Nonetheless, for those who are first seen with a balanced translocation, such as the Philadelphia chromosome, allogeneic transplantation must be considered as the treatment of choice because it offers the only opportunity for cure.

129.2 **Answer: (c)** Age is an adverse factor with respect to cancer prognosis for many specific neoplasms. The incidence of cancer may be bimodal, as with ALL, where there are two distinct peaks, one at 4 to 7 years of age and the other in persons over 50 years. The cure rate for pediatric patients with ALL is 60 to 80%. Although drug tolerance is somewhat better in younger patients, the most important reason for relatively poor results in older patients is tumor cell biologic differences. For example, hyperdiploidy, which correlates with a favorable prognosis, is more common in lymphoblasts obtained from children than adults. Conversely, balanced translocations, which are poor prognostic indicators, are more common in adults.

130.1 **Answer: (d)** CLL lymphocytes are monoclonal B cells—they are CD23+; whereas, mantle cell lymphoma (also CD19+, CD5+) cells are CD23–. CD103 is expressed on hairy cell leukemia.

130.2   Answer: (c)   Presence of somatic hypermutations in IgV genes and absence of CD38 expression on CLL cells have recently been discovered to be associated with good prognosis.

130.3   Answer: (a)   Autoimmune hemolytic anemia occurs in CLL, but it is not a common occurrence; when it is seen, it is with warm antibodies (IgG type). Although it is not clearly established, it is commonly recognized that fludarabine usage has caused an increase in the incidence of AIHA. Monthly prophylactic γ-globulin infusions did decrease the frequency of major infections, but the statement that this therapy prolongs the survival time in CLL patients is not true.

130.4   Answer: (b)   There is no evidence that CLL patients with marked hypogammaglobulinemia benefit in anyway if systemic therapy for their leukemia is started merely because of this clinical finding.

130.5   Answer: (b)   A large North American Intergroup clinical trial of previously untreated CLL patients clearly demonstrated the superiority of fludarabine over chlorambucil in the incidence of complete and partial remissions, but the trial failed to demonstrate statistically significant improvement in the overall survival time among fludarabine-treated patients.

131.1   Answer: (b)   Pancytopenia and splenomegaly are present in a great majority of patients who have HCL. Hepatomegaly and adenopathy are rare occurrences.

131.2   Answer: (d)   Atypical mycobacterial infections, lytic bone lesions, vasculitic lesions, and splenic rupture are reported in patients who have HCL. Hematuria is not a problem as the platelet count is rarely < 20,000.

131.3   Answer: (a)   CD5+ is most common in chronic lymphocytic leukemia, whereas CD11c+ and CD25+ are characteristic of HCL. CD19 is not seen in HCL.

131.4   Answer: (c)   Splenectomy reverses thrombocytopenia but does not address the bone marrow underproduction. Cladribine yields a more rapid response than interferon. Fludarabine and cytarabine can be considered after cladribine has failed but not for primary treatment.

131.5   Answer: (b)   Hypocellular marrow in patients who have HCL requires a gentle long-term treatment approach so as not to induce prolonged aplasia.

132.1   Answer: (e)   Many immune and nonimmune stimuli cause mast cell granules to fuse to the cell membrane causing release of anaphylaxis mediators. Mast cell granules contain substances that have been previously synthesized (primary mediators), which regulate the vasoactive and inflammatory processes characteristic of allergy. Primary mediators are contained in such granules include heparan sulfate, chondroitin sulfate, biogenic amines, acid hydrolases, and neutral proteases. Newly generated mediators such as platelet-activating factor and arachidonic acid and metabolites leukotrienes and prostaglandins are synthesized at the time of mast cell activation. Other substances potentially produced by mast cells include cytokines, antiogenic substances, and matrix metalloproteins.

132.2   Answer: (c)   Urticaria pigmentosa is the most common manifestation of neoplastic mast cell proliferation and is characterized by mast cell infiltration of the skin, usually presenting with an eruption of multiple discrete hyperpigmented nodular papular lesions, which portend a benign clinical course. The serum tryptase level is often elevated. Patients with systemic mast cell disease may also have an indolent course but usually have mast cells found in noncutaneous areas including marrow, spleen, and gut. Cutaneous symptoms in those with systemic disease and in patients with urticaria pigmentosa include pruritic and episodic flushing, but the most dramatic and common manifestation are urticarial wheals that result from mast cell degranulation in response to mechanical trauma; this is known as Darier's sign.

132.3   Answer: (c)   The research in cell lines and from patient samples has demonstrated that the basis for growth independence of mast cells obtained from patients with systemic mastocytosis is constitutive activation of c-*kit*. The activation is generally caused by a mutation in codon 816 in the kinase domain. The typical asparagine-to-valine mutation in codon 816 has been detected in both B cells and monocytes in patients with systemic mastocytosis, suggesting that this is a clonal disorder rising from an early hematopoietic progenitor cell. It is possible that tyrosine kinase inhibitors, which target activated c-*kit,* may be therapeutically useful in patients with systemic mastocytosis; however, the codon 816 mutation is insensitive to the c-*kit* inhibitor imatinib mesylate, which is highly useful in patients with chronic myeloid leukemia.

133.1   Answer: (c)   Postsplenectomy sepsis is highest among patients who have their spleen removed for thalassemia or other reticuloendothelial system diseases such as Hodgkin's disease. The risk of overwhelming infection is lower in patients who have a splenectomy for trauma, ITP, or hereditary spherocytosis. Typically, infections caused by encapsulated bacteria such as *Streptococcus pneumoniae, Neisseria meningitidis,* or *Haemophilus influenzae* account for approximately 75% of cases. Patients who undergo splenectomy for staging should be vaccinated before splenectomy in order to reduce the risk of overwhelming infection.

133.2   Answer: (d)   Non-Hodgkin's lymphoma, in contrast to Hodgkin's disease, is increasing in incidence, in part due to acquired immunodeficiency syndrome (AIDS) and transplantation-related immunosuppression. Patient age influences the pathology and stage of Hodgkin's disease. In persons over 40 or younger than 16 years, lymphocyte-predominant histology is more common. Hodgkin's disease has two age peaks that occur in developed countries. In developing countries, the younger age peak is predominant.

133.3   Answer: (e)   Lymphocyte-predominant Hodgkin's disease is most commonly seen in males under 15 or over 40 years of age. This subtype is often localized to a single lymph node. Patients with mixed cellularity more often have systemic symptoms and more often have advanced-stage disease. Nodular sclerosing Hodgkin's disease makes up 70% of patients in economically developed countries but is less common in developed countries. The presence of granulomatous lesions in lymph nodes increases the likelihood of coexistent Hodgkin's disease and may have favorable prognostic implications.

133.4   **Answer: (c)**   EBV may play a causal role in the development of Hodgkin's disease. There is an excess incidence of Hodgkin's disease in individuals who have previously had infectious mononucleosis. Various techniques have been used to find EBV genome fragments in RS cells of 30 to 50% of patients, especially those with mixed cellularity histology. The absence of an effective lymphocyte (polyclonal) response histologically may indicate a particularly immunosuppressed state and is predictive of a poor outcome. The lymphocyte-predominant variant with the distinctive lymphocytic and histiocyte RS variants is negative for LEU-M1 (CD15), a marker that is typically expressed in classic RS cells of the mixed cellularity and nodular sclerosing subtypes. The RS cell is clonal and may represent the true neoplastic cell. Patients who have the lymphocyte-depleted variant, which accounts for less than 5% of cases in developed countries, are usually seen with advanced disease.

133.5   **Answer: (c)**   RS cells in patients with mixed cellularity or nodular sclerosing Hodgkin's disease express CD15 in contrast to RS cells from patients with the lymphocyte-predominant subtype. CD15 (My1) reacts with normal granulocytes as well. Ki-1, also known as CD30, is commonly present on RS cells but is also expressed by activated B and T cells and large cell anaplastic lymphoma. Other B-cell activation antigens such as the IL-2 receptor and human leukocyte antigen (HLA)-DR may be expressed on RS cells. Antigen receptor gene rearrangement occurs, but rarely. The t(14;18) is characteristic of follicular, small cleaved cell B-cell lymphomas and is unusual in Hodgkin's disease. Transforming growth factor, produced by RS cells, may stimulate the fibroblastic reaction seen in the nodular sclerosing subtype.

133.6   **Answer: (e)**   The immune deficit in patients with Hodgkin's disease is present at the time of diagnosis and presumably precedes disease onset. Even in patients who achieve long-term remission with radiotherapy or chemotherapy, cellular immunologic deficits persist for years. Herpes zoster appears most commonly within the first year. Pneumococcal conjugated vaccines may be given following splenectomy but ideally should be given preceding splenectomy to optimize response.

133.7   **Answer: (e)**   The anatomic spread of Hodgkin's disease tends to involve central rather than peripheral lymph nodes. Hodgkin's disease in the early stages tends to spread by continuity to adjacent lymph nodes. In stage IV patients, however, there is evidence for hematogenous spread. Relapse at pretreatment sites of tumor after complete remission with chemotherapy is highly likely in Hodgkin's disease and substantially less likely in non-Hodgkin's lymphoma. With liver involvement, the spleen is almost always involved (but the reverse is not correct).

133.8   **Answer: (d)**   Patients who relapse after combination chemotherapy, whether it be MOPP or ABVD, have a much lower response to treatment with the original combination. ABVD is superior to MOPP in that infertility and secondary tumors are much less common. The superiority of ABVD over MOPP is probably intrinsic, although in comparative studies downward dose modification with MOPP occurs more commonly than with ABVD. So-called hybrid regimens derived from the components of MOPP and ABVD, or MOPP-ABVD alternating regimens, are not superior to ABVD in terms of overall survival.

134.1   **Answer: (b)**   The large randomized trial from Southwest Oncology Group demonstrated equivalence of options (b) and (c); however, there were excess treatment-associated deaths in the older patients treated with eight cycles of CHOP. The 5-year progression-free survival for this patient is 79%, with a 5-year overall survival of 77%.

134.2   **Answer: (d)**   CODox-M alternating with IVAC (two cycles of each) is also referred to as the Magrath regimen. This very intensive regimen developed for pediatric and young adult patients has been used for adults as well. Although patients with localized disease can have a long-term survival of 50 to 70% with this treatment, bone marrow or central nervous system disease decreases survival by 10 to 30%. CHOP alone, or with rituximab, is inadequate therapy for this disease, and there is no evidence in the literature that first remission autologous transplantation improves survival.

134.3   **Answer: (d)**   Peripheral T-cell lymphoma represents about 6% of non-Hodgkin's lymphomas with patients having a median age of 65 years. Approximately 65% of patients have stage IV disease with involvement of lymph nodes, skin, liver, spleen, and other viscera. Patients can also have eosinophilia, pruritus, and hemophagocytic syndromes. These are aggressive diseases and stage for stage, as well as with the IPI, these patients have a worse prognosis than do those with diffuse large B-cell lymphoma.

134.4   **Answer: (d)**   The response rate to CVP is very high, and not different than CHOP. Based on his symptoms owing to retroperitoneal disease, developing cytopenias, observation is not a good option. There is no evidence that adding doxorubicin hydrochloride adds significantly to the response rate or duration of response in follicular lymphoma, grade 1. Similarly, the role of rituximab, either as a single agent or in combination with chemotherapy, in the primary therapy of follicular lymphoma continues to be addressed in randomized clinical trials.

135.1   **Answer: (c)**   MF is a helper T-cell neoplasm (CD4+, CD8–, CD20–). Usually, there is a loss of mature T-cell antigens such as CD7 (CD7–).

135.2   **Answer: (d)**   Early-stage B-cell lymphomas often involve the face, scalp, or extremities; however, early-stage MF often involves the bathing trunk area.

135.3   **Answer: (c)**   Epidermotropism (cells in the epidermis) is an essential characteristic in MF. These may be scattered individual cells or clusters (Pautrier's microabscesses). A prominent grenz zone would suggest a B-cell lymphoma. Epidermal ulceration is not common in MF, and Pautrier's microabscesses are not truly abscesses. Reed-Sternberg-like cells are not seen in MF but may be seen in lymphomatoid papulosis.

135.4 **Answer: (c)** Total skin electron beam therapy achieves the highest response rates for cutaneous MF. For patients with cutaneous tumors, the depth of penetration of either PUVA or topical nitrogen mustard is insufficient to control disease adequately. Systemic chemotherapy in this setting generally achieves only a brief palliative response. Systemic retinoids achieve only minor responses in the presence of cutaneous tumors.

135.5 **Answer: (e)** The depth of penetration of total skin electron beam therapy is insufficient to cause systemic effects, and there are no risks to the bone marrow, bowel, or lungs. The complications are restricted to superficial tissues, resulting in epilation, onychoptosis (temporary nail loss), and alteration of sweat gland function.

136.1 **Answer: (c)** Understand the significance of MGUS: 2% of individuals above the age of 50 years have < 3.5 g/L monoclonal Ig, little or no proteinuria, < 5% monoclonal marrow plasma cells, and no bone lesions, anemia, hypercalcemia, or renal dysfunction. These patients should be followed up with annual SPEPs as 1% annually of these patients eventually develop MM.

136.2 **Answer: (b)** β_2-Microglobulin has been identified as the single most important independent prognostic variable in the presence of normal renal function. However, all of the above-mentioned variables have prognostic significance and are additive in predicting prognosis.

136.3 **Answer: (c)** Despite the use of combination chemotherapy and newer agents, such as thalidomide, dexamethasone or steroids remain the single most active agents in the treatment of myeloma.

136.4 **Answer: (f)** Renal failure in myeloma is multifactorial and can be corrected by aggressive hydration, treatment of underlying infection, and correction of the precipitating cause.

136.5 **Answer: (c)** Bisphosphonate therapy is an important adjunct to myeloma therapy, specifically in patients with bone disease. Although it has not consistently shown an improvement in overall or disease-free survival, randomized studies have demonstrated that treatment with pamidronate decreases the incidence of skeletal-related events such as fractures and reduces the need for radiation therapy.

137.1 **Answer: (a)** All experts in chronic myeloproliferative disorders agree that secondary as well as relative polycythemia must be considered and excluded before a diagnosis of (PV) is made. Clinical history is key in this regard. In routine clinical practice, the information from both bone marrow examination and measurement of serum erythropoietin concentration is often adequate enough to make a working diagnosis of PV. An experienced hematologist rarely needs the additional information from red cell or plasma volume measurements. The tests outlined in the other three choices are neither specific (a positive test is possible in other chronic myeloproliferative disorders) nor necessary for the diagnosis of PV. However, in equivocal cases, they might help distinguish clonal from nonclonal erythrocytosis.

137.2 **Answer: (b)** Drug therapy has not be shown, in a controlled setting, to influence survival in essential thrombocythemia (ET). However, treatment with hydroxyurea has been shown, in a randomized study, to significantly reduce the incidence of thrombosis in high-risk patients with ET. This is not the case with either aspirin or anagrelide. There is currently no evidence to support cytoreductive treatment in low-risk patients with ET (age < 60 yr and the absence of thrombosis history). Observation alone, with or without the use of low-dose aspirin, is the current treatment choice for low-risk pregnant patients with ET.

137.3 **Answer: (d)** Although marked collagen fibrosis is a typical feature of MMM, its presence is not a prerequisite for establishing the diagnosis of MMM (ie, the cellular phase of MMM). Similarly, severe bone marrow fibrosis is not specific to MMM and can also be seen in CML, MDS, chronic myelomonocytic leukemia, chronic eosinophilic leukemia, and systemic mast cell disease. Although cytogenetic studies reliably distinguish MMM from CML, the morphologic distinction between MMM and MDS with fibrosis can sometimes be problematic. On the other hand, the diagnosis of ET, by definition, requires the absence of the Philadelphia translocation, substantial myelofibrosis, and trilineage dyshematopoiesis (ie, ET is currently a diagnosis of exclusion).

NEOPLASMS IN AIDS

138.1 **Answer: (c)** This is a tumor that is highly immune responsive, and improvement in immune function with suppression of human immunodeficiency virus type 1 (HIV-1) replication can both suppress existing KS and prevent future lesion development. Therapy directed at herpesviruses has had a poor record of activity against KS. Cytotoxic chemotherapy and radiation therapy may be used but only in selected settings.

138.2 **Answer: False** KS has an extremely variable clinical course, with some patients maintaining indolent disease for years and others undergoing spontaneous regression. The responsiveness to improved immune function probably accounts for this variability and is the rationale for emphasizing control of HIV-1 as a component of care for KS.

138.3 **Answer: False** KSHV prevalence rates are estimated at under 10% in the general population in North America, although it is much more common in some subsets of individuals, particularly those from high endemic areas such as the Mediterranean basin and sub-Saharan Africa. Transmission mode is still being determined and may include salivary contact; it certainly is increased by male homosexual sexual practices.

138.4 **Answer: (e)**

UNKNOWN PRIMARY SITE

139.1   **Answer: (c)**   Women who develop peritoneal carcinomatosis and do not have an obvious primary site should be treated according to guidelines for advanced ovarian cancer. This management is appropriate even in women with normal-appearing ovaries, and in women who have previously had bilateral oophorectomy. When histology suggests ovarian cancer (ie, serous cystadenocarcinoma or papillary features), this syndrome has been termed *peritoneal papillary serous carcinoma*. Initial treatment includes laparotomy with maximal surgical cytoreduction, followed by taxane/platinum chemotherapy, as recommended for advanced ovarian cancer. Response to treatment and prognosis is similar to stage III ovarian cancer.

139.2   **Answer: (b)**   Major considerations in the differential diagnosis of this patient include lymph node metastases from squamous cancers arising in the head and neck, and various lymphomas. Lung cancer is less likely with involvement in the upper cervical lymph nodes. When squamous cancer of the head and neck is suspected, complete ENT endoscopic evaluation is indicated, with biopsy of any suspicious lesions. If no primary site is identified, needle biopsy is the preferred diagnostic method in a patient at risk of head and neck cancer. Excisional or incisional lymph node biopsy interrupts local lymphatics and is therefore problematic when subsequent surgical procedures or radiation therapy are required. Patients who present with small volume squamous cancer in cervical lymph nodes, without an identifiable head and neck primary site, have a good prognosis (60–70% 5-year disease-free survival) when treated with concurrent chemotherapy/radiation therapy, as recommended for locally advanced head and neck cancer.

139.3   **Answer: (e)**   Isolated axillary adenopathy owing to metastatic adenocarcinoma in a female should be treated following guidelines for stage II breast cancer. Primary treatment should include either modified radical mastectomy (60% result in detection of an occult breast primary) or an axillary lymph node dissection and radiation therapy of the breast. Adjuvant therapy should follow established guidelines for stage II breast cancer, with selection of treatment based on the number of involved lymph nodes and the hormone-receptor status.

139.4   **Answer: (d)**   Immunoperoxidase stains are required in the evaluation of poorly differentiated metastatic tumors. The initial light microscopic diagnosis of "anaplastic neoplasm" indicates the inability to distinguish between carcinoma, lymphoma, melanoma, or sarcoma based on histologic features. Positive stains for cytokeratin, chromogranin, and synaptophysin in this poorly differentiated tumor are diagnostic of a poorly differentiated neuroendocrine carcinoma.

139.5   **Answer: (d)**   In adults the most common high-grade neuroendocrine carcinoma is small cell lung cancer, an unlikely diagnosis in this patient who is a nonsmoker with a normal results of a chest CT scan. Further evaluation is unlikely to identify a primary site. Poorly differentiated neuroendocrine carcinoma of unknown primary site has a high response rate to combination chemotherapy using regimens similar to those established for the treatment of small cell lung cancer.

PEDIATRIC ONCOLOGY

DIRECTIONS: Numbering for questions and answers reflects the corresponding chapter in *Cancer Medicine-6*. Each question contains suggested responses. Select the best response to each question.
Answers for Pediatric Oncology begin on page 155.

PEDIATRIC ONCOLOGY

140a.1   **The most common form of pediatric cancer is**
a.   Brain tumor
b.   Wilms' tumor
c.   Acute leukemia
d.   Hodgkin's disease

140a.2   **Improved survivor rates in childhood cancer over the past three decades are owing largely to**
a.   The development of molecularly targeted therapy resulting from increased understanding of tumor biology
b.   Improved methods of early detection
c.   The development of multidisciplinary multicenter clinical trials
d.   The decreased toxicity associated with cancer therapy in children

140a.3   **Improved outcomes in childhood acute lymphoblastic leukemia (ALL) are attributed to all of the following** *except*
a.   The definition of prognostic factors
b.   The concept of risk-adjusted therapy
c.   Bone-marrow transplantation
d.   Preventive central nervous system (CNS)-directed therapy

140a.4   **The treatment approaches advanced by clinical trials in childhood cancer are equally focused on improving survival rates and**
a.   Understanding epidemiologic associations of childhood cancer
b.   Exploring the biologic mechanisms of drug resistance and treatment failure
c.   Exploring the ethical issues of clinical research in children
d.   Decreasing short- and long-term toxicities of therapy

140b.1   **When considering cancer in children under the age of 15 years, which of the following is true?**
a.   It represents approximately 10% of all cancers diagnosed in the United States.
b.   It is the leading cause of death owing to disease in this age group in the United States.
c.   It demonstrates little international variability in incidence.
d.   Approximately 85% of cases consist of leukemia or central nervous system tumors.
e.   All of the above are true.
f.   None of the above are true.

140b.2   **Leukemia in children under the age of 15 years is characterized**
a.   As predominantly acute myeloid
b.   As the second leading form of malignancy
c.   As being most common between the ages of 12 to 15 years
d.   As having a higher incidence among Blacks compared with incidence in non-Blacks
e.   In all of the above ways
f.   In none of the above ways

140b.3   **The Li-Fraumeni cancer family syndrome is characterized by inheritance of a germline mutation in the** *P53* **gene. Which childhood cancer is associated with the Li-Fraumeni syndrome?**
a.   ALL
b.   Hodgkin's disease
c.   Rhabdomyosarcoma
d.   Wilms' tumor
e.   All of the above
f.   None of the above

141a.1   **Which of the following statements does** *not* **characterize acute lymphoblastic leukemia (ALL) in childhood?**
a.   The peak incidence of childhood ALL is between 3 and 6 years of age.
b.   Treatment duration is 2 to 3 years in length.
c.   There is a male predominance in childhood ALL cases of all ages.
d.   A 9-year-old child with a white blood cell count (WBC) at presentation of 50,000 is designated to have high-risk ALL by the conventional classification.
e.   T-lineage ALL in childhood makes up 15% of all ALL cases.

141a.2 **Which of the following is *not* an adverse prognostic factor for a newly diagnosed child with ALL?**
  a. Age 10 years old or greater
  b. Presence of extramedullary leukemia
  c. Translocation (12;21)
  d. Failure to achieve remission by the end of the induction phase of chemotherapy
  e. Presenting WBC of 50,000 or higher

141a.3 **Outcome after the diagnosis of relapsed ALL in a child is dependent on all of the following *except***
  a. Age at time of relapse
  b. Steroid resistance of leukemia
  c. Duration of first remission
  d. Site of relapse
  e. Ability to achieve a second remission

141a.4 **Identify the *incorrect* statement. In childhood ALL, cranial irradiation**
  a. Has been linked to neurocognitive damage
  b. Has been linked to second malignancy
  c. Has been eliminated for most patients because of improved systemic therapy
  d. Is the only neurotoxic component of ALL treatment
  e. Is given to high-risk patients with a slow initial response to therapy and to patients with overt CNS leukemia at diagnosis

141a.5 **The evaluation of bone marrow transplantation (BMT) data for childhood ALL has been confounded by all of the following variables *except***
  a. Differences in pretransplant conditioning regimens
  b. Variability in the types of graft-versus-host disease prophylaxis used
  c. Waiting time bias
  d. Selection bias
  e. Uniformity in the types of graft-versus-host disease prophylaxis

141b.1 **Which of the following cytogenetic abnormalities confers a high probability of cure in pediatric acute myelogenous leukemia (AML)?**
  a. Hyperdiploidy
  b. Trisomy 8
  c. t(10;11)
  d. Constitutional trisomy 21
  e. t(12;21)

141b.2 **Compared with chemotherapy, bone marrow transplantation is more likely to cause which of these late complications in survivors of pediatric AML?**
  a. Impaired short-term memory
  b. Hepatic hemosiderosis
  c. Infertility
  d. Cardiac myopathy
  e. Pulmonary fibrosis

141b.3 **Randomized comparisons of maintenance to no maintenance therapy in pediatric AML have shown that maintenance therapy is associated with which of the following outcomes?**
  a. Prolonged event-free survival
  b. Reduced survival
  c. Increased second malignant neoplasms
  d. Fewer extramedullary relapses
  e. Late-onset veno-occlusive disease

141b.4 **Postremission dose intensification of which of the following chemotherapeutic agents leads to improved event-free survival in pediatric and adult patients with AML?**
  a. Cytosine arabinoside
  b. Daunorubicin
  c. Etoposide
  d. 6-Thioguanine
  e. Idarubicin

141b.5 **Which of the following agents is associated with a risk of treatment-related AML characterized by nonrandom chromosomal rearrangements?**
a. Carboplatinum
b. Procarbazine
c. Etoposide
d. Ionizing radiation
e. Cyclophosphamide

141c.1 **The most appropriate initial therapy for nondisseminated cerebellar juvenile pilocytic astrocytoma in a patient without neuro-fibromatosis type 1 (NF1) disease is**
a. Complete surgical resection and 5,500 cGy local irradiation
b. > 50% surgical resection and 5,500 cGy local irradiation with adjuvant chemotherapy
c. Complete surgical resection and 1,800 cGy craniospinal irradiation with 3,600 cGy local irradiation boost to the tumor bed
d. > 50% surgical resection and 1,800 cGy craniospinal irradiation with 3,600 cGy local irradiation boost to the tumor bed and adjuvant chemotherapy
e. Complete surgical resection and close observation

141c.2 **Which of the following is the most accurate statement regarding brain stem glioma (BSG) in children?**
a. Most BSGs arise in the midbrain or medulla, demonstrate benign pathology, and respond to radiotherapy but do not respond to chemotherapy.
b. Most BSGs arise in the pons, demonstrate benign pathology, and do not respond to either radiotherapy or chemotherapy.
c. Most BSGs arise in the midbrain or medulla, demonstrate malignant pathology, and respond to radiotherapy but do not respond to chemotherapy.
d. Most BSGs arise in the pons, demonstrate malignant pathology, and respond to radiotherapy.
e. Most BSGs arise in the pons or medulla, demonstrate malignant pathology, and do not respond to either radiotherapy or chemotherapy.

141c.3 **Which of the following is the most accurate statement regarding the stratification and current survival rate of children with standard-risk medulloblastoma?**
a. Standard-risk medulloblastoma is defined by age < 3 years, absence of brainstem involvement, and absence of metastatic disease; it has a 5-year survival rate of about 60%.
b. Standard-risk medulloblastoma is defined by age > 3 years, postoperative residual tumor < 1.5 cm^2, and absence of metastatic disease; it has a 5-year survival rate of about 80%.
c. Standard-risk medulloblastoma is defined by age < 3 years, postoperative residual tumor < 1.5 cm^2, and absence of metastatic disease; it has a 5-year survival rate of about 80%.
d. Standard-risk medulloblastoma is defined by age > 3 years, postoperative residual tumor < 1.5 cm^2, and absence of metastatic disease; it has a 5-year survival rate of about 60%.
e. Standard-risk medulloblastoma is defined by age > 3 years, absence of brainstem involvement, and absence of metastatic disease; it has a 5-year survival rate of about 60%.

141c.4 **Atypical teratoid/rhabdoid tumor (AT/RT) of the central nervous system in children is a relatively newly described entity that is believed to be distinct from primitive neuroectodermal tumor (PNET)/medulloblastoma (MB) because of which of the following clinical findings?**
a. Occurence mostly in older children and adolescents, a low propensity to spread, histology consistent with PNET but with the presence of rhabdoid cells, and association with chromosome 22 deletion
b. Occurence only in infancy, common presentation with cranial nerve VI and VII deficits, histology consistent with PNET but with the presence of rhabdoid cells, and association with chromosome 11;22 translocation
c. Rare occurence in older children and adolescents, cyst formation and hemorrhage commonly seen on computed tomography (CT), presence of rhabdoid cells with prominent nucleolus on histology, and association with *INI1* mutation
d. Rare occurence in infancy, typically nonmalignant, presence of rhabdoid cells with prominent nucleolus on histology, and association with 1;22 translocation or 17p chromosomal deletion
e. Occurence only in infancy, common presentation of cranial nerve VI and VII deficits, histology consistent with PNET but with the presence of rhabdoid cells, and association with chromosome 17p deletion

141d.1 **All of the following are performed in staging pediatric patients with Hodgkin's disease *except***
a. Chest computed tomography (CT)
b. Staging laparotomy
c. Bone marrow aspiration and biopsy for patients with advanced disease
d. Abdominal/pelvic CT
e. Gallium or positron emission tomography

141d.2 **All of the following drugs are used in front-line therapy for Hodgkin's disease** *except*
   a. Dactinomycin
   b. Procarbazine
   c. Cyclophosphamide
   d. Etoposide
   e. Doxorubicin

141d.3 **Concerning the use of radiation for pediatric patients with Hodgkin's disease, which of the following statements is** *not* **true?**
   a. High-dose radiation (> 36Gy) to the mantle field is associated with an increased risk for breast cancer.
   b. Low-dose extended field radiotherapy is often used in conjunction with chemotherapy.
   c. Low-dose radiation to the neck is associated with a significant incidence of compensated hypothyroidism.
   d. High-dose radiation alone to extended fields is not recommended as therapy for patients with early-stage disease.
   e. Patients who relapse after chemotherapy only have a better salvage rate compared with patients who relapse after chemotherapy and low-dose radiation.

141e.1 **All of the following are commonly seen pediatric non-Hodgkin's lymphomas** *except*
   a. Diffuse large B-cell lymphoma
   b. Follicular small cleaved cell lymphoma
   c. Burkitt's and Burkitt's-like lymphomas
   d. Lymphoblastic lymphoma
   e. Anaplastic large cell lymphoma

141e.2 **Systemic anaplastic large cell lymphoma (ALCL) in children is characterized by all of the following** *except*
   a. A high incidence of anaplastic lymphoma kinase (ALK) staining by immunohistochemistry
   b. A strong expression of CD30
   c. A high incidence of molecular and cytogenetic abnormalities involving the ALK locus, most commonly manifested as a t(2;5)(p23;q35)
   d. Common expression of B-cell markers CD19, CD20, and CD22
   e. The lack of expression of T- or B-cell markers (null cell)

141e.3 **For the treatment of childhood non-Hodgkin's lymphoma, radiation therapy is indicated for which of the following?**
   a. Localized resected extranodal tumors
   b. Central nervous system prophylaxis
   c. Diffuse intra-abdominal disease
   d. Cranial nerve palsy
   e. All of the above

141e.4 **Which of the following is** *not* **an effective treatment for localized lymphoblastic lymphoma?**
   a. Multiagent chemotherapy
   b. A shortened course of B-cell non-Hodgkin's lymphoma (B-NHL) therapy
   c. Treatment similar to that used for acute lymphoblastic leukemia
   d. Central nervous system prophylaxis
   e. Initial surgical resection of a single extranodal tumor

142a.1 **The following conditions have been associated with the development of hepatocellular carcinoma** *except*
   a. Hepatitis B infection
   b. Familial adenomatous polyposis
   c. Hereditary tyrosinemia
   d. Alagille syndrome
   e. Glycogen storage disease type I

142a.2 **Which of the following statements is correct?**
   a. Carcinomas account for < 1% of all pediatric cancers.
   b. Melanoma accounts for nearly one-third of all pediatric carcinomas.
   c. Thyroid carcinoma is the least common pediatric carcinoma.
   d. The majority of pediatric carcinomas affect children < 3 years of age.

142a.3 **The risk of developing retinoblastoma for the offsprings of survivors of bilateral retinoblastoma is**
   a. 45%
   b. < 1%
   c. 50%
   d. 10%
   e. 100%

142a.4 The most common type of malignant germ cell tumor in prepubertal children is
a. Choriocarcinoma
b. Embryonal carcinoma
c. Germinoma
d. Yolk sac tumor
e. Mixed malignant germ cell tumor

142b.1 Which one of the following is *not* normally in the histologic differential diagnosis for Wilms' tumor?
a. Neuroblastoma
b. Congenital mesoblastic nephroma
c. Germ cell tumor
d. Renal cell carcinoma
e. Rhabdoid tumor of the kidney

142b.2 The strongest prognostic factor for Wilms' tumor is
a. The presence of diffuse blastema
b. The presence of a pseudocapsule
c. Lymph node involvement
d. Diffuse anaplasia
e. Extrarenal extension

142b.3 Most patients with Wilms' tumor present with
a. An asymptomatic abdominal mass
b. Gross hematuria
c. Abdominal pain
d. Renal failure
e. Aniridia

142b.4 The initial work-up for patients with suspected Wilms' tumor should include all of the following *except*
a. Ultrasonography of the abdomen
b. Bone scan
c. Computed tomography (CT) scan of the chest
d. CT of the abdomen

142b.5 A radical or modified radical nephrectomy performed prior to chemotherapy is recommended because
a. Relapse-free survival is superior if gross total tumor removal is performed prechemotherapy
b. This facilitates accurate identification of histology and staging
c. Surgical morbidity is minimized
d. Second-look surgery is technically more difficult
e. This facilitates the use of immediate postoperative radiation where indicated

142c.1 Which of the following sets of variables are most important in determining the prognosis of a patient with neuroblastoma?
a. 1p36 loss of heterozygosity and *MYCN* gene copy number
b. Pathologic classification and *MYCN* gene copy number
c. Age at diagnosis and disease stage
d. Pathologic classification and disease stage
e. Age at diagnosis and deoxyribonucleic acid (DNA) index

142c.2 Which of the following statements is *not* true concerning neuroblastoma screening studies?
a. Neuroblastomas usually produce increased levels of catecholamines whose metabolites are easily detectable in the urine, making mass screening practical in young infants.
b. Mass screening allows for early detection of patients with unfavorable biologic features.
c. When young infants are screened, the prevalence of neuroblastoma is increased.
d. The majority of tumors identified by mass screening of young infants have biologically favorable features.
e. When young infants are screened, the prevalence of neuroblastoma in patients > 1 year does not change appreciably.

142c.3 What is the most sensitive method for detecting bone metastases in neuroblastoma?
a. Technetium Tc 99m (^{99m}Tc)-diphosphate scintigraphy
b. Metaiodobenzylguanidine iodine 123 (^{123}I-MIBG) scintigraphy
c. ^{131}I-MIBG scintigraphy
d. Computed tomography (CT) scanning
e. Plain radiography

142c.4   What is the recommended management of patients with stage 4S neuroblastoma with favorable biologic features?
    a.   Diagnostic biopsy and observation with moderately intensive chemotherapy for symptomatology from tumor expansion
    b.   Gross total resection of primary tumor with moderately intensive chemotherapy for symptomatology from tumor expansion
    c.   Diagnostic biopsy and observation with local radiation therapy for symptomatology from tumor expansion
    d.   Diagnostic biopsy followed by intensive induction therapy and myeloablative consolidation therapy with stem cell rescue
    e.   Diagnostic biopsy followed by moderately intensive chemotherapy

142c.5   What is the currently recommended management for neuroblastoma patients with high-risk disease?
    a.   Gross total tumor resection followed by intensive induction therapy and myeloablative consolidation therapy with stem cell rescue
    b.   Intensive induction therapy followed by nonmyeloablative consolidation therapy
    c.   Intensive induction therapy followed by myeloablative consolidation therapy with allogeneic bone marrow transplantation
    d.   Intensive induction therapy followed by myeloablative consolidation therapy with autologous stem cell transplantation followed by targeted therapy for minimal residual disease with 13-*cis*-retinoic acid

142d.1   The most common histologic type of rhabdomyosarcoma (RMS) is
    a.   Undifferentiated
    b.   Spindle cell
    c.   Alveolar
    d.   Embryonal
    e.   Botryoid

142d.2   Alveolar histology of RMS is characterized by which of the following gene fusion(s)?
    a.   *EWS-FLI1* — t(11;22)
    b.   *PAX3-FKHR* — t(2;13)
    c.   *SYT-SSX1* — t(X;18)
    d.   *PAX7-FKHR* — t(1;13)
    e.   *EWS-WT1* — t(11;22)

142d.3   Effective therapy for alveolar RMS is composed of
    a.   Surgery only
    b.   Surgery followed by irradiation if resection is incomplete
    c.   Surgery and multiagent chemotherapy
    d.   Surgery and irradiation for all tumors, regardless of resectability
    e.   Surgery, irradiation for all tumors, and multiagent chemotherapy

142d.4   For treatment purposes, the extent of disease for RMS is categorized by
    a.   Tumor resection
    b.   Lymph node involvement
    c.   Tumor site
    d.   Tumor size
    e.   Presence of metastatic disease
    f.   All of the above

142d.5   In comparing and contrasting the features of soft tissue sarcomas occurring in adults with those features of the non-RMS soft tissue sarcomas occurring in children, which of the following statement(s) is (are) *incorrect*?
    a.   Soft tissue sarcomas in both adults and children often are biologically similar.
    b.   Histologic grading of soft tissue sarcomas is important in predicting outcome.
    c.   Size and invasiveness are important prognostically in both children and adults with soft tissue sarcomas.
    d.   Complete surgical resection is the mainstay of treatment.
    e.   Infantile fibrosarcoma is less sensitive to chemotherapy than is fibrosarcoma occurring in adults.

143a.1   An example of a pediatric tumor with unique morphologic features that are not shared with adult ones is
    a.   Clear cell sarcoma of the kidney
    b.   Thyroid carcinoma
    c.   Clear cell sarcoma of soft tissue
    d.   Osteosarcoma
    e.   Renal cell carcinoma

143a.2   All of the following tumors resemble embryonal tissue *except*
    a.   Embryonal rhabdomyosarcoma
    b.   Retinoblastoma

    c.   Sialoblastoma
    d.   Wilms' tumor
    e.   Fibrolamellar variant of hepatocellular carcinoma

143a.3 Which of the following in situ lesions is most commonly associated with pediatric neoplasms?
    a.   Low-grade squamous intraepithelial lesion
    b.   Ductal carcinoma in situ
    c.   Nephroblastomatosis
    d.   Actinic keratosis
    e.   Adenomatous polyp

143a.4 The fusion gene most characteristic of alveolar rhabdomyosarcoma is
    a.   *EWS/FLII*
    b.   *EWS/WTI*
    c.   *SYT/SSXI*
    d.   *PAX3/FKHR*
    e.   *PML/RAR*

143a.5 Which of the following pediatric tumors is typically undifferentiated?
    a.   Embryonal rhabdomyosarcoma
    b.   Ewing's sarcoma
    c.   Wilms' tumor
    d.   Neuroblastoma
    e.   Fibrolamellar carcinoma

143b.1 The most common types of cancer during the second decade of life are
    a.   Hodgkin's disease, non-Hodgkin's lymphoma, thyroid cancer
    b.   Hodgkin's disease, germ cell tumors, acute lymphoblastic leukemia
    c.   Hodgkin's disease, thyroid cancer, acute lymphoblastic leukemia
    d.   Hodgkin's disease, central nervous system tumors, non-Hodgkin's lymphoma
    e.   Hodgkin's disease, germ cell tumors, central nervous system tumors

143b.2 Which one of the following statements is *not* true about Americans between 15 and 45 years of age?
    a.   Females are far more likely than males to develop thyroid cancer.
    b.   Females are far more likely than males to develop melanoma.
    c.   African Americans are far more likely than white Americans to develop osteosarcoma.
    d.   Whites are far more likely than African Americans to develop Ewing's sarcoma.
    e.   Whites are far more likely than African Americans to develop malignant melanoma.

143b.3 Which of the following statements about Americans between 15 and 45 years of age is known to be true?
    a.   The cause of cancer in most patients is related to environmental carcinogens.
    b.   A majority of cancers have been attributed directly to single environmental or inherited factors.
    c.   Clear cell adenocarcinoma of the uterus is an example of transplacental carcinogenesis owing to aflatoxin.
    d.   Cancer control efforts to reduce teenage exposure to environmental carcinogens are unlikely to affect rates of cancers in adolescents but should decrease rates in adults.
    e.   The majority of cancers are second malignant neoplasms in patients previously treated for cancer.

143b.4 Which one of the following is *not* true about Americans between 15 and 30 years of age?
    a.   There is an abundance of literature that addresses the psychosocial needs of older adolescents and young adults with cancer.
    b.   The malignant diseases in this age group are not unique; they are examples of cancer in younger or older patients and not age-specific biologic types that occur predominantly, if not exclusively, during late adolescence or early adulthood.
    c.   Most of the cancers that are managed in patients within this age group are nonepithelial malignancies.
    d.   The examiner who is not aware of the prominence of sarcomas, thyroid and testicular cancers, and melanoma in this age group may overlook these possibilities when taking the history and performing the physical examination.
    e.   Sun exposure, exposure to other environmental carcinogens including tobacco, recreational drugs, alcohol, and sexually transmitted diseases begins or intensifies during this age period.

143b.5 Clinical trial participation is lower in 15- to 40-year-olds than in younger and older patients; this is directly correlated with less survival prolongation and less mortality reduction in patients with cancer diagnosed during this age range. Which one of the following is *not* a reasonable explanation for the low clinical trail participation rate?

a. Young adults are less likely to have health insurance.

b. Oncologists (surgeons, radiotherapists, medical oncologists, gynecologists) in private practice may retain these patients rather than refer them to a tertiary-care facility or cooperative group member institution.

c. Providers, patients, and/or parents may be unaware of opportunities for participation for adolescents and young adults with cancer in clinical trials.

d. The existing national cancer cooperative groups do not have a mechanism for protocol development for patients in this age range.

e. A clinical trial may not be available.

ANSWERS

PEDIATRIC ONCOLOGY

140a.1 **Answer: (c)**   Acute leukemia accounts for one-third of all childhood cancer. Brain tumors are the most common solid tumor, but account for only 15 to 20% of childhood cancers.

140a.2 **Answer: (c)**   The improvements in childhood cancer survival rates paralleled the cooperative clinical trials groups and widespread, nearly universal, accrual to clinical trials.

140a.3 **Answer: (c)**   Recognition of the importance of CNS-specific therapy and the use of therapy of increased intensity in patients at greatest risk of relapse have had the greatest impact on outcome in ALL.

140a.4 **Answer: (d)**   Given the improved success rates, clinical trials in pediatric oncology are appropriately focused on risk reduction of morbidity and long-term sequelae.

140b.1 **Answer: (b)**   In the United States, cancer diagnosed under the age of 15 years represents only 1 to 2% of all cancers seen in the population. Internationally, there are marked differences in the observed incidence rates for many of the childhood malignancies. In general, leukemia and malignancies of the central nervous system comprise approximately half of the cancers in children. Although there have been remarkable improvements in the survival rates for most childhood cancers, it still remains the leading cause of death owing to disease in the United States.

140b.2 **Answer: (f)**   Leukemia, the most common malignant diagnosis in children, is predominantly acute lymphoblastic, with acute myeloid leukemia representing only approximately 15% of the leukemias diagnosed in this age group. The age-specific incidence of leukemia is highest in the younger age groups, with a characteristic peak between 2 and 6 years of age for acute lymphoblastic leukemia (ALL) and the highest incidence of acute myelogenous leukemia occurring in the first several years of life. The incidence of leukemia is significantly lower among Blacks and is driven primarily by the differences within ALL. The reason for this observed difference in incidence among Blacks remains unclear.

140b.3 **Answer: (c)**   The initial characterization of the Li-Fraumeni syndrome was based on a proband with the diagnosis of rhabdomyosarcoma. It is well accepted that rhabdomyosarcoma and other soft tissue sarcomas during childhood are a common characteristic of this cancer family syndrome. Other childhood cancers have been associated with the Li-Fraumeni syndrome including bone sarcomas and brain tumors.

141a.1 **Answer: (c)**   There is a male predominance in childhood ALL cases of all ages except in infancy. During infancy, defined as children < 12 months of age, there is a female predominance. All of the other statements are correct characterizations of childhood ALL.

141a.2 **Answer: (c)**   Translocation (12;21) carries a favorable prognosis in childhood ALL. This translocation is also known as the *TEL-AML1* translocation. The *TEL* transcription factor gene is found on chromosome 12, whereas the *AML1* oncogene is located on chromosome 21. All of the other statements provide examples of adverse prognostic factors in childhood ALL.

141a.3 **Answer: (a)**   Although age at time of the initial diagnosis of ALL is an important prognostic factor regarding the projections for disease outcome, the age at time of relapse does not have a similar prognostic factor. Other factors, such as how long the first remission lasted, the relative sensitivity (or resistance) of the leukemia to steroids or even other drugs, site(s) of disease at time of relapse, and whether a second remission is actually achieved, significantly influence long-term disease outcome.

141a.4 **Answer: (d)**   The neurotoxicity of cranial irradiation is well documented; however, it is not the only component of treatment that may cause neurologic sequelae. Intrathecal medications and high-dose methotrexate are two examples of other potentially neurotoxic therapies.

141a.5 **Answer: (e)**   Comparative evaluations of the impact of BMT as a treatment modality are complicated by the lack of uniformity in the treatment of pediatric ALL patients from center to center. It is also complicated by the exclusion, in most cases, of patients who are not BMT candidates, perhaps because of relapse or the inability to obtain a new remission. This introduces bias in study population assessments. Therefore, uniformity in the types of graft-versus-host disease prophylaxis is the only variable listed that does not adversely affect the data for a comparative analysis.

141b.1 **Answer: (d)**   Constitutional trisomy 21 by definition occurs in children with Down syndrome. They experience a > 80% cure rate with low- to moderate-intensity AML therapy.

141b.2 **Answer: (c)**   Infertility occurs in over 90% of young patients treated with busulfan and cytoxan or cytoxan and total body irradiation prior to marrow or stem cell transplantation. Infertility is uncommon in survivors treated with chemotherapy alone. There is no significant difference in the frequency of the other complications.

141b.3 **Answer: (b)** Randomized trials conducted in both France and the United States have shown that maintenance therapy in AML significantly reduces overall survival and confers no significant benefits with respect to relapses of any type, and no significant increase in any other major complications.

141b.4 **Answer: (a)** Trials in the Children's Cancer Group and in Cancer and Leukemia Group B have shown that high-dose cytosine arabinoside in postremission therapy improves event-free survival and overall survival. Intensification of none of the others has consistently shown benefits in any phase of therapy.

141b.5 **Answer: (c)** Etoposide is an inhibitor of deoxyribonucleic acid topoisomerase II. This group of agents is associated with treatment-related AML characterized by t(11q;23), t(8;21), t(15;17), and others.

141c.1 **Answer: (e)** Total surgical resection is curative in 95 to 100% of cases. Juvenile pilocytic astrocytomas are benign World Health Organization grade I tumors that do not undergo malignant transformation and may stabilize for long periods of time or even spontaneously regress. However, the behavior of cerebellar astrocytomas in children with NF1 may be more aggressive. Those children whose lesions are inoperable because of brainstem involvement may require additional therapy, although residual tumor may remain quiescent for years; thus, irradiation and/or chemotherapy should be reserved for tumors that demonstrate clear growth or symptomatic change.

141c.2 **Answer: (d)** BSGs most commonly arise in the pons (diffuse intrinsic), in which location they typically resemble adult glioblastoma multiforme and have an almost uniformly dismal prognosis. In contrast, those arising from midbrain or medulla are likely to be low-grade lesions that have a more indolent course and improved outcome. Treatment is local irradiation to 5,500 to 6,000 cGy. Over 90% of patients with diffuse intrinsic lesions transiently respond, but ultimately succumb to disease progression within 18 months of diagnosis. Neither hyperfractionated radiotherapy nor chemotherapy has been shown to add benefit. Low-grade lesions are treated with similar irradiation doses but overall respond less favorably than do their counterparts in other locations.

141c.3 **Answer: (b)** Treatment groups designated as high risk and standard risk are created based on the criteria of age > or < 3 years, residual tumor > or < 1.5 cm^2, and the presence or absence of metastatic disease on neuroimaging or cerebrospinal fluid sampling (CSF). Age < 3 years is predictive of a poor outcome. This fact is difficult to separate from the finding that younger children more commonly present with metastatic disease, are less likely to be treated with conventional doses of radiotherapy, and are more likely to have subtotal tumor resection. Extent of resection was found to correlate with better survival for patients without metastatic disease in the Children's Cancer Group study 921. Metastatic disease at the time of diagnosis has been repeatedly correlated with poor survival, the exception being M1 disease, defined as CSF cytology positive for medulloblastoma cells. A Children's Cancer Group protocol reduced the craniospinal dose from the standard 3,600 cGy to 2,340 cGy with the addition of adjuvant chemotherapy consisting of vincristine, cisplatin, and lomustine for standard-risk medulloblastoma. The progression-free survival was 86% at 3 years and 79% at 5 years.

141c.4 **Answer: (c)** AT/RT is an aggressively malignant primitive tumor most often arising in children < 2 years of age. Approximately half of AT/RTs arise in the infratentorial compartment with a propensity to invade the cerebellopontine angle. Because of its association with chromosome 22 deletion and *INI1* mutation, analysis of these markers in infants with presumed PNET/MB should be considered for all children who are < 1 year of age. Focal findings related to cranial nerve involvement, especially nerves VI and VII, are common. The ability of these tumors to disseminate along CSF pathways is well known. Heterogeneous enhancement, cyst formation, and hemorrhage are common findings on CT imaging. The histologic hallmark of AT/RT is the presence of rhabdoid cells. These cells are characterized by a variable size eccentric nucleus with a prominent nucleolus.

141d.1 **Answer: (b)**

141d.2 **Answer: (a)**

141d.3 **Answer: (b)**

141e.1 **Answer: (b)** The vast majority of childhood non-Hodgkin's lymphomas are high-grade tumors with aggressive clinical behaviors, in contrast to adult non-Hodgkin's lymphomas, which tend to be indolent to intermediate grade. The four major subtypes of childhood non-Hodgkin's lymphomas include the small cleaved cell (Burkitt's and non-Burkitt's) lymphomas, lymphoblastic lymphomas, large cell lymphomas, and anaplastic large cell lymphomas. Follicular lymphomas may rarely be seen in children and usually occur in extranodal sites; they are much more commonly seen in the adult population.

141e.2 **Answer: (d)** Systemic pediatric ALCL is usually considered to be a peripheral T-cell neoplasm, which has strong expression of CD30 and is composed of large anaplastic cells. The majority of ALCLs have T-cell markers on the cell surface (CD2, CD3, CD5, CD7, CD45RO, or CD43) or may fail to demonstrate staining with either T- or B-cell markers (null cell type). Under the current World Health Organization and Revised European American Lymphoma classifications, a B-cell phenotype for anaplastic large cell lymphomas is not recognized. Some diffuse large B-cell lymphomas may express CD30, but there has not been convincing demonstration of characteristic molecular abnormalities involving the ALK locus in these cases. Greater than 90% of pediatric ALCLs stain with ALK, which is very specific for systemic ALCL. This staining demonstrates the product of specific cytogenetic and molecular abnormalities associated with ALCL; this involves the ALK locus on chromosome 2, including t(2;5)(p32;q35), which transposes the ALK locus next to an ALK tyrosine kinase gene. The ALK gene may also be translocated to partner genes on chromosome 1, 2, 3, and 17, causing dysregulation of ALK expression. ALK translocations are usually absent in cutaneous ALCLs and are seen with lower frequency in adults.

141e.3 Answer: (d) The primary modality of treatment for all histologic types and stages of childhood non-Hodgkin's lymphoma is multiagent chemotherapy. Radiotherapy is occasionally required as emergency treatment of acute central nervous system (CNS) involvement and/or for superior vena caval obstruction. The prophylactic use, however, of radiation in limited-stage disease and/or active CNS involvement has been demonstrated recently to provide no advantage to current multiagent chemotherapy approaches.

Similarly, although the role of surgery is critically important in establishing a diagnosis, it is not a primary treatment modality in childhood non-Hodgkin's lymphoma. Surgery can be beneficial in specific situations, including exploratory laporatomy in patients with acute abdominal disease and surgical resection during acute emergencies. There is, however, little role for surgery in tumor debulking or for second-look surgery.

141e.4 Answer: (b) Because of reports of treatment failures after shortened courses of B-NHL chemotherapy, many international cooperative groups have now adopted histology-specific treatment strategies for localized lymphoblastic lymphoma. These treatment regimens are similar or identical to the treatment approaches used for advanced-stage (III or IV) lymphoblastic lymphoma and include CNS prophylaxis.

142a.1 Answer: (b) Hepatoblastoma *not* hepatocellular carcinoma has been associated with familial adenomatous polyposis. Acquired mutations of the *APC* gene have been reported in hepatoblastoma, and up to 50% of hepatoblastomas have associated β-catenin mutations.

142a.2 Answer: (b) Pediatric melanoma accounts for 1.3% of all cases of melanoma and for 31% of all "carcinomas" in the pediatric population. Thyroid cancer is the most common pediatric carcinoma, and most cases of carcinoma occur in patients ages 15 to 19 years.

142a.3 Answer: (a) Patients with bilateral retinoblastoma carry a germline mutation for the retinoblastoma gene. Therefore, the inheritance pattern is autosomal dominant. However, the penetrance of the mutation is not complete, and the risk for the offspring is therefore less than 50%.

142a.4 Answer: (d) Yolk sac tumor is the most common malignant germ cell tumor in prepubertal children. It is usually the malignant component in sacrococcygeal and infantile testicular tumors. Ovarian germinomas are very common in pubertal and postpubertal girls and in extragonadal sites such as the central nervous system. Embyonal carcinoma and choriocarcinoma are very rare.

142b.1 Answer: (c) Monomorphic blastemal Wilms' tumor may be difficult to distinguish from other small round blue cell tumors, and monophasic stromal Wilms' tumor may simulate mesoblastic nephroma, whereas the purely tubular and papillary varieties may be difficult to distinguish from papillary renal cell carcinoma. Primary germ cell tumor is usually histologically distinct.

142b.2 Answer: (d) The presence of diffuse anaplasia defined as markedly enlarged nuclei and the presence of multipolar or polyploid mitotic figures is associated with a dramatically worse outcome. Although extrarenal extension and lymph node involvement are adverse prognostic factors used in the staging system, their effect is not as strong as the presence of anaplasia. A pseudocapsule is typical of Wilms' and is not a prognostic factor.

142b.3 Answer: (a) Most commonly Wilms' tumors present as an asymptomatic abdominal swelling or abdominal mass often detected by a family member. Although there may be associated abdominal pain and gross or microscopic hematuria, these are less common. Renal failure would be an extraordinary initial finding, even for bilateral Wilms' tumor, and aniridia is present in < 1% of Wilms' tumor patients with the associated congenital syndrome.

142b.4 Answer: (b) A CT scan of the chest allows assessment for pulmonary metastases, and a CT scan of the abdomen provides the surgeon with information regarding resectability and the possibility of adjacent organ involvement. Ultrasonography of the abdomen additionally provides information on possible involvement of the inferior vena cava. Bone scan is not usually indicated for patients with favorable-histology Wilms' tumor as part of the initial work-up, unless there are specific symptoms to suggest bone metastasis. Patients found on histologic assessment to have clear cell sarcoma of the kidney should have a bone scan postoperatively.

142b.5 Answer: (b) The presence of diffuse anaplasia is the most critical prognostic factor for Wilms' tumor, whereas other renal tumor variants such as rhabdoid tumor of the kidney and clear cell sarcoma require different and specific therapies. The accurate identification of histology and staging allows the optimum targeting of treatment by risk of recurrence. No difference in outcome has been demonstrated between this approach and that advocated in Europe—the use of postchemotherapy nephrectomy. Surgical morbidity is not reduced by performing initial nephrectomy, nor has it been shown that outcome is affected by radiation administered pre- or postchemotherapy.

142c.1 Answer: (c) The most important variables predictive of disease outcome in neuroblastoma are the conventional clinical features, age of the patient, and stage of disease at diagnosis. These variables are of proven prognostic utility and are the cornerstone of the current risk stratification schema. Biologic variables such as histopathologic classification and genetic features including DNA index and *MYCN* gene copy number have also been shown to be prognostically important and lend important information to that gained from age and stage. Because no study to date has examined all biologic variables together in a large set of patients, it is difficult to say which single biologic variable or combination of variables is the most powerful predictor of outcome in addition to patient age and disease stage.

142c.2   Answer: (b)   Data from screening studies of infants 6 months of age or less show an overall increased prevalence of neuroblastoma but no appreciable change in the prevalence of neuroblastoma in patients > 1 year of age. In addition, the clinical and biologic features of the tumors identified as a result of mass screening are typically consistent with low-risk disease. This suggests that screening is detecting tumors in a substantial number of patients who would likely never develop symptomatic disease because their tumors would regress or mature without therapy. When screening is done at an older age, the prevalence of overdiagnosis is less, and there may be a greater number of patients with unfavorable disease features. However, it is unlikely that screening makes any substantive impact on outcome for a population of patients with high-risk disease.

142c.3   Answer: (b)   CT scanning is generally used in neuroblastoma to evaluate the primary tumor and solid organs for metastatic disease but not bony disease. Plain radiography can detect some cortical bone metastases, and this method can be used in young infants with localized tumors and favorable biologic features who are therefore at a very low risk of bony metastases. ^{99m}Tc-diphosphate scintigraphy is more sensitive for detection of occult bony metastases but can be nonspecific. MIBG scintigraphy has the greatest sensitivity and specificity for detecting bone metastases, and response at metastatic sites as judged by MIBG may be of prognostic importance. It is therefore recommended in the diagnostic evaluation of patients with high-risk disease features and may be performed with either ^{131}I or ^{123}I isotopes. The ^{123}I isotope provides better resolution and sensitivity.

142c.4   Answer: (a)   For infants with stage 4S neuroblastoma, a diagnostic biopsy is indicated for evaluation of tumor biologic features, but resection of the primary tumor does not appear to influence outcome. Patients with favorable biologic features should be observed closely for symptomatology from tumor expansion and be given moderately intensive chemotherapy if respiratory compromise becomes evident. Radiation therapy should be reserved for patients who progress despite chemotherapy. The rare stage 4S patient with unfavorable biologic features should be treated using either intermediate- or high-risk strategies as indicated by tumor biology.

142c.5   Answer: (d)   Historically, high-risk neuroblastoma patients have had long-term survival probabilities of < 15%; but with the advent of comprehensive treatment approaches that include intensive induction chemotherapy, myeloablative consolidation therapy with autologous stem cell rescue, and targeted therapy for minimal residual disease, overall survival rates have improved. Gross total resection of tumors prior to therapy in patients with high-risk disease is often not feasible without injury to vital structures and does not improve overall prognosis. An intent-to-treat analysis of a recent Children's Cancer Group study showed a significant improvement in 3-year event-free survival for patients treated with a myeloablative consolidation compared with those who underwent nonmyeloablative consolidation. Bone marrow rescue with peripheral blood stem cells provides superior engraftment kinetics and likely decreases transplantation-related morbidity. Despite this comprehensive approach, immediate and long-term morbidity and mortality rates are clearly suboptimal.

142d.1   Answer: (d)   Spindle cell and botryoid are subtypes of embryonal histology tumors. Alveolar histology tumors comprise about 25% of all RMSs. Over one-half of all tumors are of embryonal histology.

142d.2   Answer: (b) and (d)   The *PAX3-FKHR* and *PAX7-FKHR* gene fusions characterize alveolar RMS. For patients with metastatic disease at diagnosis, those with the *PAX7* fusion have a better outcome. *EWS-FLI1* occurs in the vast majority of cases of the Ewing's sarcoma family of tumors (~ 90%). *SYT-SSX1* characterizes synovial sarcoma; *EWS-WT1* is found in desmoplastic small round cell tumors. There is no specific gene fusion identified in embryonal histology tumors.

142d.3   Answer: (e)   All three treatment modalities are required to maximize cure rates in alveolar RMS. If a tumor can be completely resected, this is almost always preferable; however, these patients still need local irradiation. If the tumor is not resectable, then local irradiation is mandatory. All patients need aggressive multiagent chemotherapy; the standard three-drug chemotherapy used in the national cooperative group is VAC (vincristine, dactinomycin [actinomycin D], and cyclophosphamide). For patients with embryonal histology tumors, complete resection obviates the need for local irradiation. Lower-stage/-group patients can be treated effectively with just a two-drug therapy (vincristine and dactinomycin).

142d.4   Answer: (f)   Appropriate treatment planning is based on both the International Rhabdomyosarcoma Study Group (IRSG) Clinical Grouping system and an IRSG-modified tumor, node, metastasis (TNM) system. Clinical group is dependent on completeness of resection. Group I denotes tumors that are completely excised with negative tumor margins; group II are tumors that are grossly resected with microscopic residual disease; and group III are localized tumors that are unresected or have gross residual disease after initial surgery. The modified TNM system is based on tumor site and size and the presence of clinical lymph node involvement. The presence of metastatic disease denotes both group IV and stage 4 disease.

142d.5   Answer: (e)   Although the proportion of certain histologies is somewhat different in children and adults, most histologies of soft tissue sarcoma occur in both the pediatric and adult population and share similar histologic, biologic, and molecular features. Histologic grading of tumors, as well as size and tumor invasiveness, are prognostically important, with high-grade, large, and invasive tumors having the worst outcome. In both children and adults, surgical resection is key for effective tumor control. Infantile fibrosarcoma is a unique histology occurring in young children, with a distinct cryptic translocation involving *TEL* (chromosome 12) and *TRKC* (chromosome 15). This tumor is much more sensitive to chemotherapy than the typical fibrosarcoma that occurs in adults and older children and adolescents.

143a.1 **Answer: (a)** Clear cell sarcoma is a distinctive pediatric renal neoplasm that differs morphologically from Wilms' tumor and is associated with poor outcome. The other listed tumors can occur in both pediatric and adult populations.

143a.2 **Answer: (e)** Fibrolamellar carcinoma is a variant of hepatocellular carcinoma that occurs most frequently in adolescents and morphologically does not resemble the embryonal liver. The other tumors usually resemble embryonic muscle, retina, salivary gland, and kidney, respectively.

143a.3 **Answer: (c)** Nephroblastomatosis, or the presence of so-called nephrogenic rests, is a well-known example of a pediatric precursor lesion that is associated with Wilms' tumor and is present in about 1% of neonatal autopsies. The other examples are in situ lesions more typically associated with adult tumors.

143a.4 **Answer: (d)** *PAX3/FKHR* and *PAX7/FKHR* are the fusion genes most commonly associated with alveolar rhabdomyosarcoma. The others are associated with Ewing's sarcoma, desmoplastic small cell tumor, synovial sarcoma, and promyelocytic leukemia, respectively.

143a.5 **Answer: (b)** Ewing's sarcomas are, by definition, undifferentiated childhood tumors by routine light microscopy. Although rhabdomyosarcomas, Wilms' tumors, and neuroblastomas may appear undifferentiated, they usually contain at least an occasional focus that resembles embryonic cytodifferentiation into muscle, kidney, or ganglia, respectively. Fibrolamellar carcinoma usually presents as a recognizably hepatocytic lesion.

143b.1 **Answer: (e)** In rank order, and with proportion of all cancers that occur in the 15- to 19-year age group, the three most common malignancies are Hodgkin's disease (16%), germ cell tumors (15%), and central nervous system tumors (10%). The next most common cancers are non-Hodgkin's lymphoma (8%), thyroid cancer (7%), malignant melanoma (7%), and acute lymphoblastic leukemia (6%).

143b.2 **Answer: (c)** A bone tumor in an African American is much more likely to be osteosarcoma than Ewing's sarcoma. African Americans rarely develop Ewing's sarcoma or melanoma; this is one of the major reasons why cancer is less common in persons between 15 and 45 years of age. In this age range, thyroid cancer and melanoma are more common in females than in males.

143b.3 **Answer: (c)** Given that the duration of exposure to potential environmental carcinogens is directly proportional to age, it is not surprising that tobacco-, sunlight-, or diet-related cancers are more likely in older adolescents and young adults than in younger persons. Nonetheless, these environmental agents known to be carcinogens in older adults have not been demonstrated to cause cancer with any significant frequency in adolescents. In most persons, it appears to take considerably longer than one or two decades for these environmentally related cancers to become manifest.

143b.4 **Answer: (a)** There is remarkably little literature on cancer in the older adolescent and in the young adult. Increasingly, the cancers of older adolescents and young adults are being found to be biologically distinctive and unique. A majority of the cancers in this age group are not carcinomas; this contrasts occurrence in adults over age 50 years, in whom 80 to 90% of cancers are carcinomas. Leukemia, lymphoma, Hodgkin's disease, sarcomas, melanomas, and brain tumors account for two-thirds of the tumors in 20- to 29-year-olds. Delays in diagnosis are common in this age group, in part because internists, family practitioners, generalists, and many nononcologic specialists do not think of malignant disease when evaluating young adult patients. The majority of environmentally induced cancers become clinically detectable later in life but often have their onset during early adulthood, as lifestyles with increased cancer risk are assumed.

143b.5 **Answer (a)** The National Cancer Institute, the adult cooperative groups (eg, Southwest Oncology Group, Eastern Cooperative Oncology Group, Cancer and Leukemia Group B, Radiation Therapy Oncology Group, American College of Surgeons Oncology Group, Gynecologic Oncology Group), and the pediatric cooperative group, Children's Oncology Group, have procedures that allow young adult patients to be treated in clinical trials. A mechanism for intergroup protocol development exists.

COMPLICATIONS

DIRECTIONS: Numbering for questions and answers reflects the corresponding chapter in *Cancer Medicine-6*. Most questions contain suggested responses. Select the best response to each question. Answers for Complications begin on page 172.

COMPLICATIONS OF CANCER AND ITS TREATMENT

144.1   Which of the following cytokines is *not* implicated as a mediator of cancer cachexia?
a.   Tumor necrosis factor-α (TNF-α)
b.   Interleukin-2 (IL-2)
c.   IL-6
d.   IL-10
e.   Interferon-γ

144.2   Central nervous system neuropeptides known to be associated with anorexia include all of the following *except*
a.   Neuropeptide Y
b.   Leptin
c.   Corticotropin-releasing hormone
d. α-Melanocyte-stimulating hormone
e.   Cocaine- and amphetamine-regulated transcript

144.3   Regarding the metabolic derangements considered as mechanisms of cancer cachexia, which of the following statements is (are) *not* true?
a.   High rates of glucose use with the production of lactic acid are characteristic features of tumor cells. Hexokinase, which catalyzes the first step of the glycolytic pathway, is found to be highly overexpressed in tumor cells. The end product of the hexokinase reaction, glucose-6-phosphate, serves as a key intermediate for cell growth and proliferation.
b.   The cyclic metabolic pathway in which glucose is converted to lactic acid by glycolysis in tumor tissue, and then reconverted back to glucose in the liver, is referred to as the Cori cycle. Conversion of glucose to lactate in cancer cells yields two molecules of adenosine triphosphate (ATP), whereas lactate to glucose in the liver requires six ATPs. Therefore, cancer cells act as an energy parasite.
c.   Tumors are effective nitrogen traps, and nitrogen is translocated from host to tumor, producing nitrogen depletion in the host. Therefore, selective parasitism of the host by the tumor in the form of successful competition for nutrients is the major cause of cancer cachexia.
d.   The role of TNF-α/cachectin in the development of cancer cachexia in humans has been established. Thus, administration of recombinant TNF-α/cachectin produced demonstrable cachexia. TNF-α/cachectin serum levels were shown to be elevated in cachectic cancer patients.
e.   The metabolic manifestations of cancer cachexia are different from those of healthy subjects undergoing starvation. The alterations in metabolism in cancer patients more closely resemble that of patients with sepsis or polytrauma. Thus, almost all cancer patients exhibit increased resting energy expenditure and elevated basal metabolic rates.

144.4   Which agent(s) is (are) effective in improving appetite and preventing weight loss in cachectic cancer patients?
a.   Cyproheptadine
b.   Hydrazine sulfate
c.   Megestrol acetate
d.   Pentoxifylline
e.   Ranitidine

144.5   The following clinical conditions are known to be associated with cancer cachexia or an advanced stage of cancer *except*
a.   Gastric stasis and delayed gastric emptying
b.   Idiopathic steatorrhea or villous atrophy
c.   Nonbacterial thrombotic (marantic) endocarditis
d.   Deep vein thrombosis (DVT)
e.   Decubitus

144.6   In which of the following conditions is total parenteral nutrition (TPN) indicated? (More than one may be correct.)
a.   A 65-year-old man with a diagnosis of laryngeal carcinoma is receiving radiation therapy. He has dysphagia and has lost 4.5 kg during the past 3 weeks.
b.   A 70-year-old man with a 4-month history of progressive dysphagia for liquid and solid food and weight loss of 9 kg was diagnosed as having squamous cell carcinoma in the middle one-third of the esophagus.
c.   A 62-year-old woman with a diagnosis of pancreatic carcinoma is about to receive a 5-fluorouracil infusion and local radiotherapy. She has frequent diarrhea and has lost 7.5 kg over 3 months.
d.   A 45-year-old woman with ovarian carcinoma presents with a large amount of ascites and evidence of partial intestinal obstruction.
e.   A 5-year-old boy with a diagnosis of Wilms' tumor is about to undergo an intensive combined chemotherapy and radiotherapy program. He has good appetite and is well nourished.

145.1 A 66-year-old patient who has chronic lymphocytic leukemia is about to begin chemotherapy with chlorambucil and prednisone. Which of the following antiemetics would you recommend?
   a.   Intravenous metoclopramide (1–2 mg/kg)
   b.   Oral tetrahydrocannabinol (dronabinol) (10 mg/m^2)
   c.   Intravenous granisetron (10 µg/kg)
   d.   Oral ondansetron (8 mg)
   e.   No antiemetic

145.2 Which of the following anticancer drugs is most likely to cause significant nausea and vomiting?
   a.   Cisplatin
   b.   Bleomycin
   c.   Tamoxifen
   d.   Vinblastine
   e.   Fluorouracil

145.3 Ondansetron and granisetron have been proved to be safe and effective for which of the following vomiting syndromes?
   a.   Delayed emesis
   b.   Motion sickness
   c.   Anticipatory emesis
   d.   Bowel obstruction emesis
   e.   Radiation-induced emesis

146.1 The first seizure can be a presenting symptom of
   a.   Brain metastasis
   b.   Sagittal sinus thrombosis
   c.   Leptomeningeal metastasis
   d.   Hyponatremia
   e.   All of the above

146.2 Peripheral neuropathy from which chemotherapeutic agent commonly progresses after discontinuing the drug?
   a.   Vincristine
   b.   Taxol
   c.   Cisplatin
   d.   Suramin

146.3 Epidural spinal cord compression is diagnosed by
   a.   Bone scan
   b.   Unenhanced magnetic resonance imaging (MRI)
   c.   Spine films
   d.   Enhanced MRI
   e.   Myelography

146.4 Metabolic encephalopathy is a common complication of which chemotherapeutic agent?
   a.   Ifosfamide
   b.   Irinotecan
   c.   Vinblastine
   d.   Taxol
   e.   Cyclophosphamide

146.5 Treatment for brain metastases can include
   a.   Whole brain radiotherapy
   b.   Stereotactic radiosurgery
   c.   Surgical resection for chemotherapy
   d.   All of the above

147.1 The most common mucocutaneous reaction associated with cancer chemotherapy is
   a.   Acral erythema
   b.   Extravasation reactions
   c.   Neutrophilic eccrine hidradenitis
   d.   Stomatitis
   e.   Alopecia

147.2 The class of chemotherapeutic agents that is associated with the most common and potent vesicant reactions is
   a.   Alkylating agents
   b.   Antimetabolites
   c.   Antibiotics
   d.   Vinca alkaloids
   e.   Enzymes

147.3 During the intravenous infusion of vincristine in a cancer patient, the nurse reports that the infusion site has become very ery-thematous and tender. Choose the steps of action that should be taken in the most appropriate order.
   a.   Tell the nurse it is just common irritation and to continue administration.
   b.   Apply cold, consider antidote, discontinue infusion, aspirate drug, and remove catheter.
   c.   Apply heat, consider antidote, discontinue infusion, aspirate drug, and remove catheter.
   d.   Discontinue infusion, aspirate drug, remove catheter, apply cold, and consider antidote.
   e.   Discontinue infusion, aspirate drug, remove catheter, apply heat, and consider antidote.

147.4 In a bone marrow transplant patient who has undergone chemotherapy, which of the following cutaneous reactions often mimic acute graft-versus-host disease (GVHD) clinically and histologically: (1) neutrophilic eccrine hidradenitis, (2) eruption of lym-phocyte recovery (ELR), (3) acral erythema, or (4) eccrine squamous syringometaplasia?
   a.   1 only
   b.   3 only
   c.   2 and 3
   d.   1 and 4
   e.   1, 2, 3, and 4

147.5 Which of the following reactions are often associated with interferon-α and interleukin-2 infusions?
   a.   Psoriasis exacerbation
   b.   Seborrheic dermatitis exacerbation
   c.   Telogen effluvium
   d.   Cutaneous ulceration
   e.   All of the above

148.1 Lytic destructive bone lesions in metastatic breast carcinoma are usually caused by which of the following cells?
   a.   Macrophages
   b.   Stromal fibroblasts
   c.   Osteoclasts
   d.   Mast cells
   e.   Langerhans' cells

148.2 The type of bone destruction seen in metastatic renal cell carcinoma is
   a.   Osteoblastic
   b.   Osteolytic
   c.   Permeative associated with a high incidence of pathologic fracture
   d.   Osteolytic and permeative associated with a high incidence of pathologic fracture
   e.   All of the above

148.3 With respect to the incidence and location of skeletal metastases, which of the following is true?
   a.   Metastatic lesions are more common in the axial skeleton.
   b.   The proximal femur is the most common site for pathologic fracture.
   c.   The thoracolumbar spine represents the most common site for metastases.
   d.   Metastases below the elbow and knee are relatively rare.
   e.   All of the above are true.

149.1 The pathogen most frequently causing transfusion-transmitted disease is
   a.   Hepatitis A virus (HAV)
   b.   Hepatitis B virus (HBV)
   c.   Hepatitis C virus (HCV)
   d.   Human immunodeficiency virus (HIV)
   e.   Bacteria

149.2 Recipients of minor ABO-incompatible stem cell transplants are at increased risk of
   a.   Delayed red cell reconstitution
   b.   Increased graft rejection

c. Hemolysis 1 to 3 weeks after transplantation
d. Severe graft-versus-host disease (GVHD)
e. Early mortality

149.3 Blood products are leukoreduced for all of the following reasons *except*
a. Prevention of febrile nonhemolytic transfusion reactions
b. Prevention of transfusion-associated GVHD
c. Prevention of platelet alloimmunization
d. Prevention of cytomegalovirus (CMV) transmission

150.1 A 65-year-old male with a past medical history significant for ulcerative colitis is diagnosed with stage III colon cancer (T2N1M0). He is treated with chemotherapy and radiation therapy. His course is complicated with significant nausea, vomiting, and diarrhea. In addition, he also develops hematemesis. Laboratory evaluation reveals a hemoglobin of 7.5 g/dL, a hematocrit (Hct) of 22%, a mean corpuscular volume of 78, and a red cell distribution width of 17. The platelet count is 160,000; the white count is 12,000. The activated partial thromboplastin time (aPTT) is 58 seconds, and the international normalized ratio (INR) is 1.1. The patient is transfused with packed red blood cells and fresh frozen plasma. After transfusion his hemoglobin increases to 9.4 g/dL; however, he is noticed to have several subcutaneous hematomas. A repeat aPTT is 52 seconds. What would be the most appropriate laboratory management at this time?
a. Repeat aPTT, INR, complete blood count, peripheral blood smear, fibrinogen, D dimer, and fibrin degradation products
b. Transfuse more fresh frozen plasma and packed red blood cells
c. Perform aPTT mixing studies
d. Do a lupus anticoagulant test

150.2 A 53-year-old male 40 pack/year smoker with history of coronary artery disease, for which he required coronary stent placement, is now diagnosed with metastatic pancreatic cancer. He is treated with gemcitabine chemotherapy. Four months later, he presents with progressive edema and tenderness of the right lower extremity (RLE). A duplex/Doppler ultrasonography of the RLE demonstrates absent flow extending from the popliteal vein to the common femoral vein, consistent with a deep vein thrombosis.

The patient is hospitalized and started on anticoagulation with unfractionated heparin (UFH). Warfarin is begun on the third day after initiation of heparin. Monitoring of the complete blood count (CBC) reveals a progressive decrease in the platelet count from 156,000/mm^3 to 83,000/mm^3 after 6 days of exposure to UFH; the aPTT is 60 seconds, and the INR is 1.4. The diagnosis of heparin-induced thrombocytopenia (HIT) is considered. What would be the most appropriate management at this point?
a. Continue warfarin and use low molecular weight heparin (LMWH) instead of UFH
b. Discontinue UHF and warfarin and place an inferior vena cava (IVC) filter
c. Continue UFH and warfarin and request a heparin-platelet factor 4 enzyme-linked immunosorbent assay to confirm a diagnosis of HIT
d. Continue warfarin, discontinue UFH, and start a direct thrombin inhibitor until the INR is 2 or > 2 for 2 consecutive days

150.3 A 30-year-old male with chronic myelogenous leukemia undergoes an allogeneic stem cell transplantation. He is managed with immunosuppression with cyclosporine. On day 35 post-transplantation, he presents with fever of 38°C and mild confusion associated with a headache. Physical examination is remarkable for pale conjunctiva and mucosa and icterus. A CBC reveals an Hct of 15%, an absolute reticulocyte count of 120,000, and a platelet count of 20,000/mm^3. Urinalysis reveals microscopic hematuria and proteinuria. What would be the best next step?
a. Order a prothrombin time (PT)/INR, aPTT, fibrinogen, and D dimer to exclude disseminated intravascular coagulation (DIC)
b. Perform a bone marrow aspiration and biopsy to evaluate for the possibility of graft failure
c. Evaluate the peripheral blood smear
d. Transfuse platelet concentrates and packed red blood cells

150.4 A 51-year-old female is referred to you for thrombophilia evaluation. She had a previous history significant for systemic lupus erythematosus but has been in remission for the past 20 years. At age 35 years, she had an idiopathic cerebrovascular accident with residual minimal right-sided weakness.

At age 38 years, she was diagnosed with left breast invasive adenocarcinoma (T2N1M0); the estrogen receptors (ER) and progesterone receptors (PR) receptors were negative. She was treated with a modified radical left mastectomy (MRM) and axillary lymph node dissection. Subsequently she received six cycles of chemotherapy and was in complete remission.

Three years ago, in a routine physical examination, she was found to have a small lump in the right breast. A biopsy revealed a T1aN0M0 infiltrating adenocarcinoma. The sentinel lymph node biopsy was negative for tumor. The ER/PR receptors were positive. The patient had a right MRM and was started on tamoxifen. What would be your best advice for this patient regarding the use of selective estrogen receptor modulators?
a. Continue tamoxifen if all of the thrombophilia evaluation is negative
b. Continue tamoxifen and start on warfarin 1 mg (preventive dose)
c. Discontinue tamoxifen
d. Discontinue tamoxifen and start on an aromatase inhibitor

150.5 **What is the most likely mechanism by which patients with acute promyelocytic leukemia (APL) have a high incidence of hemorrhagic complications?**
a. Severe thrombocytopenia
b. Dysfibrinogenemia
c. DIC
d. Increased fibrino(geno)lysis because of overexpression of annexin II on APL cells

152.1 **Radiation to the mediastinum is most likely to cause**
a. Advanced coronary artery disease with myocardial infarction as a late complication
b. Severe mitral regurgitation owing to destruction of the anterior mitral leaflet
c. Constrictive pericarditis as a late complication
d. Congestive cardiomyopathy owing to primary myocyte destruction
e. Acute pericarditis occurring during the procedure or the early post-treatment period

152.2 **As a tool to follow anthracycline cardiac effects, cardiac ejection fraction determinations**
a. Are generally reliable—even small decreases should trigger a change in therapy to prevent irreversible cardiac damage
b. Established via nuclear cardiac blood-pool scans (multiple gated acquisition scans) are presently universally preferred over those obtained from cardiac ultrasonographic examinations (echocardiography)
c. Established via cardiac ultrasonographic examinations are presently universally preferred over those obtained from nuclear scans
d. Are less likely to represent a false-positive result the closer a patient is to his/her maximal cumulative dosage
e. Are more sensitive and specific than are cardiac biopsies in following patients with early anthracycline cardiac changes

152.3 **Each of the following has been used to effectively reduce the cardiotoxicity of doxorubicin** *except*
a. Liposomal delivery systems
b. High-dose vitamin C
c. Limiting the cumulative dose to 400 mg/m^2 or less
d. Dexrazoxane (Zinecard)
e. Schedule modification

152.4 **Which of the following is a true statement regarding cardiac biopsy?**
a. Cardiac changes associated with trastuzumab (Herceptin) can be readily detected.
b. Cardiac biopsy does not detect changes associated with mitoxantrone, as mitoxantrone is not an anthracycline.
c. Cardiac biopsy changes are similar for patients who have received either 200 mg/m^2 of doxorubicin or 200 mg/m^2 of mitoxantrone.
d. Cardiac biopsy changes in patients who have alcoholic cardiomyopathy are indistinguishable from those of patients with cardiotoxicity following anthracycline administration.
e. Cardiac biopsy changes are detectable at cumulative dosages below those associated with clinical evidence of cardiac dysfunction.

152.5 **Trastuzumab cardiotoxicity**
a. Is subclinical and only of theoretic concern
b. Is analogous to anthracycline cardiotoxicity, in that it has a similar mechanism, morphology, and clinical course
c. May represent a sequential stress following subclinical doxorubicin damage
d. Is always seen when the drug is administered following an anthracycline
e. Has been studied extensively

152.6 **A patient has received four cycles of doxorubicin. The cycle dose was 50 mg/m^2 by rapid infusion. The patient's regimen is being changed to mitoxantrone. To avoid an increased risk of cardiotoxicity, the dose of mitoxantrone should not exceed**
a. 160 mg/m^2 as the toxicity of each of the two cardiotoxic drugs is independent from each other, and 160 mg/m^2 is the acceptable maximum mitoxantrone cumulative dose
b. 550 mg/m^2 as this is the acceptable anthracycline maximal cumulative dose
c. 80 mg/m^2 as the patient has been exposed to about half of the acceptable dose of doxorubicin, and would be expected to tolerate about half of the maximal recommended cumulative dose of mitoxantrone
d. 0 mg/m^2—mitoxantrone should not be used in this setting as cardiotoxicity would be excessive
e. 104 mg/m^2 as the patient has received about 35% of the maximal doxorubicin dose of 550 mg/m^2 and would therefore be expected to tolerate about 104 mg/m^2 of mitoxantrone

153.1 **Respiratory infections in non-neutropenic patients with cancer commonly include all of the following** *except*
a. *Haemophilus influenzae*
b. *Pseudomonas aeruginosa*
c. *Streptococcus pneumoniae*
d. Respiratory syncytial virus
e. Adenovirus

153.2 **The use of prophylactic antibiotics and early empiric antibiotic coverage for gram-negative organisms has led to**
- a. A high rate of *Haemophilus* sepsis during neutropenic periods
- b. The emergence of the SPACE *(Serratia, Pseudomonas, Acinetobacter, Citrobacter,* and *Enterobacter)* organisms during the first week of severe neutropenia
- c. The need for empiric antifungal therapy after the first 3 days of neutropenic fever
- d. The emergence of catheter-related and mucositis-related bacteremia as the major form of gram-positive infections
- e. A significant increase in *Candida* sepsis, which can be diagnosed nearly always by blood culture

153.3 **Optimal palliation of a malignant pleural effusion includes all of the following *except***
- a. Complete drainage of the pleural space and re-expansion of the lung at the time of tube thoracostomy
- b. Waiting until the drainage of fluid just prior to pleurodesis has dropped to 50 to 100 cc/24 h
- c. Removal or reduction of loculations, if present, during thoracoscopy
- d. Pleurodesis with any of a number of sclerosing agents
- e. Systemic chemotherapy for cancers likely to be highly responsive to therapy

153.4 **Which of the following are true statements concerning patients with pericardial effusions and cancer?**
- a. Almost any cancer can cause a malignant pericardial effusion.
- b. Approximately 40% of patients with cancer and a pericardial effusion have a benign etiology for the effusion.
- c. Physical examination is not a reliable way to diagnose a significant pericardial effusion.
- d. All of the above are true.
- e. None of the above is true.

153.5 **Radiation and chemotherapy can individually and collectively cause serious lung toxicity. Which of the following statements is true?**
- a. Radiation pneumonitis is essentially always excluded if it occurs outside a radiation portal.
- b. Radiation fibrosis develops over a period of several months to 2 years.
- c. The newer chemotherapy agents (taxanes, gemcitabine, vinorelbine) have not been associated with pulmonary toxicity, unlike earlier compounds such as bleomycin and mitomycin.
- d. Drug-induced pulmonary toxicity is almost always seen in the presence of high-dose therapy.
- e. Diffuse alveolar hemorrhage can occur in up to 50% of patients undergoing allogeneic transplantation and is often associated with a gram-negative infection.

154.1 **The diagnosis of sinusoidal obstruction syndrome (hepatic veno-occlusive disease) is usually based on results of**
- a. Doppler ultrasonography
- b. CT angiography
- c. Percutaneous liver biopsy
- d. Clinical criteria
- e. Magnetic resonance imaging

154.2 **The most common side effect of chemotherapy on the liver is**
- a. Clinically apparent liver injury
- b. Transient liver test abnormalities
- c. Frank cholestasis
- d. Fibrosis

156.1 **Oral mucositis is one of the most common acute side effects of radiation therapy for cancers of the head and neck. Which of the following statements is *incorrect*?**
- a. The initial clinical appearance of radiation-induced mucositis can be seen with cumulative radiation doses of between 10 and 20 Gy.
- b. Ulceration with pseudomembrane formation is a typical manifestation of mucositis and is seen with cumulative doses of 30 to 40 Gy.
- c. It is likely that mucositis represents a biologic process limited to epithelial stem cell injury.
- d. For patients' quality of life, mucositis is one of the most significant negative outcomes associated with radiation therapy.

156.2 **The risk of osteoradionecrosis of the mandible can be markedly reduced by which of the following? (More than one may be correct.)**
- a. Preradiation dental evaluation and elimination of questionable teeth
- b. The aggressive use of topical fluorides during and following radiation
- c. Deferring tooth extraction for 1 year after radiation therapy
- d. Prophylactic antibiotic administration during radiation therapy
- e. All of the above

156.3 **Radiation-induced xerostomia is a common chronic side effect of radiation therapy. Which major salivary glands are most susceptible?**
- a. Parotid glands
- b. Submandibular glands
- c. Sublingual glands

156.4 Which of the following anatomic sites are generally *not* susceptible to chemotherapy-induced mucositis? (More than one may be correct.)
    a.   Floor of mouth
    b.   Buccal mucosa
    c.   Soft palate
    d.   Hard palate
    e.   Gingiva

156.5 Myelosuppressed patients are at risk of viral infections in the mouth. Which all the following viruses most often cause oral infections in granulocytopenic cancer patients? (More than one may be correct.)
    a.   Herpes simplex virus 1
    b.   Varicella-zoster virus
    c.   Human papillomavirus
    d.   Epstein-Barr virus
    e.   Cytomegalovirus

156.6 Granulocytopenic patients are at risk of oral fungal infections. The most common of these is candidiasis. However, on occasion, these individuals may develop deep fungal infections in the mouth. Which one is the most common?

157.1 Exposure to a moderate-dose alkylating drug would be most likely to induce permanent sterility in which of the following?
    a.   A 9-year-old boy
    b.   A 9-year-old girl
    c.   A 25-year-old woman
    d.   A 25-year-old man

157.2 The combination chemotherapy most likely to induce permanent sterility in a 25-year-old man is
    a.   MOPP (mechlorethamine, vincristine [Oncovin], procarbazine, prednisone)
    b.   ABVD (doxorubicin [Adriamycin], bleomycin, vinblastine, dacarbazine)
    c.   PVB (cisplatin, vinblastine, bleomycin)
    d.   PEB (cisplatin, etoposide, bleomycin)

157.3 A 26-year-old woman conceives a pregnancy 8 years after completing standard-dose chemotherapy for AML. She should be advised
    a.   Of the high risk of fetal wastage in this setting
    b.   That congenital anomalies are common and she should consider therapeutic termination of this pregnancy
    c.   That most pregnancies in this setting successfully produce healthy babies with no clear health or developmental problems anticipated
    d.   That this child will be at high risk of cancer as he/she matures

157.4 The best option for preserving fertility after chemotherapy for lymphoma in a 42-year-old man would be
    a.   Semen cryopreservation before chemotherapy administration
    b.   Gonadotropin-releasing hormone (Gn-RH) analogue administration prior to chemotherapy administration
    c.   Careful selection of treatment options to include the least alkylating drug possible
    d.   Testicular sperm extraction at the time conception is desired

157.5 Options for preservation of fertility in a 23-year-old woman who will undergo total nodal radiation for Hodgkin's disease include
    a.   Gn-RH analogue administration to suppress ovulation
    b.   Embryo cryopreservation
    c.   Ovarian transposition
    d.   All of the above

158.1 Paraneoplastic endocrine syndromes are caused by neoplasm production of
    a.   Steroid hormones
    b.   Thyronines
    c.   Catecholamines
    d.   Peptides/proteins
    e.   Antibodies

158.2 Breast cancer produces hypercalcemia predominantly by
    a.   Widespread bony metastatic disease
    b.   Tumor production of 1,25-dihydroxy vitamin D
    c.   Tumor production of parathyroid-related protein (PTH-RP)

    d. Tumor production of parathyroid hormone (PTH)

    e. Tumor production of osteoclastic-activating factors (OAF)

158.3 Cancer-caused Cushing's syndrome is commonly associated with

    a. Increased circulating adrenocorticotropic hormone (ACTH) precursor molecules

    b. Failure to suppress cortisol production with high-dose dexamethasone treatment

    c. Much higher plasma ACTH than in Cushing's disease (pituitary-dependent)

    d. Hypokalemia

    e. All of the above

158.4 Which of the following is *not* chorionic gonadotropin (CG) production by cancers?

    a. Nonmalignant normal tissues also produce CG.

    b. The presence of a malignancy may be diagnosed when CG is detected in urine or blood of nonpregnant subjects.

    c. CG is secreted in small amounts by the normal pituitary.

    d. Desialated CG is metabolized more rapidly than fully sialated CG.

    e. In normal pregnancy, beta-core is the predominant form of CG in urine.

158.5 Increased serum titers of anti-Hu are associated with which of the following neurologic disorders?

    a. Encephalitis

    b. Subacute sensory neuropathy

    c. Cerebellar degeneration

    d. Lambert-Eaton myasthenic syndrome

    e. Visual paraneoplastic syndrome

158.6 Which of the following chemotherapy drugs is/are associated with hypothyroidism: (1) L-asparaginase, (2) paclitaxel, (3) interleukin-2, or (4) doxorubicin?

    a. 1, 2, and 3

    b. 1 and 3

    c. 2 and 4

    d. Only 4

    e. 1, 2, 3, and 4

158.7 Which axis of hypothalamic-pituitary function is the most likely to be impaired by radiation to the brain?

    a. The thyrotropic axis (responsible for TSH)

    b. The gonadotropic axis (responsible for luteinizing hormone, follicle-stimulating hormone [LH/FSH])

    c. The adrenocortical axis (responsible for ACTH)

    d. The somatotropic axis (responsible for growth hormone [GH])

158.8 A patient who has acute lymphoblastic leukemia develops neutropenic fever after the fourth cycle of hyperfractionated cyclophosphamide, vincristine, doxorubicin, and dexamethasone (hyper-CVAD). On presentation to the emergency center, the patient is alert but diaphoretic, tachycardic, and hypotensive with systolic blood pressure about 70 mm Hg. Which of the following medications should be administered urgently: (1) hydrocortisone succinate 100 mg intravenously (IV); (2) a large volume of crystalloid IV fluid to try to maintain adequate systolic blood pressure; (3) broad-spectrum antibiotics (eg, imipenem/cilastatin with vancomycin) after obtaining cultures; or (4) synthetic ACTH (cosyntropin) 1 µg intravenously?

    a. 1, 2, and 3

    b. 1 and 3

    c. 2 and 4

    d. Only 4

    e. 1, 2, 3, and 4

158.9 Which of the following chemotherapy drugs are associated with renal sodium and magnesium wasting: (1) mithramycin, (2) cisplatin, (3) doxorubicin, or (4) cyclophosphamide?

    a. 1, 2, and 3

    b. 1 and 3

    c. 2 and 4

    d. Only 4

    e. 1, 2, 3, and 4

158.10 A 45-year-old woman who has no evidence of disease after breast cancer treatment by surgery and external beam radiation 5 years ago complains of a lump in her neck. Examination reveals no lymphadenopathy or hoarseness, but there is a 2 cm nodule in the left lobe of the thyroid gland. She denies dysphagia and dyspnea. Fine-needle aspiration biopsy of the thyroid nodule shows a follicular neoplasm. Which of the following will be most appropriate?
   a.   Perform a radioiodine scan of the thyroid.
   b.   Perform a radioiodine ablation of the thyroid.
   c.   Reassure the patient that thyroid nodules are very common after radiation exposure and the nodules are predominantly benign.
   d.   Perform total thyroidectomy.
   e.   Perform left thyroid lobectomy.

159.1 The most common cause of a second malignancy overall is
   a.   Genetic family syndromes
   b.   Random chance
   c.   Radiation therapy
   d.   Combined radiation and chemotherapy
   e.   Tobacco use

159.2 A 50-year-old woman is diagnosed with stage I breast cancer; she undergoes lumpectomy and radiation therapy, as well as adjuvant chemotherapy. Which of the following screening/early detection strategies would you *not* recommend?
   a.   Annual mammography and clinical breast examination
   b.   Annual carcinoembryonic antigen (CEA) level
   c.   Annual sigmoidoscopy or colonoscopy
   d.   Annual gynecologic examination
   e.   Annual Hemoccult (modification of guaiac test for occult blood)

159.3 The incidence of multiple primary cancers has been increasing dramatically. Which of the following states the reason for this increase?
   a.   Cancer patients are more likely to survive their initial malignancy and hence have the opportunity to develop a second malignancy.
   b.   There are fewer competing causes of mortality such as heart disease.
   c.   Increased use of screening tests, such as prostate cancer screening, are picking up more occult or less aggressive tumors.
   d.   Generally the cancer population is aging.
   e.   All of the above are reasons for the increase.

159.4 Which of the following syndromes is associated with an increased risk of developing several malignant neoplasms?
   a.   Neurofibromatosis type 1 (NF1)
   b.   Bloom syndrome
   c.   Beckwith-Wiedemann syndrome
   d.   Familial adenomatous polyposis (FAP)
   e.   All of the above

159.5 It is generally accepted that individuals who are genetically susceptible to cancer are more likely to develop secondary cancers. What percentage of individuals who develop cancer are predisposed by virtue of a genetic condition?
   a.   < 1%
   b.   1 to 5%
   c.   5 to 15%
   d.   15 to 25%
   e.   > 25%

159.6 Radiation therapy in the treatment of primary cancers imparts a risk of developing *all but* which of the following cancers?
   a.   Sarcomas of soft tissue and bone
   b.   Breast cancer
   c.   Acute leukemia
   d.   Embryonal tumors
   e.   Thyroid cancer

159.7 Which of the following statements about secondary leukemia is *incorrect*?
   a.   Secondary leukemias usually develop within 10 years of primary therapy.
   b.   Secondary leukemias are associated with the use of high-dose alkylating agents.
   c.   The most common type of secondary leukemia is acute myeloid leukemia (AML).
   d.   Secondary leukemias associated with epipodophyllotoxins are schedule dependent.
   e.   Secondary AML is usually curable with allogeneic bone marrow transplantation.

INFECTION IN THE CANCER PATIENT

160.1 Bacterial infections are common in patients with severe neutropenia. Which of the following is the organism *least likely* to cause significant bacterial infections in this patient population?
a. Viridans streptococci
b. Vancomycin-resistant enterococci (VRE)
c. *Pseudomonas aeruginosa*
d. *Stenotrophomonas maltophilia*
e. *Listeria monocytogenes*

160.2 Which of the following statements is true?
a. Gram-negative infections (particularly those caused by *P. aeruginosa*) are being documented less often in neutropenic patients. Potent antipseudomonal coverage is therefore not an essential component of empiric antibiotic regimens.
b. Gram-positive organisms are the predominant pathogens in neutropenic patients and are associated with increasing antimicrobial resistance, morbidity, and mortality, making agents such as vancomycin, quinupristin and dalfopristin (Synercid), and linezolid an essential component of empiric regimens.
c. Both are true.
d. Neither is true.

160.3 Empiric antifungal therapy is often administered to febrile neutropenic patients who fail to respond to antibacterial therapy. Which of the following is the agent of choice for empiric antifungal therapy?
a. Fluconazole
b. Itraconazole
c. Caspofungin
d. Amphotericin B (lipid preparations)
e. Flucytosine
f. Voriconazole

ONCOLOGIC EMERGENCIES

161.1 The most common cause of spinal cord compression in cancer patients is
a. Extradural tumor metastasis involving the lumbosacral spine
b. Extradural tumor metastasis involving the thoracic spine
c. Extradural tumor metastasis involving the cervical spine
d. Epidural abscesses
e. Direct tumor invasion of the spinal cord

161.2 Imaging studies that may be used in the diagnostic work-up of a pulmonary embolus include
a. Ventilation-perfusion (V/Q) scan
b. Spiral computerized tomography (CT)
c. Pulmonary angiography
d. V/Q scan and pulmonary angiography
e. All of the above

161.3 Factors predisposing cancer patients to hemoptysis include
a. Thrombocytopenia
b. Fungal infections
c. Liver involvement by the malignancy
d. Thrombocytopenia and liver involvement by the malignancy
e. All of the above

161.4 Which of the following statements about a carcinoid crisis is (are) true?
a. The crisis may be precipitated by anesthesia, biopsy, surgery, chemotherapy, or adrenergic drugs (eg, dopamine, epinephrine).
b. These patients may develop refractory hypotension, arrhythmias, and bronchospasm owing to massive release of serotonin and other vasoactive peptides from the tumor.
c. The carcinoid crisis can be aborted or treated effectively with octreotide acetate (Sandostatin), a somatostatin analogue.
d. All of the above are true.
e. None of the above are true.

161.5   **Emergency treatment of torsades de pointes may entail which of the following?**
   a.   Intravenous magnesium
   b.   Electrical overdrive pacing or pharmacologic overdrive with isoproterenol
   c.   Intravenous phenytoin or lidocaine
   d.   Defibrillation
   e.   All of the above

161.6   **Which of the following cytokines or antibody-derived pharmaceutic agents are associated with fever, hypotension, and dyspnea during or after administration?**
   a.   Interleukin-2 (IL-2)
   b.   Rituximab (Rituxan)
   c.   Denileukin diftitox (Ontak)
   d.   Gemtuzumab ozogamicin (Mylotarg)
   e.   Rituximab and gemtuzumab ozogamicin
   f.   IL-2 and denileukin diftitox
   g.   All of the above

ANSWERS

COMPLICATIONS OF CANCER AND ITS TREATMENT

144.1 **Answer: (d)** IL-10 has not been implicated as a mediator of cancer cachexia. IL-10 counteracted cachexia in animals bearing IL-6-produced tumors.

144.2 **Answer: (b)** Leptin is produced by peripheral fat tissues.

144.3 **Answer: (c), (d), and (e)** In patients with cancer, cachexia may appear when the tumor weight is < 0.01% of total body weight, and in the majority of cancer patients the tumor mass seldom exceeds 500 g at autopsy. Therefore, it is unlikely that simple competition of available nitrogen between tumor and host is responsible for the development of cachexia, especially in early-stage cancer.

TNF-α was rarely detected in patients with clinical cancer cachexia, and administration of recombinant TNF-α did not produce demonstrable cachexia.

Several studies show that patients with cancer are not necessarily hypermetabolic. In one study, measurements of resting energy expenditure in 200 hospitalized cancer patients showed that only 26% of them were hypermetabolic; 33% were hypometabolic and the rest were normometabolic. In another study, resting energy expenditure was measured in 68 patients: 23 were hypermetabolic, 10 were hypometabolic, and 35 were normometabolic. Patients with pancreas cancer tend to be hypometabolic, whereas patients with lymphoma or lung cancer tend to be hypermetabolic.

144.4 **Answer: (c)** Several randomized studies showed that megestrol acetate produced appetite stimulation, increased food intake, and weight gain. Body weight gain was mainly from accumulation of fat and water.

Cyproheptadine is a serotonin antagonist. A randomized study in patients with various malignancies showed that cyproheptadine decreased nausea and mildly enhanced appetite, but it did not abate progressive weight loss in these patients.

Two randomized studies by a cooperative study group assessing the effects of hydrazine sulfate did not show that the agent improved appetite, body weight, quality of life, or survival.

In a randomized controlled trial in patients with solid tumors, pentoxifylline failed to provide improvement in appetite or body weight compared with that in a placebo group.

Ranitidine has not been investigated to determine whether it has any activity in patients with anorexia or with documented tumor-associated gastroparesis.

144.5 **Answer: (d)** DVT is common in patients with cancer; however, DVT may occur in an early stage of cancer. DVT can be the initial sign of cancer. Occurrence of DVT during treatment with tamoxifen in patients with breast cancer is well known.

144.6 **Answer: (d) and (e)** With debulking surgery and combination chemotherapy, the patient with ovarian carcinoma is expected to do well. Therefore, TPN should be inaugurated in this patient to maintain/improve nutritional status.

Because of limited nutritional reserve, children with cancer develop malnutrition more often than do adult cancer patients. Therefore, combined chemotherapy-radiotherapy protocols for children with neuroblastoma and Wilms' tumor routinely incorporate parenteral nutritional support. Prolonged parenteral nutrition given concurrently with chemotherapy and radiotherapy has resulted in significant improvements in arm muscle area and increases in serum albumin.

For patients with laryngeal carcinoma and esophageal carcinoma with dysphagia, placement of a gastrostomy feeding tube should be considered first.

The symptoms of the patient with pancreatic carcinoma are most likely owing to the lack of secretion of pancreas enzymes. The patient should first be treated with pancreas enzyme preparations. TPN has not been proven to enhance effects of chemotherapy and/or radiotherapy or to improve survival in these patients.

145.1 **Answer: (d)** Daily chlorambucil by mouth is only mildly emetogenic. It is reasonable to offer oral ondansetron and then to withdraw it after 1 or 2 days. If chlorambucil is being given as a single large dose at infrequent intervals, oral ondansetron may need to be repeated with each dose of chemotherapy.

145.2 **Answer: (a)** Cisplatin is the most emetogenic chemotherapeutic agent, causing predictable and severe vomiting. Young adults are particularly susceptible during the first 4 to 6 hours after administration. It is recommended that prophylactic antiemetics be given before the chemotherapy. The other drugs listed, especially vinblastine, tamoxifen, and bleomycin, rarely cause vomiting.

145.3 **Answer: (e)** Ondansetron and granisetron are potent and specific antagonists of the serotonin receptor, which exists in both central and peripheral sites. These drugs are the most effective agents for suppression of chemotherapy-induced or radiotherapy-induced emesis. Unfortunately, these safe drugs have limited effectiveness in other causes of vomiting.

146.1 **Answer: (e)** Brain and leptomeningeal metastasis can cause structural damage to the brain resulting usually in focal seizures. Superior sagittal sinus thrombosis can cause cortical venous infarction resulting in either focal or generalized convulsions. Severe hyponatremia, particularly when acquired acutely and with a severe drop in serum sodium, can present with seizures.

146.2 **Answer: (c)** Cisplatin neuropathy may begin after the treatment is completed and may progress for several months thereafter.

146.3 **Answer: (b)** Extension of tumor into the epidural space cannot be visualized on either bone scan or plain films. The best test is MRI, and it should be unenhanced. Gadolinium can obscure the identification of tumor, and, therefore, an unenhanced image is optimal. An enhanced scan is used to detect leptomeningeal and parenchymal spinal metastases. Myelography should be used only in those patients who cannot undergo MRI.

146.4 **Answer: (a)** Ifosfamide can cause an acute toxic encephalopathy, which usually resolves, but in some patients it can result in permanent damage.

146.5 **Answer: (d)** All of these modalities can be employed in patients with brain metastases. Resection and stereotactic radiosurgery are particularly suitable for patients with single or few brain metastases. Systemic chemotherapy is useful for chemosensitive primaries, such as small cell lung cancer or choriocarcinoma.

147.1 **Answer: (e)** Alopecia is the most common dermatologic complication associated with cancer chemotherapy due to effects of chemotherapy on the highly mitotic follicular matrix cells during the anagen phase of hair growth. Alopecia is seen with the use of most antineoplastic agents, as approximately 90% of hair cells are in the anagen phase at any one time. Certain agents such as doxorubicin often cause severe and complete alopecia. Among other types of reactions, stomatitis and extravasation reactions are also commonly seen.

147.2 **Answer: (c)** Antibiotics such as doxorubicin, dactinomycin, daunorubicin, and mitomycin are the most common and potent vesicants. Infusion of these agents should be monitored closely.

147.3 **Answer: (e)** When extravasation is suspected during administration of a known vesicant, action is necessary as it is estimated that approximately 30% of such extravasations will ulcerate. The drug infusion should be discontinued promptly, followed by an attempt at aspiration of residual drug through the catheter. The catheter may then be removed. Although cold may be applied to sites of injuries caused by other chemotherapeutic agents, heat is required with the extravasation of vinca alkaloids, as cold application may actually worsen the reaction. Antidotes may then be considered, especially hyaluronidase for vinca alkaloid extravasation.

147.4 **Answer: (c)** Both acral erythema and the eruption of lymphocyte recovery may mimic acute GVHD in the bone marrow transplant patient. Like acral erythema, acute GVHD may also be limited to the hands and is also indistinguishable from acral erythema histologically during the first 3 weeks. The erythematous exanthem of ELR may also mimic acute GVHD clinically and histologically, especially with regard to time of onset after bone marrow transplantation.

147.5 **Answer: (e)** Use of interferon (IFN)-α and interleukin (IL)-2 immunotherapy is associated with a wide variety of dermatologic reactions. They share the ability to induce telogen effluvium alopecia, cutaneous ulcerations, and exacerbations of seborrheic dermatitis and psoriasis.

148.1 **Answer: (c)** The mechanism of bone resorption is primarily osteoclast mediated. Several known osteoclastic factors play a significant role in the process of bone resorption. Osteoclasts are the principal bone-resorbing cells.

148.2 **Answer: (d)** Bone metastases from renal cell carcinoma are destructive lytic permeative radiolucent lesions releted to osteoclastic bone resorption. These lesions are highly vascular and may cause extensive bleeding at the time of open biopsy. In such cases arteriographic embolization should be considered preoperatively.

148.3 **Answer: (e)** Within the skeleton the site of a metastatic lesion is correlated to the activity of the bone marrow. The axial skeleton contains active hematopoietic marrow, whereas the peripheral skeleton contains relatively avascular fatty marrow. The thoracolumbar spine represents the most common site for metastases; this is partly related to the paravertebral venous plexus system described by Batson.

149.1 **Answer: (e)** Because there is no carrier state for HAV, transfusion-transmitted infections are extremely rare. The current per-unit risk of HBV is estimated to be approximately 1:200,000. With nucleic acid testing now being done routinely for both HIV and HCV, the per-unit risks for both of these agents is now estimated to be approximately 1:2,000,000. Because platelets must be stored at room temperature, bacterial contamination remains a serious problem. It is estimated that 1:12,000 platelet units may be associated with bacterial sepsis.

149.2 **Answer: (c)** Delayed red cell reconstitution is a rare complication of major ABO-incompatible transplants (eg, group A donor and group O recipient). In minor ABO-incompatible transplants (eg, group O donor and group A recipient), the donor has isoagglutinin versus recipient red blood cells. Hemolysis of circulating host red cells may occur 1 to 3 weeks after transplantation as mature lymphocytes in the stem cell product engraft in the host, proliferate, and produce anti-A and/or anti-B antibodies. Minor ABO-incompatible transplants have not been associated with increased graft rejection, more frequent or severe GVHD, or increased overall mortality.

149.3 **Answer: (b)** A subset of febrile nonhemolytic transfusion reactions appears to be triggered by recipient antibody binding to donor leukocytes; leukoreduction prevents these reactions. Leukoreduction performed prior to component storage additionally prevents febrile reactions caused by an accumulation of leukocyte-derived cytokines in the product. Currently, the only approved method to prevent transfusion-associated GVHD is irradiation. Leukoreduction has clearly been demonstrated to reduce the frequency of alloimmunization to human leukocyte antigen (HLA)-A and HLA-B. CMV is present in monocytes and other leukocytes. Providing leukoreduced blood products is approximately as effective as providing CMV-seronegative blood products for preventing CMV transmission.

150.1   Answer: (c)   We already observe in the question that, in spite of the patient receiving fresh frozen plasma, the aPTT does not correct. Moreover, he has also spontaneous subcutaneous hematomas. These findings are suggestive of the presence of a specific acquired coagulation factor inhibitor. Therefore, the next step in the evaluation of this patient is to do mixing studies of the aPTT. In the case of an acquired coagulation factor inhibitor, the aPTT remains prolonged when normal plasma is added to the patient's plasma.

150.2   Answer: (d)   Option (a) is incorrect as LMWH has approximately a 30% cross-reactivity with UFH; therefore, this may worsen the clinical situation. Choice (b) is also incorrect. There is no indication for an IVC filter. This device would be indicated in cases of absolute contraindications for anticoagulation, such as active bleeding, the presence of nontreated brain metastases, or a history of central nervous system bleeding or intraocular hemorrhage. Option (c) is wrong as it may take several days to get the results of the test, and in clinical practice the HIT diagnosis is considered highly probable when the platelet count drops at least 30% from the baseline measurement, usually by days 5 to 10 on exposure to heparin. The decrease in the platelet count may occur earlier if there is a history of a previous exposure to heparin. The correct answer is (d). As the INR is not therapeutic yet, the patient should be covered with an antithrombotic medication that does not have any cross-reactivity with heparin until the INR is therapeutic. This includes direct thrombin inhibitors.

150.3   Answer: (c)   The patient has clinical symptoms of a thrombotic thrombocytopenic purpura (TTP), which can be seen in patients taking immunosuppressive therapy after bone marrow or stem cell transplantation. The peripheral blood smear would demonstrate the presence of schistocytes, polychromasia, and a markedly decreased platelet count. The PT/aPTT should be normal in TTP. If graft failure was the etiology, there would be reticulocytopenia. Platelet transfusions are contraindicated in TTP unless there are signs of bleeding.

150.4   Answer: (d)   The first choice would not be adequate because, even if the thrombophilia evaluation is negative, this patient has an increased risk of thrombosis in view of her past medical history of a thromboembolic event. Moreover, not all the thrombophilic conditions have been identified. In the second choice, the warfarin dose may not be sufficient to prolong the INR to the level required to prevent a thromboembolic event. The third option would not be adequate because, if tamoxifen is discontinued, the patient would not receive the additional hormonal benefits that would decrease her risk of recurrence of breast cancer.

Choice (d) would be the best route as the aromatase inhibitors are not associated with an increased risk of thromboembolic complications, and the patient would receive the additional adjuvant hormonal benefits.

150.5   Answer: (d)   Although these patients usually present with severe thrombocytopenia, this is not the main reason for the typical bleeding diathesis of this leukemia. Dysfibrinogenemia is usually seen in patients with severe liver disease. DIC is common in APL; however, after treatment with all-*trans* retinoic acid, DIC may persist in vivo for several weeks without any bleeding manifestations. Abnormally high levels of expression of annexin II on APL cells increase the production of plasmin. Overexpression of annexin II appears to be a mechanism for excessive fibrino(geno)lysis and the hemorrhagic less complications of APL.

152.1   Answer: (e)   Radiation in high doses affects all cardiac structures, and any of the phenomena in the choices can theoretically occur if exposure is sufficiently high. Patients may experience premature coronary artery disease, and both angioplasty and bypass surgery may be more difficult in patients who have undergone irradiation. Myocardial infarction is fortunately an unusual occurrence. Likewise, mitral leaflet thickening can occur, but it is not usually associated with significant valvular dysfunction. Constrictive pericarditis is a serious complication seen months or years following radiation. If not treated aggressively it can be fatal. With modern radiation techniques, constriction is unusual. Congestive cardiomyopathy following irradiation is also rare. Some degree of pericarditis is often seen following radiation and may manifest itself with low-grade fever, pericardial friction rubs, chest pain, and electrocardiographic changes that are often typical. Most patients respond to nonsteroidal anti-inflammatory agents such as ibuprofen.

152.2   Answer: (d)   Both nuclear and echocardiographic ejection fraction determinations are imperfect; additionally, many noncardiac factors influence a patient's ejection fraction. Some of these factors include shunting of blood, hormonal effects, body temperature, and the degree of anemia. Neither ultrasonographic estimations nor nuclear techniques are inherently superior to the other for estimating ejection fractions. Some patients can be studied better by one or the other technique—patients with extensive radiation may be studied better by nuclear imaging, whereas children and patients who cannot remain still may be studied more advantageously with ultrasonography. Because cardiotoxicity is unusual at low cumulative doses of an anthracycline, false-positive decreases in ejection fraction may exceed true-positive results. Cardiac biopsies are more sensitive and specific for determining cardiac damage than are ejection fraction determinations. The biopsies are not usually needed in following patients clinically, especially in the era of cardioprotection, but have been of tremendous value in establishing safe cumulative anthracycline dosages and in comparing the relative toxicities of various cardiotoxic agents and administration schedules.

152.3   Answer: (b)   Liposomal delivery systems are approved for the treatment of a number of tumors, and the use of such agents has been shown to be clearly cardioprotective. Dexrazoxane is also cardioprotective, but there is some controversy surrounding a possible reduction in efficacy of the oncologic regimen, and this may limit the overall use of this agent. Continuous infusion schedules, with infusion times ranging from 48 to 96 hours, are also clearly cardioprotective and do not alter efficacy; stomatitis is increased with prolonged infusion schedules. Interestingly, liposomal delivery systems, dexrazoxane, and continuous infusion result in comparable protection, which allows up to twice the cumulative dose of doxorubicin that can be safely given by rapid-infusion administration. Dose limitation keeps the risk of cardiotoxicity acceptable by avoiding cumulative dosages likely to be associated with cardiac damage. Vitamin C is not used for cardioprotection.

152.4 **Answer: (e)** Trastuzumab has not been shown to exhibit characteristic changes, and the biopsy material is often normal even in the face of significant cardiac dysfunction. Changes are similar for mitoxantrone and for doxorubicin, but they reflect a cardiotoxic dose rather than the actual number of milligrams administered. The changes associated with the toxic dose of 200 mg/m^2 of mitoxantrone would be much greater than those associated with the relatively low cumulative dose of 200 mg/m^2 of doxorubicin. The biopsy changes associated with anthracyclines are quite specific and would not be confused with changes associated with chronic alcoholism. Biopsy changes are detectable at cumulative dosages that are quite low and considerably lower than the cumulative dosages associated with clinical cardiac dysfunction.

152.5 **Answer (c)** Trastuzumab cardiotoxicity is an interesting phenomenon. Early reports have suggested that patients treated with an anthracycline and who are then exposed to trastuzumab have a significant chance of developing clinically relevant cardiotoxicity. The mechanism is unknown and is under investigation. Cardiac biopsies have not been adequately undertaken, but anecdotally typical anthracycline-like changes have not been found. Cardiotoxicity is seen in as many as 27% of the sequentially treated patients, making a sequential stress phenomenon a strong possibility.

152.6 **Answer: (c)** The recommended maximal dose of doxorubicin is about 400 mg/m^2, and this patient has received half of this acceptable exposure. Such a patient would be expected to tolerate half of the recommend mitoxantrone dose of 160 mg/m^2, or about 80 mg/m^2. When crossing over from one cardiotoxic drug to another, the burden of prior regimens is kept, and the cumulative dose of the subsequent drug or drugs must be adjusted accordingly. When doxorubicin was initially introduced, a maximal cumulative dose of 550 mg/m^2 was considered safe, but this recommendation has been reduced and most authorities now consider 400 mg/m^2 to be the recommended maximum. Although the cumulative dose of mitoxantrone must be reduced by about 50% because of the prior doxorubicin exposure, it is not contraindicated in this setting.

153.1 **Answer: (b)** The other infections are all community-acquired organisms common in all adults.

153.2 **Answer: (d)** SPACE and fungal infections arise later in neutropenia; *Candida* is only diagnosed by culture in 50% of cases, and *Haemophilus* is a rare cause of sepsis.

153.3 **Answer: (b)** Waiting for a diminution of presclerosis outflow may increase the risk of loculations and reduce palliation.

153.4 **Answer: (d)** Although statements (a), (b), and (c) are individually correct, it is the sum of all three that is important. The key issue is recognizing the substantial number of cancer patients with benign etiologies for their effusions.

153.5 **Answer: (b)** Radiation pneumonitis can occur outside a port and seems to be immunologic in origin. The newer drugs and standard doses of chemotherapy can often cause drug-related pulmonary toxicity, and diffuse alveolar hemorrhage is much less common (5–15%) and is noninfectious.

154.1 **Answer: (d)** The diagnosis of sinusoidal obstruction syndrome is usually based on clinical features, notably hyperbilirubinemia, painful hepatomegaly, fluid retention, and time of onset of symptoms relative to the time of drug exposure. Doppler ultrasonography may be supportive of the diagnosis, but it is not diagnostic. Percutaneous liver biopsy is rarely needed to differentiate sinusoidal obstruction syndrome from hyperacute graft-versus-host disease in the first few weeks following hematopoietic stem cell transplantation.

154.2 **Answer: (b)** Chemotherapeutic agents most commonly cause transient increases in liver test abnormalities without clinical evidence of liver impairment. The reason for the relative infrequency of significant injury is unknown, but it may be related to the relative strength of the detoxification pathways within the hepatocyte or that chemotherapeutic drugs tend to target rapidly proliferating cells, whereas liver cells have a slow turnover.

156.1 **Answer: (c)**

156.2 **Answer: (a), (b), and (c)**

156.3 **Answer: (a)**

156.4 **Answer: (d) and (e)**

156.5 **Answer: (a) and (b)**

156.6 **Answer: Mucormycosis**

157.1 **Answer: (d)** Permanent infertility seems to be both dose and to some extent age related. Men fare worse than do women. In both sexes children do better than adults, perhaps because the germ cells in the prepubertal gonad are mitotically less active.

157.2 **Answer: (a)** Alkylating agents are associated with the highest risk of permanent infertility. Both the mechlorethamine (nitrogen mustard) and the procarbazine in MOPP are highly toxic to germinal epithelium. ABVD is clearly the choice for treatment of Hodgkin's disease when fertility is an issue; reports indicate it is only rarely associated with sterility. Both PEB and PVB have been used in young men treated for testis cancer, and although sterility is seen in up to one-quarter of patients, it is not the rule.

157.3 **Answer: (c)** Large series of offspring of cancer patients have now been published and indicate that the rates of congenital anomalies are similar to those in the general population. Fetal wastage is probably slightly more common in the early period after chemotherapy but is still uncommon, and at 8 years after treatment it would not be a major concern. Follow-up of these children indicates that they develop normally and seem to have no excess risk of cancer themselves.

157.4 **Answer: (a)** Careful selection of chemotherapy options is an important concern in preserving fertility, but dose response and other factors determining ultimate fertility are uncertain enough that this is an unreliable approach to preventing sterility. Gn-RH analogue treatment is likewise unreliable and has not been shown to be of much benefit. Testicular sperm extraction after treatment remains an option, but cost is significant and the technique is not universally effective. Sperm banking should be recommended to all men in this setting. Although many men are oligospermic at presentation, semen cryopreservation remains the mainstay of fertility preservation for young men.

157.5 **Answer: (d)** Although Gn-RH analogue administration can be cumbersome and fraught with side effects, it has been offered to women anticipating ovarian toxins (chemotherapy and radiation). Its results are mixed. Embryo cryopreservation is a viable option for women with stable partners willing to fertilize an egg, but it is costly, poses ethical issues, and is not appropriate for many women. Ovarian transposition is useful for women who will undergo pelvic radiation, but it is time consuming in urgent settings and costly (insurance coverage is not universal). Procedures of oocyte or ovarian tissue cryopreservation are in early stages of development, but they are technically difficult and have rarely preserved fertility.

158.1 **Answer: (d)** Paraneoplastic syndromes are caused by tumor production and secretion of peptides or proteins. Although differentiated cancers arising from steroid synthesizing tissues (ie, adrenal, ovary, or testis) may retain the ability to synthesize steroids, or thyroid cancer may retain thyronine-synthesizing properties, cancers arising from other tissues do not synthesize thyronines, steroids, or catecholamines. Small amounts of many protein hormones, or prohormones, are produced by many normal tissues and presumably act in paracrine signal systems. When produced in large amounts by cancers, these may produce distant endocrine effects resulting in clinically recognizable paraneoplastic endocrine syndromes. Paraneoplastic neurologic syndromes are associated with tumor protein-induced antibody production, an immune reaction to exposed immunogens. Direct tumor production of antibodies is not known to occur except with myeloma.

158.2 **Answer: (c)** PTH-RP is produced by the normal breast and is secreted into milk. It presumably acts in calcium secretion and is a paracrine hormone in the normal breast, as well as in many other normal tissues of the body. Re-evaluation of the cause of hypercalcemia, so commonly seen in breast cancer, both metastatic and nonmetastatic, reveals that PTH-RP is very commonly produced by breast cancers and is probably the cause of the hypercalcemia. Breast cancer production of PTH has been described in a single case. Even in patients with bony metastases from breast cancer, production of excess PTH-RP is likely to be the cause of hypercalcemia.

158.3 **Answer: (e)** Many or most normal tissues produce precursor ACTH molecules, which presumably act in paracrine control systems. Cancers produce increased quantities of these proteins and a small percentage convert the precursors to bioactive ACTH. Thus, the paraneoplastic Cushing's syndrome is associated with often dramatically increased circulating ACTH precursors along with increased ACTH. Pituitary-dependent Cushing's disease is associated with high normal or slightly above normal ACTH concentrations without normal diurnal variation. Very high ACTH concentrations appear to inhibit the conversion of cortisol to cortisone, a normally required control system to prevent cortisol from binding to the renal mineralocorticoid receptor. With such inhibition, cortisol itself acts as a mineralocorticoid. Thus, hypokalemia is common in the paraneoplastic Cushing's syndrome and unusual in Cushing's disease.

158.4 **Answer: (b)** Small amounts of CG are extractable from most or all normal tissues. The normal pituitary secretes small amounts of CG, and this secretion is stimulated by hypothalamic gonadotropin-releasing hormone (Gn-RH) and inhibited by long-acting Gn-RH antagonists and by androgens and estrogens. Thus, differentiation of CG production by cancers from normal production and secretion is a quantitative process; the presence of CG in blood or urine does not indicate a cancer is present.

158.5 **Answer: (b)** Paraneoplastic neurologic disorders are usually associated with tumor immunogen stimulation of antibody production. Different circulating antibodies are more likely to be associated with specific syndromes, although these syndromes and antibodies may also be seen in individuals without cancers. The anti-Hu antibody is strongly associated with the subacute sensory syndrome, but not with the other syndromes listed. It remains controversial whether the particular antibody is the cause of the syndrome.

158.6 **Answer: (b)** L-asparaginase inhibits thyroid hormone-binding proteins and decreases serum levels of thyroid hormones without true hypothyroidism. L-asparaginase can also inhibit the synthesis of thyroid-stimulating hormone and lead to central hypothyroidism in some cases. Interleukin-2 can enhance autoimmunity against the thyroid gland and lead to hypothyroidism.

158.7 **Answer: (d)** The somatotropic axis (GH) is the most likely to be impaired by radiation to the brain.

158.8 **Answer: (a)** This patient with neutropenic fever may be suffering from sepsis and possibly secondary adrenal insufficiency (given the history of recent high-dose glucocorticoid administration). The appropriate urgent treatments of this patient include resuscitation with crystalloid intravenous fluid, broad-spectrum antibiotics, and stress doses of glucocorticoid.

158.9 **Answer: (c)** Cisplatin and cyclophosphamide are associated with renal sodium and magnesium washing.

158.10   **Answer: (d)**   Follicular neoplasms can be benign adenomas or malignant follicular carcinomas. The diagnosis of adenoma versus carcinoma requires histologic examination of the resected specimen. Given the history of prior exposure to radiation, which increases the risk of thyroid malignancies, we believe total thyroidectomy should be performed.

159.1   **Answer: (b)**   Genetic family syndromes, although they are extremely important and are major causes of multiple cancers for those who bear those genetic mutations (eg, hereditary retinoblastoma), are relatively rare occurrences in the overall population. Radiation therapy and/or chemotherapy also contribute overall to the second malignancy problem but not to an exceedingly large fraction of cases. Tobacco is an important cause of second malignancies, particularly in those with a tobacco-related malignancy, but this still does not reach the level of simple chance.

159.2   **Answer: (b)**   A breast cancer survivor has an elevated risk of developing of contralateral breast cancer and should undergo breast cancer screening. In addition, any adult > age 50 years should have routine colon cancer screening on an annual basis, including fecal occult blood testing and endoscopy with either sigmoidoscopy or colonoscopy. Some evidence, in fact, suggests that breast cancer survivors are at increased risk of colon cancer; therefore, colon screening is even more important. In addition, breast cancer survivors are at elevated risk both for endometrial and ovarian cancers—a routine gynecologic examination seems appropriate. Certainly if the patient was treated with tamoxifen, with its elevation in risk of endometrial cancer, this would be an even more appropriate recommendation. Most experts no longer consider serum CEA levels a useful test in screening for colorectal cancer; as a result there would not appear to be an indication for its use from a screening perspective.

159.3   **Answer: (e)**   Since the most critical factor contributing to cancer generally is age, and since cancer patients are now surviving for longer periods, their potential for developing other malignancies is increased. Fewer competing causes of death also contribute to the longevity enjoyed by cancer survivors. Screening for occult neoplasms has increased for the general population, and as cancer survivors are seen more often in follow-up, the likelihood of detecting tumors elsewhere is also increased. Not mentioned above, but especially important to long-term survivors of pediatric cancer, is the prolonged latent period associated with radiation-associated neoplasms.

159.4   **Answer: (e)**   Many inherited syndromes are associated with benign and malignant tumors. In many cases the clinical manifestations of the syndrome are obvious long before the development of a benign or malignant neoplasm. Each of the syndromes predisposes to a spectrum of tumors and is specific to the syndrome, with little, if any, overlap. For example, in NF1, gliomas and neurofibrosarcomas predominate, whereas in FAP, colon cancer, desmoid tumors, and hepatoblastoma are increased. Knowledge of the tumors to which individuals are predisposed can assist the practitioner in providing appropriate follow-up.

159.5   **Answer: (b)**   Cancer occurs because of mutations in the tissue of origin. These somatic mutations are rarely present in the individual's germline. About 1 to 5% of cancers reported arise in individuals with a hereditary condition that predisposes to cancer, and some of these individuals are at increased risk of second cancers. Not all of these predisposing conditions are identified before the affected patient is diagnosed with a first cancer, but a good review of the patient's past medical history and the family history may reveal such a hereditary cancer syndrome; this would alert the clinician to perform a more focused follow-up.

159.6   **Answer: (d)**   Embryonal tumors such as neuroblastoma, Wilms' tumor, and hepatoblastoma are not seen as secondary cancers following radiation therapy, probably because of their origins in developing tissues in utero. Sarcomas of the bone and soft tissue are the most frequent second neoplasms following radiation therapy, with a greater risk following exposure to doses > 4,000 cGy. On the other hand, thyroid neoplasms and leukemias are usually seen following considerably lower doses. Other tissues within the radiation field, such as breast, thyroid, and skin, are also at risk.

159.7   **Answer: (e)**   Secondary or treatment-related AML has a very low cure rate with < 10% of patients surviving at 5 years. Although secondary acute lymphocytic leukemia is more curable, rates of cure are < 50%. Secondary leukemias are associated with radiation, which is usually combined with chemotherapy, or with chemotherapy alone, primarily alkylating agents, and epipodophyllotoxins. There is some suggestion that schedule rather than total dose influences the risk of epipodophyllotoxin-associated leukemia.

INFECTION IN THE CANCER PATIENT

160.1   **Answer: (e)**   The spectrum of bacterial infections in neutropenic patients continues to change and depends on multiple factors, including local hospital microflora, use of prophylactic and therapeutic regimens, use of vascular access devices, and environmental exposure. Currently gram-positive organisms such as coagulase-negative staphylococci, *Staphylococcus aureus*, viridans streptococci, and the enterococci (including VRE) are the most frequently isolated gram-positive organisms. Although gram-negative bacilli are isolated less frequently than in the past, they are still important pathogens, and many institutions are describing increased rates of gram-negative infections with organisms such as *Escherichia coli, Klebsiella* spp, *P. aeruginosa, Enterobacter* spp, *Citrobacter* sp, and *Stenotrophomonas maltophilia. L. monocytogenes* causes infections primarily in patients with defects in cell-mediated immunity (ie, not in neutropenic patients).

160.2 **Answer: (d)** Although it is true that gram-negative bacilli are being isolated less frequently from febrile neutropenic patients (FNP), *P. aeruginosa* remains an important pathogen in this setting, and potent antipseudomonal coverage is essential for empiric therapy. Gram-positive organisms are being isolated with increasing frequency from FNP, and some of these are associated with increased morbidity and mortality, but most studies have shown no difference in mortality associated with gram-positive infections in regimens such as vancomycin at the onset of empiric therapy compared with the addition of such agents later in the course of febrile neutropenia.

160.3 **Answer: (d)** The spectrum of fungal infections has widened appreciably in the past decade or so and includes *Candida albicans,* non-albicans *Candida* spp, *Aspergillus* spp, *Fusarium, Trichosporon, and Zygomycetes* among others. Many *Candida* spp are less susceptible (or resistant) to the azoles fluconazole and itraconazole. Fluconazole is inactive against most molds. Flucytosine is associated with the rapid development of resistance and substantial toxicity. Caspofungin and voriconazole may have a role to play in this setting but need to be fully evaluated. Amphotericin B (or its lipid formulations) remains the agent of choice.

ONCOLOGIC EMERGENCIES

161.1 **Answer: (b)** In 95% of cases, spinal cord compression is caused by extradural metastases from tumors involving the vertebral column, most commonly the thoracic spine (70%; lumbosacral, 20%; cervical spine, 10%). Thoracic spine metastasis is frequently more significant because of a vulnerable blood supply and a narrowing of the spinal canal in the thoracic region compared with the lumbar and cervical canals.

161.2 **Answer: (e)** The V/Q scan is the initial test usually performed in the diagnostic work-up of a pulmonary embolus. Unfortunately, V/Q scans are often read as intermediate probability, and usually further testing is required. Other testing that may be used for diagnosis is spiral CT, magnetic resonance imaging (MRI), and pulmonary angiography. Spiral CT and MRI are newer modalities, each with sensitivities and specificities of about 80 and 90%, respectively. The gold standard for diagnosis is pulmonary angiography.

161.3 **Answer: (e)** Factors predisposing cancer patients to hemoptysis include hematologic abnormalities secondary to cancer treatments or infiltration of the bone marrow, and coagulopathy owing to decreased hepatic production of clotting factors because of extensive liver involvement by the malignancy. For hematologic and bone marrow transplantation patients, the risk is increased by infection with angio-invasive fungal infections (aspergillosis, mucormycosis). Factors contributing to fatal hemoptysis include diffuse alveolar damage, thrombocytopenia, coagulopathy, viral and bacterial infections, sepsis, radiation lung injury, and lung injury owing to chemotherapeutic agents.

161.4 **Answer: (d)**

161.5 **Answer: (e)** Defibrillation is in the standard protocol for pulseless ventricular tachycardia. Emergency treatment of torsades de pointes may vary from the standard algorithms for other types of ventricular tachycardia, and it entails expedient use of intravenous magnesium, electrical overdrive pacing or pharmacologic overdrive with isoproterenol, and the administration of phenytoin or lidocaine.

161.6 **Answer: (g)** All of these agents can cause the cytokine-release syndrome.

NOTES

NOTES